"*Sync & Savor* is more than a cookbook; it's a guide to feeling at home in your body. Paige beautifully unpacks the complexity of the female cycle while offering simple, delicious recipes that make every phase feel nourished, supported, and, most of all, celebrated."

—ELLA HENRY, CREATOR OF @GLOWWITHELLA

"Paige has spent years sharing fun, delicious, and easy recipes on her social channels that help nourish the body. Learning to honor the body with menstrual cycle–synced food items is a game changer for overall energy and vitality. *Sync & Savor* is full of tasty yet nourishing recipes to help you feel your best at all times of the month, all while supporting your health and hormones. Every woman should have a copy!"

—HANNAH MUEHL, PA-C, MS, RDN,
CREATOR OF @THECONSCIOUSNUTRITIONIST

Sync & Savor

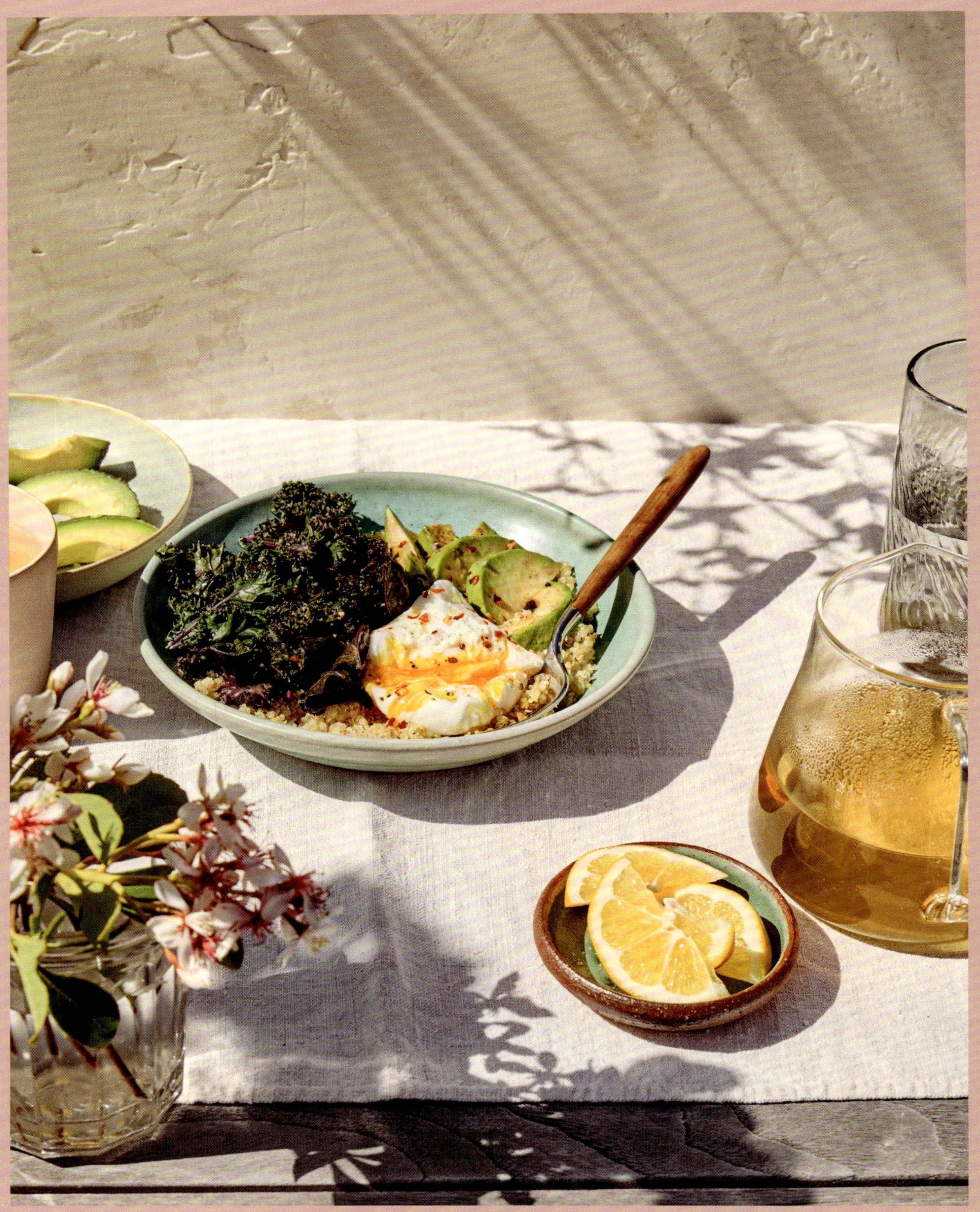

Sync & Savor

Cycle-Based Nutrition *for* Hormone Health *and* Balance

Paige Lindgren

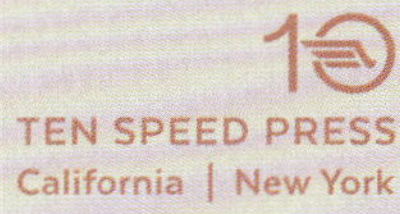

Photography by
Kristin Teig

Contents

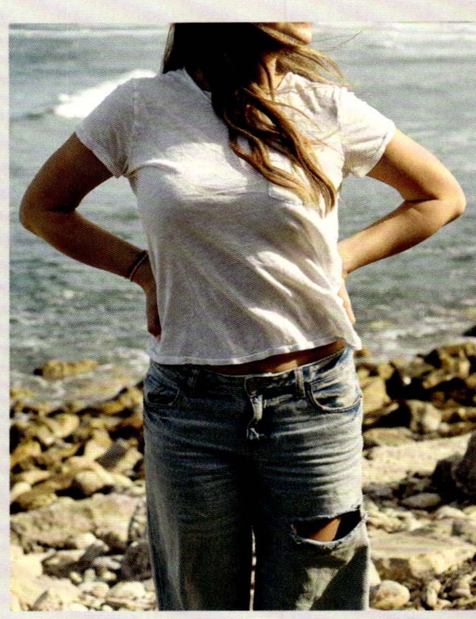

Follicular Phase: Energizing Your Body 83

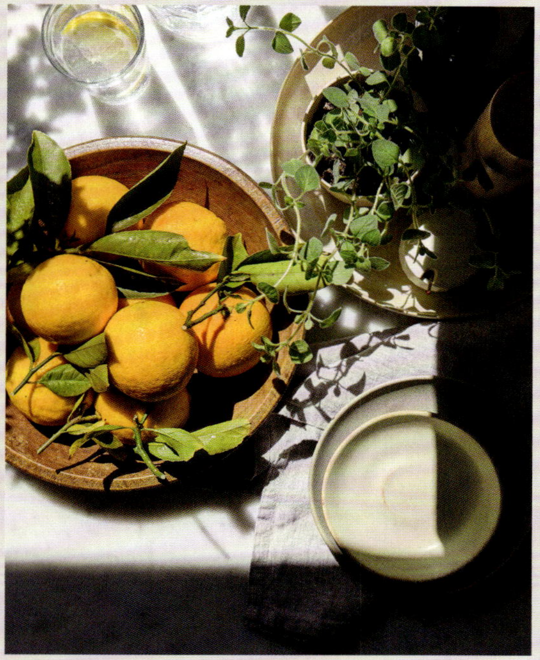

Ovulatory Phase: The Peak of Your Cycle 133

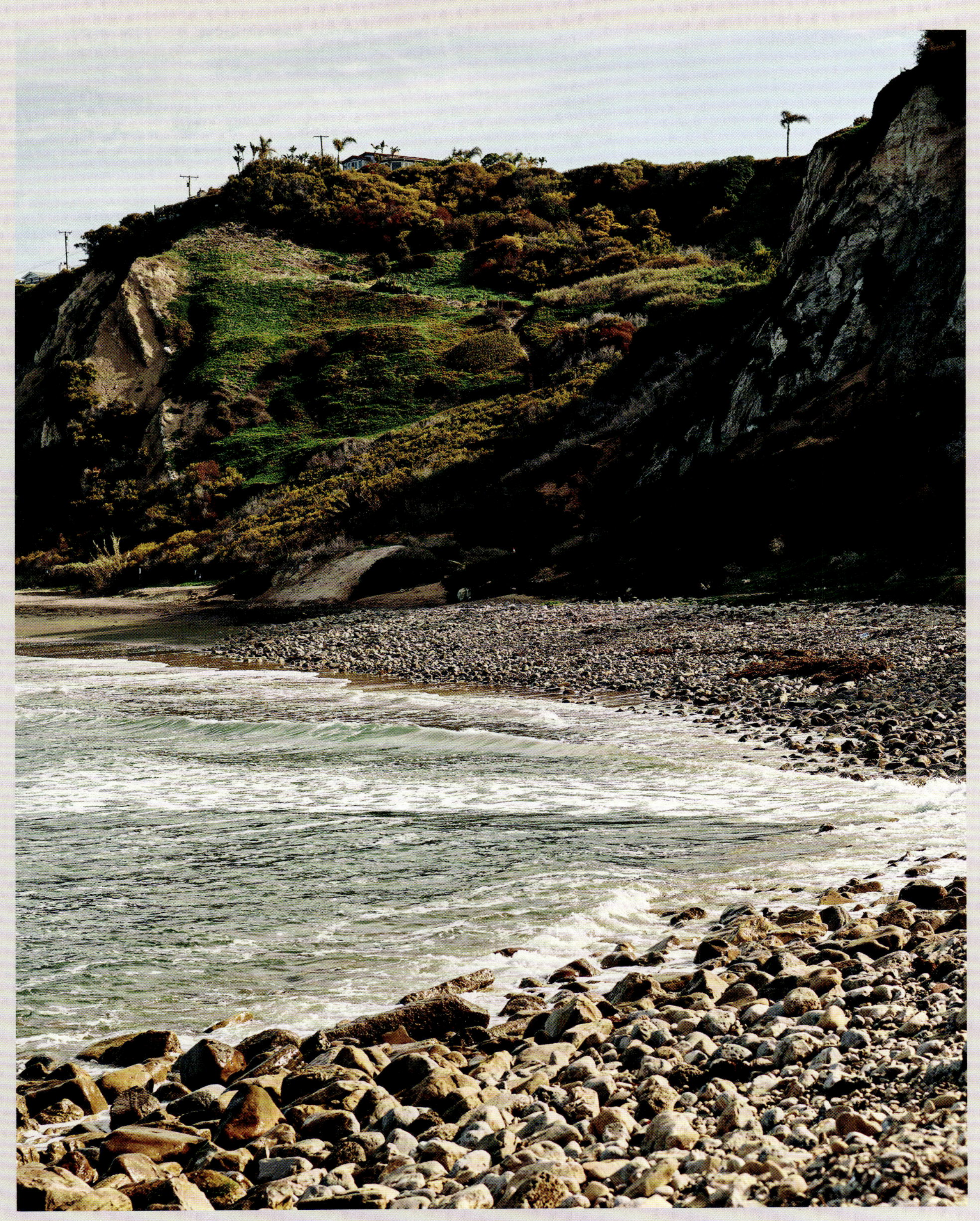

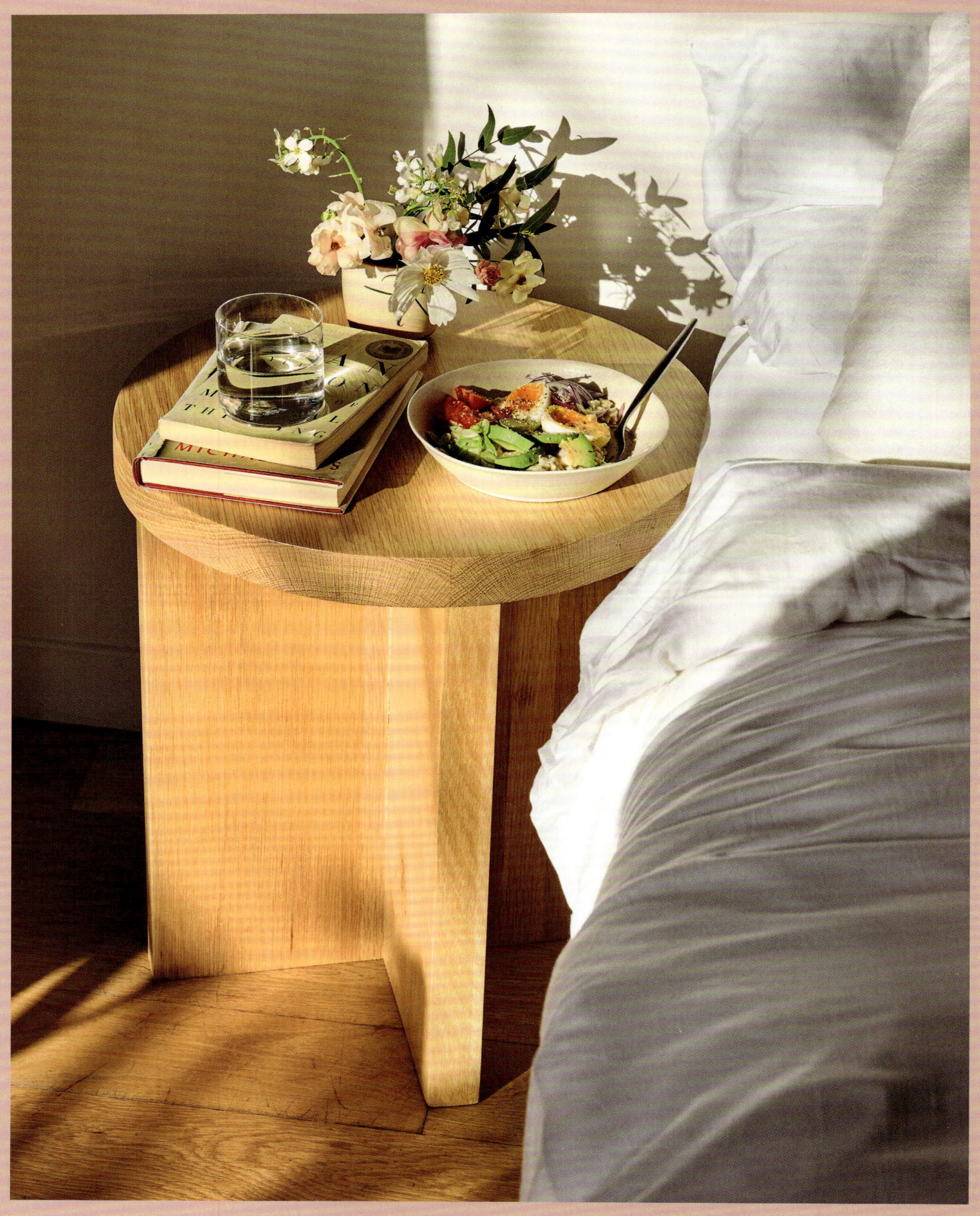

Foreword

In my years working in women's health, I've witnessed firsthand the disconnect so many women feel from their bodies and their unique hormonal cycle. We're often conditioned to view our cycles as burdensome or inconvenient or simply a marker for fertility rather than as a powerful barometer of our health and well-being. The truth is, when we understand how our hormones shift throughout the month and how to work *with* those rhythms rather than against them, everything changes.

Sync & Savor is a beautiful invitation to do just that. This book isn't just a collection of recipes but is also a road map for nourishing your body in sync with its natural hormonal flow. With each phase of the menstrual cycle, Paige offers gentle yet practical guidance through recipes that are not only supportive but also deeply satisfying.

What I love most about eating in flow with your cycle is there's no rigid dogma here. Just encouragement to listen, to nourish, and to create a safe haven for your hormones. In a wellness world that can sometimes feel overwhelming or restrictive, *Sync & Savor* is refreshingly empowering. It reminds us that food isn't just fuel but instead a form of self-care, of connection, of tuning in.

If you've ever felt confused about your hormones, overwhelmed by health advice, or simply wanted to feel more grounded in your body, this book is for you. I'm honored to share space in these pages and can't wait for you to experience the healing that unfolds when we sync with our bodies and savor the process.

Dr. Paria Vaziri,
Naturopathic doctor and
hormone health expert

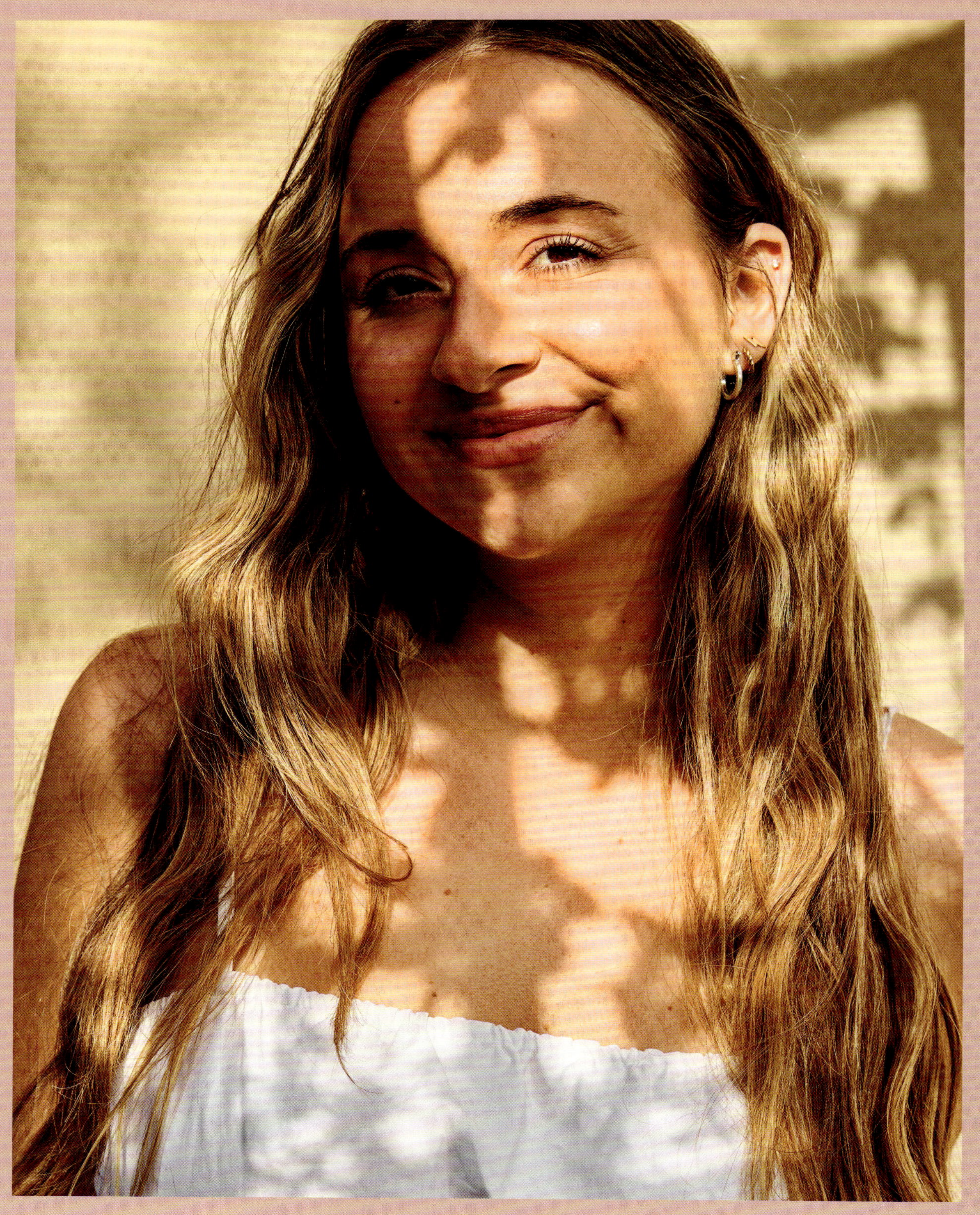

Introduction

Understanding Your Cycle and Its Power

As women, we're taught to resent our cycle, to feel shame around that time of the month, and to suppress the natural rhythm of our bodies through hormonal birth control. We're encouraged to ignore our need for rest and nourishment in order to keep up with the demands of a male-dominated society and workplace. We slog through punishing workouts, believing they'll provide the results we're looking for, not knowing that we may be causing our cortisol to spike and deliver the opposite outcome. We visit the doctor or gynecologist only to be told there's nothing wrong, or that our pain is normal; we're made to believe we don't even know our own bodies.

For years, my body felt like an unsolvable puzzle. For reasons I still don't really understand, I lost my period at age 22, and when it came back about a year and a half later, it was painful and irregular. I remember lying in bed with a heating pad on full blast, canceling plans because I felt so awful. My face was swollen, my stomach was bloated, and my mood swung so wildly that I sometimes felt like a stranger to myself. On top of that, I was battling Hashimoto's, an autoimmune disease that affects the thyroid and makes all things hormone-related even harder.

Like many of you, I turned to the internet for answers. I was following "healthy" trends, eating "clean," and working out intensely, but nothing seemed to help. I felt so lost—like I was battling my own body—which only led to more stress and anxiety.

That was when, through my integrative medicine doctor, I discovered hormone-aligned nutrition, and everything changed.

Hormone-aligned nutrition is the act of eating in tune with the four phases of your cycle to support your unique hormonal needs and honor the body's rhythms throughout the natural menstrual cycle. Cyclical living acknowledges the fact that you're going to feel vastly different on day 2 of your cycle than you will on day 25, and *that's okay*! It recognizes that your body needs a variety of nutrients, exercise, and rest at different times of the month. And most important, it empowers you to listen to your body and understand what it's asking you for—whether it's an extra hour of sleep or that chocolate you've been craving all day.

When I first started living in alignment with my cycle, I kept it super simple. I began with small shifts, like changing up my breakfast or swapping a workout for a walk during my luteal phase, and built from there. I quickly noticed that certain times of the month felt easier with these small adjustments. My energy started to come back, my mood stabilized, and I felt less inflamed and bloated. One of the biggest game-changers for me was learning how to work out *with* my cycle rather than against it. I used to force myself through high-intensity workouts even when my body was screaming for rest. Now I move in a way that supports where I am in my cycle—and not only do I feel better but I also see better results. I have polycystic ovary syndrome (PCOS), too, which adds another layer to all this. But syncing with my cycle has helped me manage symptoms naturally: fewer flare-ups, more regular cycles, and more energy overall.

We're all busy, and revolutionizing your life to accommodate your cycle can sound like a lot to take on, but that's the beauty of this practice: It can be whatever you make it. Perhaps for you, it simply means you avoid scheduling too many social events the week before your period to honor the alone time your body is so desperately asking you for. Maybe you incorporate just a few more fresh veggies into your diet toward the middle of the cycle. Or maybe you simply keep note of what day you're on so that when you suddenly want to scream in traffic on a random Thursday, you give yourself a bit of grace because you know you're at the height of your PMS.

I started sharing my health journey during my senior year of high school. I was just trying to figure out what made me feel good, experimenting with recipes and documenting the process along the way. It was super casual: I'd snap a photo of my meals or write a quick caption about how I was feeling. Over time, I got more confident and started posting videos, sharing what I was learning and recipes I was trying; I was also opening up about my struggles with hormone health. That's when my account slowly started to grow.

Wanting to help more women heal through food the way I had, but also wanting to feel confident about sharing more than just my journey, I went on to become a certified Hormone Specialist in 2021 and a certified Holistic Nutritionist in 2024. Since then, I've had the privilege of supporting thousands of women through their hormone and health journeys to help them feel at home in their bodies again and be educated about their cycles and what their body goes through every month! Whether it's through one-on-one guidance or daily tips and recipes on social media, my mission has always been to make hormone health feel accessible, empowering, and doable. It still blows me away that something that began as a personal outlet turned into a full-blown community. The absolute best part of what I do is hearing from people who say one of my tips helped them feel better, or getting tagged in photos and videos of someone making one of my recipes. Those messages mean the world to me. They make all the ups and downs of my own health journey feel so worth it.

I wrote this book to be a catch-all guide for anyone looking to learn more about living in tune with their cycle. The recipes in these pages are all intentionally simple and easy to pull together on a busy weeknight, and they will slot easily into your life whether you're just starting to get curious about living in alignment with your cycle or are already a pro just looking to incorporate some fresh recipes into the mix. I've also provided advice for exercise and lifestyle adjustments that will empower you through each phase.

Many women have also found this method to be an incredible resource for mitigating symptoms of PCOS, endometriosis, premenstrual dysphoric disorder (PMDD), and other conditions we as women face. Honoring your cycle and focusing on these nutrient-dense meals can also support fertility for those looking to start or support that journey. While I always recommend speaking with your ob-gyn or health professional, learning to live in tune with your body through lifestyle and nutrition shifts can be an amazing way to honor your body's needs, find body peace, and feel empowered.

Ultimately, the advice in this book is meant as a resource for you to use in whichever way serves you. If you're just starting out, maybe you will just try one recipe per week from the book and see how you feel, then slowly move on to adopting some of the lifestyle changes I recommend. The goal is for you to deepen your understanding of your own body's beautifully unique needs, so you can feel empowered all month long.

Following, I've included some basic education about the menstrual cycle as it relates to nutrition and syncing, with the help of my friend Dr. Shamsah Amersi, one of the country's leading ob-gyns and an advocate for holistic gynecology. I highly recommend doing your own research into other aspects of hormonal health if you're interested in learning more: Alisa Vitti, Dr. Jolene Brighten, Maisie Hill, and Lisa Hendrickson-Jack have all written incredible books that provide essential deep dives into various aspects of the period and female hormones.

Your Body's Built-In Guide

Hormones. We often blame them for everything from mood swings, to bloating, to fatigue, as if they were working against us. But what if we've been looking at them all wrong? The truth is, hormones aren't the enemy. Your endocrine system is an incredible tool that keeps your body running smoothly. When you understand the building blocks of that system, you can work with your body instead of feeling like you're constantly fighting against it.

Unfortunately, factors such as chronic stress, endocrine disruptors in our environment, and conditions like endometriosis, PCOS, PMDD, uterine fibroids, and sexually transmitted infections (STIs) can disrupt your body's natural rhythms and affect your cycle. In today's world, there are a lot of factors working against us; luckily, simple changes can make all the difference in bringing your hormones back into balance and working for you, not against you.

This book is here to shift how you think about your body and your cycle. By the time you finish, my hope is that you'll know exactly what your body needs, and how to give it the support it deserves.

HORMONAL BIRTH CONTROL AND YOUR CYCLE

*A note about HBC**: Research has shown that many forms of HBC are in fact some of the most powerful endocrine disruptors out there, and they can have long-lasting effects on your hormonal health, even after you choose to come off them. Fortunately, cycle-attuned living can be a powerful tool in rebalancing your hormones after coming off HBC. For more information, I highly recommend reading Dr. Jolene Brighten's *Beyond the Pill*, as well as discussing the matter further with a trusted gynecologist.

I think it's important to note here that you will not feel the benefits of tracking your cycle if you are currently on hormonal birth control. I still welcome you to use this book as simply a collection of body-loving, nutrient-dense recipes, or as a way to feel empowered as a woman, but it's worth noting that, as HBC disrupts your natural cycle, the relevance of this information to your hormones will be minimal.

* Hormonal birth control is an incredible tool that represents a pivotal development in the women's liberation and empowerment movement, allowing women to decide when and if they want to get pregnant, so they can in turn have careers, earn their own money, and live life on their own terms. I don't want to downplay the importance of this medication in enabling women to choose for themselves, nor do I want to shame anyone who is currently choosing to take it.

The Science of Your Cycle

Hormones are chemical messengers that influence everything from energy and mood to digestion and skin health. Throughout our cycle, these hormones fluctuate in predictable ways, and each phase brings its own set of strengths and challenges. Let's dive into the female sex hormones and how to care for them. I always encourage you to speak to your doctor or gynecologist about your body's unique symptoms. The internet can be a great place to find guidance, but it's important to make sure you're making lifestyle and nutrition choices based on trusted, accredited sources.

Key Hormones and Their Role

Estrogen

Estrogen is the primary sex hormone in women. It plays a role in ovulation and it thickens the uterine lining to prepare you for pregnancy. Estrogen peaks right before ovulation, falls, and then begins a sustained rise in the luteal phase.

Progesterone

Progesterone prepares the body for pregnancy. If the egg is not fertilized, progesterone levels drop, triggering a new menstrual cycle. Progesterone has a calming effect, which is why relaxation feels so aligning during the luteal phase.

Testosterone

Though often thought of as a male hormone, testosterone plays a key role in female hormone balance, too. It supports libido, confidence, energy, and muscle strength. Testosterone tends to peak just before ovulation, contributing to that mid-cycle burst of motivation, flirtiness, and drive. A dip in testosterone can leave you feeling sluggish or less interested in intimacy.

Cortisol

Cortisol is our main stress hormone, controlling how well all the other hormones function. I bet many of you can relate to the following: waking up feeling exhausted despite a full night's sleep, craving sugar and caffeine just to get through the day, and experiencing stubborn weight gain despite eating and exercising well. These can all be signs of cortisol imbalance. It is impossible to have high cortisol levels and balanced hormones at the same time, as the body cannot properly digest food, maintain energy, regulate weight, or support regular cycles under constant stress.

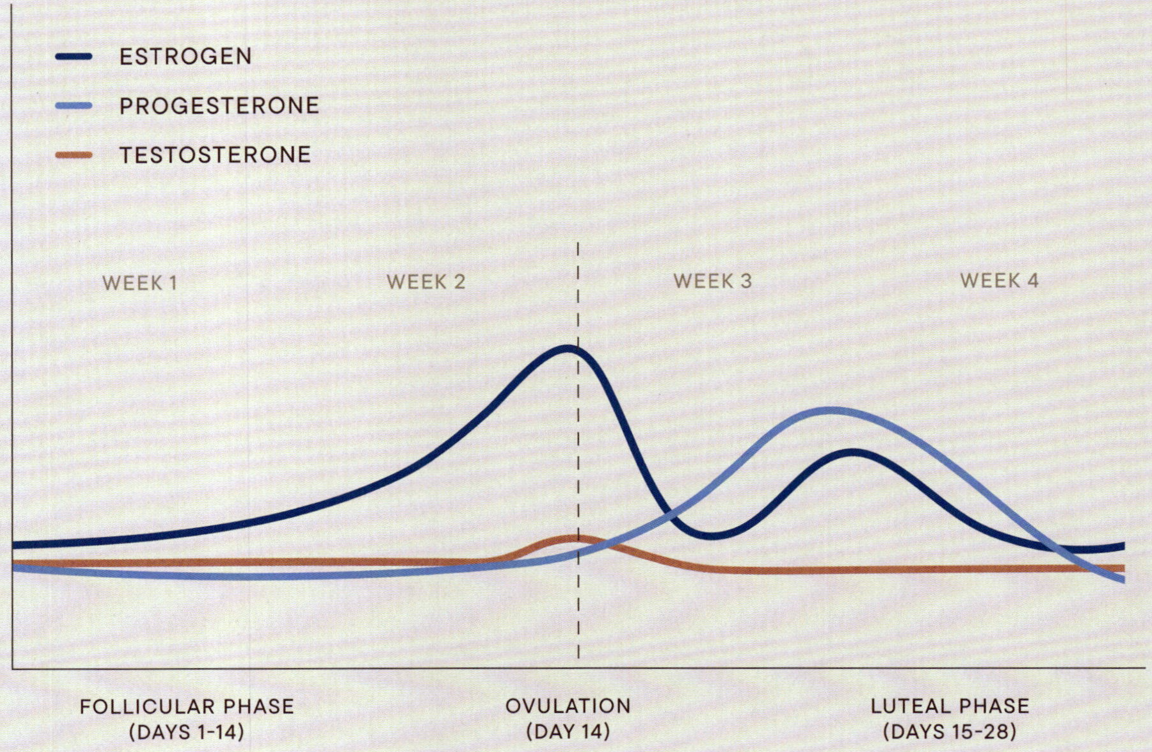

Dr. Amersi has shared the tip that cortisol levels tend to be higher in the second half of the cycle, from ovulation until the beginning of the next period. This is why finding ways to recharge during the luteal phase is extra important. Here are some ways to support healthy cortisol levels:

- Prioritizing sleep
- Walking often
- Eating protein with every meal
- Limiting caffeine on an empty stomach
- Getting morning sunlight
- Practicing deep breathing and journaling
- Avoiding harsh or high-intensity workouts

Understanding Your Body's Rhythm

Ever feel like your body is running on a completely different schedule than everyone else's? Turns out, it kind of is. Our society is built on a 24-hour circadian rhythm, but women follow an infradian rhythm—a 28-day cycle that governs our hormones. This is why what works for men doesn't always work for us! Understanding the phases of your cycle can help you know how to eat, move, and rest at the right times. By syncing with your natural rhythm, you can prevent common issues like PMS, digestion problems, and burnout. We'll get more into the four phases in each individual chapter, but here is the breakdown:

- MENSTRUAL PHASE Starts the first day of your bleed and generally lasts 3 to 7 days. This phase is marked by the most "prominent" or "visible" part of your cycle, your period.
- FOLLICULAR PHASE Starts the day your bleed ends, generally lasts 7 to 10 days.
- OVULATORY PHASE Marks the 3 to 4 days around ovulation.
- LUTEAL PHASE The longest phase, largely known for the PMS symptoms that show up during this time, runs for roughly the 10 to 14 days leading up to the first day of your period.

GENERAL HORMONE TIPS

- 7 to 9 hours of sleep per night
- Morning sunlight
- Daily movement
- More healthy fats (coconut, olive oil, ghee)
- Emotional release practices (journaling, therapy, meditation)

WHAT TO AVOID FOR HEALTHY HORMONES

- Caffeine on an empty stomach
- Plastic water bottles and BPAs
- Conventional perfumes and toxic beauty products
- Over-exercising and under-eating
- Excess refined sugars and processed foods
- Stress and toxic relationships

A note about your cycle: The standard woman's cycle is roughly 28 days long, but everyone is unique. Your phases may differ greatly from what's listed here, particularly if your cycle is irregular. I recommend looking into cycle-tracking methods or journals if you're curious to learn more about your exact cycle length, and Alisa Vitti provides an excellent blueprint for getting an irregular cycle back on track in her book *In the Flo.*

Some women with irregular periods may also find that adopting a 28-day cycle-based routine helps their periods become more regular. Please consult with a gynecologist before making any lifestyle changes that may affect your cycle.

Food and Your Cycle

Not surprisingly, what we put into our bodies greatly affects our hormones. But here's something that's often overlooked: Our bodies respond differently to food depending on where we are in our cycle. A crisp salad or spring roll might hit the spot during the ovulatory phase, but that same meal could leave you bloated and uncomfortable during the luteal or menstrual phase.

When I spoke with Dr. Amersi, she explained that our body chemistry shifts daily and weekly with our hormones. It makes sense that the foods we eat interact differently depending on what our body is experiencing at any given time.

When I began paying attention to these changes—swapping out generic health advice for nutrition tailored to each phase—everything shifted. The constant bloating I had been dealing with eased, my mood stabilized, and most important, I started to feel like myself again.

In today's wellness landscape, we're often sold on quick fixes, detox teas, or pricey supplements as the answer to our symptoms. But I've found that small, intentional changes can go so much further. My goal here is to help you feel just how powerful everyday ingredients can be. A carrot. Chickpeas. A pot of chili, or a cozy harvest bowl. These are the things that bring us back to balance.

You'll also notice that I place a strong emphasis on protein throughout the recipes. Protein is essential for hormone production, blood sugar balance, and satiety, and most women simply aren't getting enough of it. By making protein the foundation of each meal, you'll support stable energy, reduced cravings, and better overall hormone health.

I intentionally kept every recipe simple and approachable. Most meals require ten ingredients or fewer and can be made in about 30 minutes. I chose ingredients you can find at your local grocery store or Trader Joe's; there's no need to fill your pantry with expensive powders or exotic superfoods to feel the effects of hormone-happy nutrition.

MY TOP 5 PCOS TIPS

Although I absolutely recommend consulting a gynecologist if you have (or believe you have) PCOS, I often get asked for advice on this topic. Here are my top tips for those of you living with symptoms.

1 — Prioritize Protein + Fiber at Every Meal

This combo is foundational for blood sugar balance, something women with PCOS absolutely need. It supports steady energy, fewer cravings, improved insulin sensitivity, and more balanced hormones. Think eggs with veggies in the morning or salmon with a quinoa and greens bowl at dinner.

2 — Start Your Day with a Blood Sugar–Friendly Breakfast

Eating a high-protein breakfast (25–30g) within 60–90 minutes of waking can dramatically improve blood sugar, cortisol rhythms, and reduce hormone-related symptoms like fatigue, mood swings, and cravings.

3 — Strength Train (and Don't Overdo Cardio)

Building lean muscle improves insulin sensitivity, supports metabolism, and balances hormones. Strength-based workouts a few times a week, paired with gentle movement like walking and rest, are far more supportive than long, intense cardio sessions.

4 — Support Your Body with Inositol

Inositol (especially a 40:1 blend of myo- and d-chiro-inositol) is one of the most researched supplements for PCOS. It supports regular cycles, ovulation, egg quality, and insulin resistance, and it can be a game-changer for many.

5 — Focus on Real, Anti-Inflammatory Foods

PCOS is closely tied to inflammation. Prioritize whole, unprocessed foods: colorful vegetables, omega-3s from salmon and chia, antioxidant-rich berries, and spices like turmeric and cinnamon. These ingredients help soothe inflammation and support hormonal harmony from the inside out.

Remember: PCOS isn't a one-size-fits-all diagnosis and healing doesn't happen overnight. But small, consistent shifts like these add up. The recipes in this book are built to help you feel nourished, supported, and empowered every step of the way.

A quick note on servings: Most breakfasts are made to serve 1 to 2 people, while lunches and dinners are designed to serve 2 to 4. I chose to combine lunches and dinners into a single section within each phase for a reason: While traditional cookbooks often save the most involved recipes for dinner, every recipe in this book is designed to be quick and easy. That means your "dinner" recipes can double as lunch the next day, and vice versa. Flexibility is key, especially when you're busy and trying to stay consistent in nourishing yourself well.

This book is divided into sections, each one focused on a different phase of the menstrual cycle. Every section begins with a deeper look into what's happening in your body during that phase, how best to support it, and the kinds of foods that will leave you feeling grounded, nourished, and at your best.

Nutrition for the Four Phases of the Menstrual Cycle

The four phases of the menstrual cycle closely mimic the seasons, each with its own energy and needs:

- MENSTRUAL PHASE (WINTER) A time for rest and replenishment. Focus on warming foods like soups and stews.
- FOLLICULAR PHASE (SPRING) A fresh start, ideal for creativity and new beginnings. Think light, fresh foods.
- OVULATORY PHASE (SUMMER) A time for confidence and connection. Enjoy vibrant fruits and refreshing salads.
- LUTEAL PHASE (AUTUMN) Encourages reflection and grounding. Opt for warming spices, tea, and roasted veggies.

Dr. Amersi notes that what fuels your energy in the first half of your cycle may leave you feeling sluggish in the second half. The key is learning to work with your cycle, recognizing these shifts and adjusting your food choices accordingly.

Seed Cycling: A Simple Yet Powerful Hormone-Boosting Practice

Seed cycling is a natural and easy way to support hormone balance throughout your menstrual cycle. By incorporating specific seeds into your diet during its different phases, you provide essential nutrients that help stabilize hormonal fluctuations.

- MENSTRUAL, FOLLICULAR, OVULATORY PHASE (DAYS 1 TO 14) Flax and pumpkin seeds support estrogen metabolism.
- LUTEAL PHASE (DAYS 15 TO 28) Sesame and sunflower seeds promote progesterone production.

Simply rotate these seeds each week, adding a tablespoon per day to your meals (smoothies, salads, yogurt bowls, baked goods). While some women notice benefits like improved cycles and reduced PMS within a few weeks, it typically takes about three months to really feel the difference with new nutrition swaps, supplements, or lifestyle adjustments for hormones.

A Guide to Clean Products, Pantry Staples, and Kitchen Essentials

As you begin your journey with these hormone-supportive recipes, I share a few of my favorite things that make nourishing your body feel simple, approachable, and enjoyable. From the clean beauty brands I trust, to the pantry staples I always keep stocked, to the essential kitchen tools I use every day, this list is designed to support you without overcomplicating things.

Clean Skincare and Beauty Brands I Love

Hormone health isn't just about what you eat; what you put on your skin and hair matters, too. These are some of my go-to clean beauty and skincare brands that prioritize non-toxic, hormone-safe ingredients. Look for products that are free from endocrine-disrupting chemicals like parabens, phthalates, synthetic fragrances, and formaldehyde-releasing preservatives. I always check the ingredient labels or use resources like the Environmental Working Group's Skin Deep database or the Think Dirty app to make sure a brand aligns with hormone-safe standards.

- OSEA
- Cocokind
- Araza Beauty
- Ilia
- Tower 28
- Westman Atelier
- Saie, RMS Beauty
- Honey Girl Organics
- Innersense Haircare
- Living Libations

Tried-and-True Pantry Staples

These are the brands of everyday staples I rely on in my own kitchen. They're simple, clean, and make it easy to build balanced, supportive meals.

- LENTIL PASTA Tolerant Organic or Trader Joe's
- OATS One Degree Organics Sprouted Oats
- PROTEIN POWDER Truvani (plant-based) and Be Well by Kelly (beef isolate)
- COLLAGEN Further Food Collagen Peptides
- GRANOLA Purely Elizabeth
- COCONUT YOGURT Culina and CocoJune
- NUT BUTTERS Artisana Organics; Trader Joe's and Costco also have great organic almond and peanut butters
- BONE BROTH Fond Bone Broth
- CRACKERS Simple Mills Almond Flour Crackers, Mary's Gone Crackers
- DARK CHOCOLATE Hu Kitchen and Evolved
- HERBAL TEAS Organic India, Traditional Medicinals, Pique Tea
- SUPERFOODS I USE OFTEN Navitas Maca Powder, Beeya Seed Cycling Blends, Ceylon cinnamon, ground flaxseed

These ingredients show up often in the recipes throughout this book. Keeping them on hand will help you feel more prepared and less stressed at mealtimes.

Kitchen Basics (Non-Toxic Edition)

You don't need a full kitchen makeover to eat well, but having a few high-quality, non-toxic tools makes a big difference. Look for brands that are transparent about their materials—like stainless steel, cast iron, or ceramic—and avoid coatings like Teflon or anything labeled "nonstick" unless it's clearly PFAS free. I usually do a quick ingredient or material check online and look for certifications or third-party testing to make sure a product is truly safe.

As a rule, I try to avoid single-use plastics in the kitchen and I always store or reheat my food in glass containers. And it's not just about what you cook with; hormone-disrupting scents from conventional cleaners, or even candles and air fresheners, can also impact your endocrine system. I opt for fragrance-free or naturally scented products using essential oils, and I always read the labels for hidden toxins.

These are the essentials I recommend:

Cookware

- NON-TOXIC SKILLET OR FRY PAN Caraway or GreenPan
- CAST-IRON SKILLET Lodge
- LARGE POT OR DUTCH OVEN Xtrema or Our Place Perfect Pot

Bakeware

- BAKING DISH (9 × 13-INCH) Caraway or Our Place
- BAKING SHEETS Nordic Ware Natural Aluminum
- MUFFIN TIN USA Pan

Appliances

- BLENDER Vitamix
- MINI FOOD PROCESSOR Cuisinart
- IMMERSION BLENDER Mueller
- TOASTER OVEN OR AIR FRYER Breville Smart Oven or Our Place Wonder Oven

Utensils and Storage Containers

- SPATULAS AND SPOONS Food-grade silicone or bamboo
- CUTTING BOARDS Maple or bamboo
- GLASS STORAGE CONTAINERS Ello or Pyrex
- MASON JARS For dressings, smoothies, or overnight oats
- REUSABLE SILICONE BAGS Stasher

Clean-Living Extras

- WATER FILTER Berkey or AquaTru
- AIR PURIFIER AirDoctor or Mila
- LAUNDRY DETERGENT Clean People or Molly's Suds
- UNBLEACHED PARCHMENT PAPER for baking without toxins

Your Journey Starts Here

Living in alignment with your cycle isn't just about easing cramps or reducing bloating (though those are welcome benefits). It's also about building a deeper connection with your body, honoring its rhythms, and providing it with the nutrients it needs to thrive. Your body does so much for you, it's time to give back!

By syncing your nutrition with your cycle, you'll regain a sense of control and empowerment. No more feeling like your body is an unpredictable force. Instead, you'll have the tools to navigate each phase confidently, supporting your hormones in a sustainable, realistic way.

In the sections that follow, we explore each phase of your cycle, dive into the nutrients that support it, and provide simple, approachable recipes that make hormone-aligned nutrition easy and enjoyable. You don't need to completely overhaul your life to make this work; these recipes are designed to fit into your busy schedule and nourish you from the inside out.

Your body knows what it needs. Lean into that guidance. No two days are the same, so take what resonates and trust yourself!

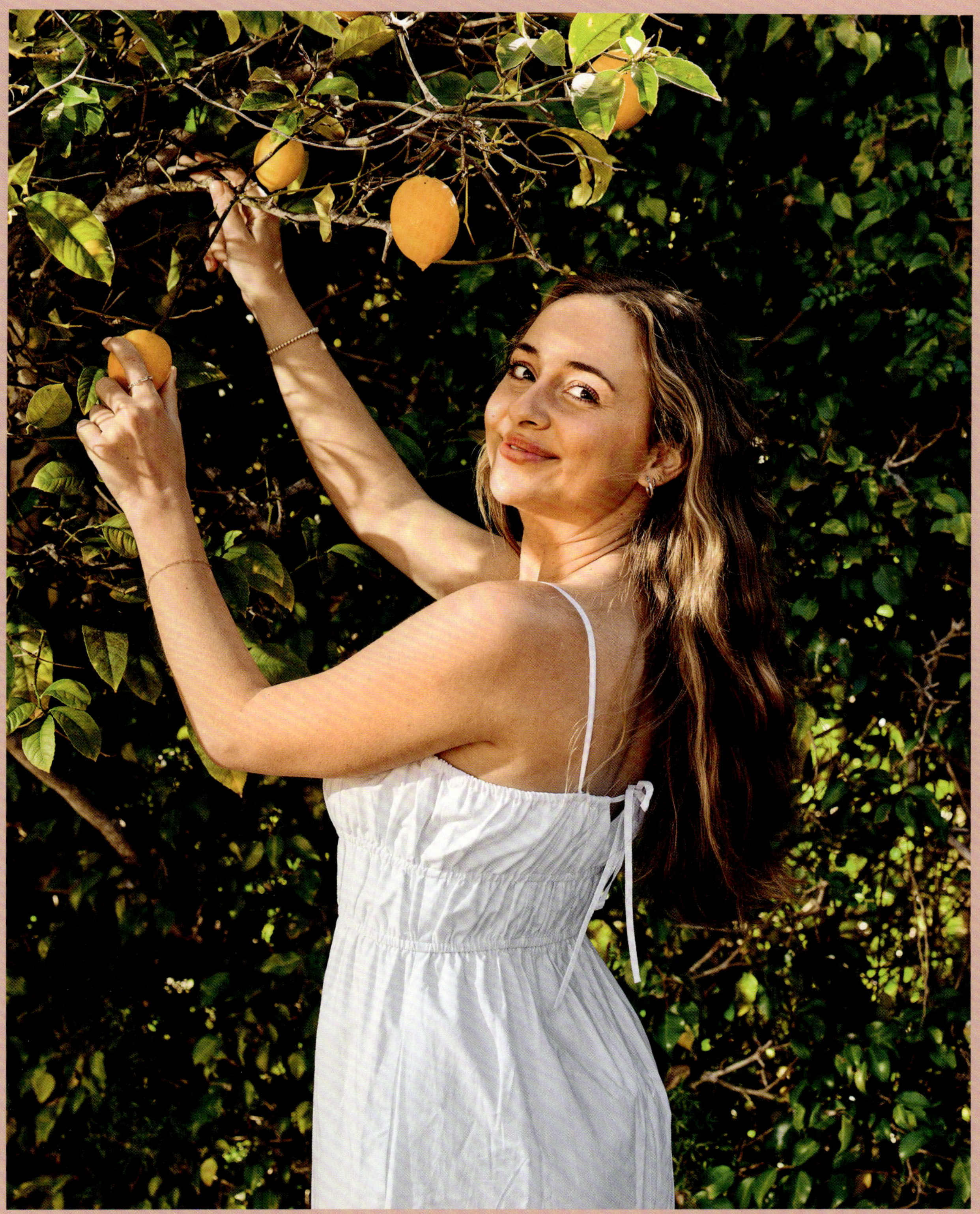

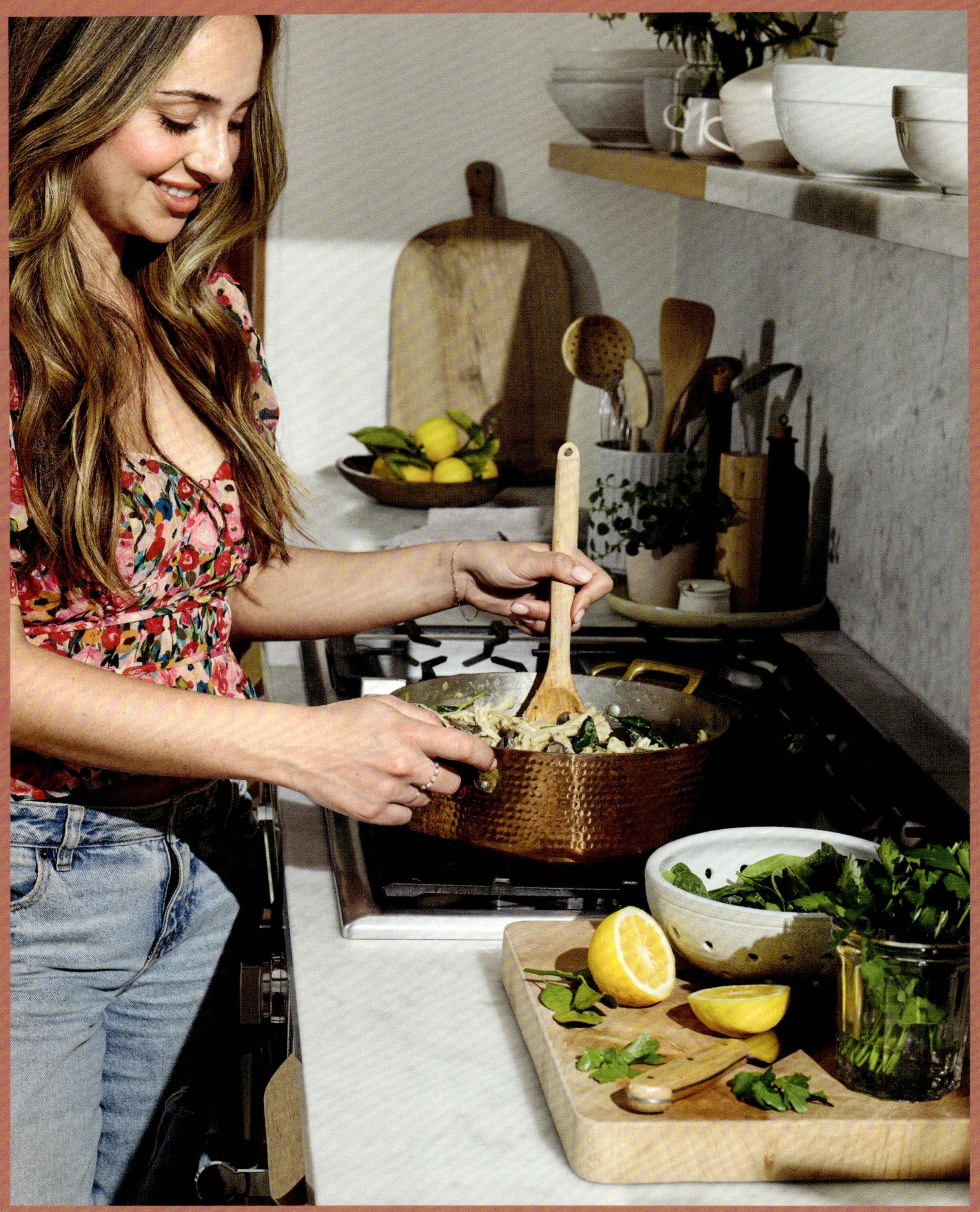

Menstrual Phase

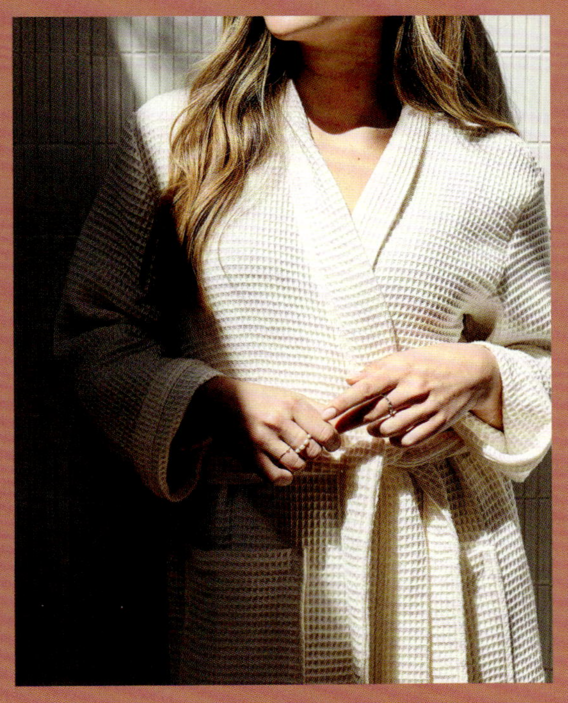

Nurturing Your Body

The menstrual phase marks the beginning of your cycle, starting on day 1 when your period begins and typically lasting three to seven days. During this time, your body is hard at work shedding the uterine lining, which triggers significant hormonal shifts. As both estrogen and progesterone hit their lowest levels at the start of your period, it's common to feel low on energy and more inward-focused, and to experience mood swings or physical symptoms like cramps, bloating, and backaches. Toward the end of your period, the estrogen and progesterone begin to rise again, which can gradually improve your energy and mood. In the meantime, focusing on nourishing foods and self-care can help ease many of these symptoms and give your body the support it needs to get through this phase a little more comfortably.

Hormonal Breakdown: What's Happening?

Let's talk hormones:

- ESTROGEN AND PROGESTERONE ARE AT THEIR LOWEST POINT This drop is what triggers menstruation. As your hormone levels dip, your energy may follow suit—so if you're feeling a little more tired, tender, or inward, you're not imagining it. This is your body's cue to rest and reset.
- PROSTAGLANDINS ARE ON THE RISE These are hormone-like compounds that help the uterus contract to shed its lining. But when they spike too high, they can cause cramps, headaches, and digestive discomfort.

This is your body's natural detox phase—shedding the old and getting ready for a new cycle. It's the perfect time to lean into nourishing comfort foods, keep your blood sugar steady, and focus on gentle movement or rest. Your body is doing a lot behind the scenes, so go easy on yourself and prioritize warmth, minerals (like iron and magnesium), and replenishment.

How Food Can Support You

As your uterine lining is shed, the body loses iron, which can contribute to feelings of fatigue. Focusing on warming, nutrient-dense, and easy-to-digest foods is crucial for replenishing lost minerals and helping you feel more energized. Think of meals like hearty lentil soup rich in iron, warm quinoa bowls with roasted veggies and avocado for magnesium and healthy fats, or slow-cooked beef stew for easily digestible protein and iron. These nutrients are key to reducing inflammation, easing cramps, and restoring energy. Dr. Amersi notes it's a good idea to avoid heavily processed foods, alcohol, spicy foods, and sugar, which can contribute to inflammation that can in turn cause even more severe period cramps. She also shares that this stage is most associated with high levels of food cravings, but offers encouragement to try to be gentle with yourself and listen to what feels good for your body and emotional needs.

Top Nutrition Tips for the Menstrual Phase

1 — Focus on Iron

During menstruation, your body loses iron, which can lead to feelings of fatigue and low energy. Replenishing iron is crucial to help combat these symptoms. Opt for iron-rich foods like spinach, grass-fed red meat, lentils, and chickpeas to restore your levels. To maximize iron absorption, pair these with vitamin C–rich foods such as citrus fruits, bell peppers, tomatoes, or berries. The vitamin C helps your body absorb non-heme iron (the type found in plant-based sources) more effectively!

2 — Boost Magnesium Intake

Magnesium is known as the "relaxation mineral" because it helps relax muscles, which can be particularly helpful in easing menstrual cramps. Including magnesium-rich foods like cacao, almonds, pumpkin seeds, and dark leafy greens can make a difference in reducing the tension in your body. Magnesium also plays a role in stabilizing your mood and supporting restful sleep, both of which are essential during this phase when your body might feel more depleted.

3 — Healthy Fats for Hormone Support

Omega-3 fatty acids are particularly beneficial during menstruation because they help reduce inflammation, a common side effect of menstruation. Inflammation can exacerbate cramps, joint pain, and discomfort during this time. Incorporating omega-3-rich foods like salmon, walnuts, chia seeds, flax seeds, and avocado can help soothe these symptoms by supporting hormone regulation and reducing inflammatory responses. These healthy fats also provide long-lasting energy and support hormone production, keeping you balanced throughout your cycle.

4 — Emphasize Warming, Nourishing Foods

During the menstrual phase, your body tends to crave warmth and comfort, for both physical and emotional support. Warm foods like soups, stews, and broths can be easier to digest and help promote circulation. Adding anti-inflammatory spices like ginger, turmeric, and cinnamon not only enhances flavor but also supports digestion and reduces bloating. These spices are also known for improving circulation and keeping your body feeling balanced and comfortable as it slows down.

5 — Prioritize Hydration

Staying well hydrated is key for preventing bloating and helping your body flush out toxins more effectively. Drinking plenty of water throughout the day can also reduce the likelihood of headaches, improve digestion, and support overall energy levels. Herbal teas, such as peppermint or ginger tea, can be particularly soothing, helping with cramps and digestion while providing warmth and hydration.

6 — Start Strong

Eating breakfast is especially important during this phase. Studies have shown that skipping breakfast can increase cortisol, trigger reproductive hormone dysregulation, cause brain fog, and lead to blood sugar spikes that may cause you to reach for more salty and sugary foods as the day goes on.

Exercise and Lifestyle Tips

The menstrual phase is often a time when your body signals the need to slow down, and it's important to honor that. Even if you're someone who usually likes to push through, listening to your body and taking things easier during this phase can actually set you up for a more balanced, energized cycle. This phase is all about restoration, so embracing gentle movement and self-care can be powerful ways to support your energy, mood, and overall well-being.

Gentle Movement

Your body is naturally lower on energy during this phase as it focuses on shedding the uterine lining, and it's normal to feel more fatigued. Opt for light, low-impact activities like walking, Pilates, gentle stretching, or restorative yoga. These movements help ease cramps, boost circulation, and release endorphins without overburdening your body. Keeping movement light will help balance these stress hormones and avoid overexertion.

Rest and Rejuvenation

Your body is working hard during your period, and it's important to honor that by giving yourself permission to rest. This is not the time to push through intense workouts or mentally demanding tasks. Prioritizing extra sleep and relaxation allows your body to recover and prepare for the next phase of your cycle. Think of it as a reset button: By resting now, you're setting yourself up for more energy and productivity later on. Rest is your best friend during this phase!

Heat Therapy

Using heat is one of the simplest, most effective ways to ease menstrual cramps and discomfort. A heating pad or a warm bath can help relax the muscles around your uterus, reduce inflammation, and provide comfort. The warmth also stimulates blood flow, which can alleviate tension in your lower abdomen. It's not just about soothing cramps; heat therapy can also be a great way to decompress and recharge emotionally.

Herbal Teas

Certain herbal teas are perfect during the menstrual phase, helping to soothe common discomforts. Chamomile tea is known for its calming properties, easing both cramps and stress. Peppermint can help with bloating and digestive issues, while ginger is a great anti-inflammatory that also supports digestion and can ease nausea. Sipping on these teas throughout the day can provide hydration, warmth, and relaxation!

Self-Care Practices to Support Your Menstrual Phase

- JOURNALING AND REFLECTION This phase is ideal for turning your attention inward and processing your emotions, thoughts, and experiences. During this time, the connection between the right and left sides of the brain becomes more integrated, which can enhance your ability to both reflect creatively and think logically. This balanced brain state makes it a great time to journal, as you may find it easier to express your emotions while gaining clarity on problem-solving and goal-setting. Journaling during your period can help you identify any patterns or recurring thoughts, and offers an opportunity to plan ahead with a clear, focused mind. By allowing yourself this quiet space for introspection, you're also creating the foundation for more balanced decision-making and mindfulness throughout the rest of your cycle.
- GENTLE BREATHWORK Practices like deep belly breathing, box breathing, or alternate nostril breathing help regulate the nervous system, lowering cortisol levels and reducing stress, which is the foundation for hormonal balance. Engaging in these practices during this phase can also help support you throughout the rest of your cycle by promoting a more resilient nervous system. When your body is calm and centered, it's better equipped to handle the natural energy fluctuations that occur in later phases, allowing you to stay grounded and connected.

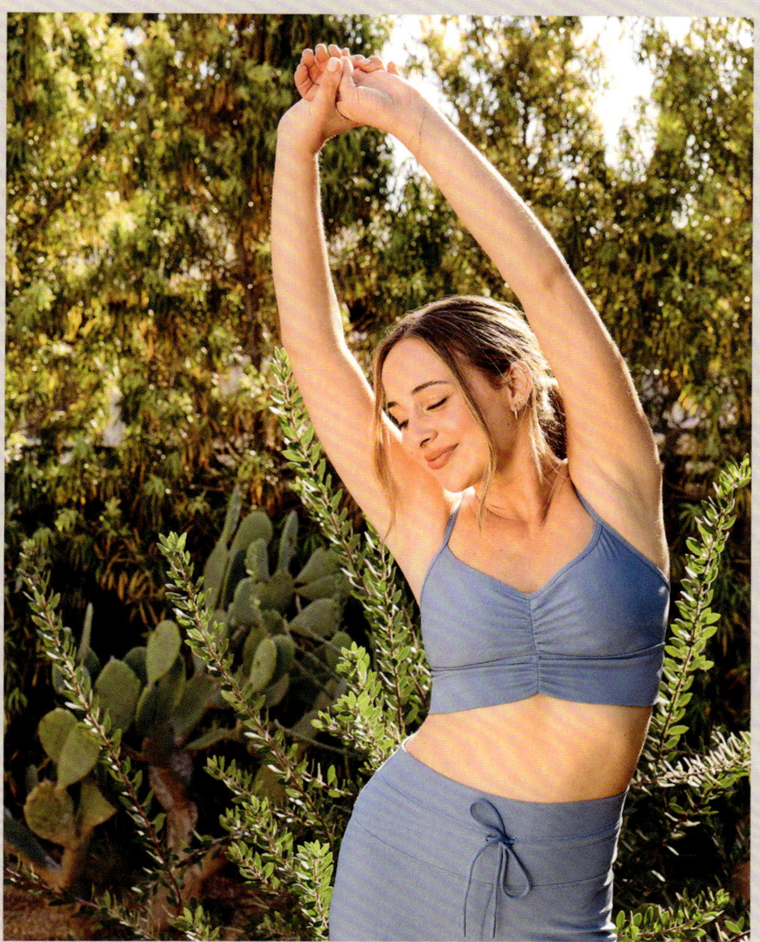

Incorporating breathwork in your menstrual phase helps set you up for more productive, energetic, and balanced days ahead.

— **NOURISHING RITUALS** Create comforting rituals that soothe both your body and your mind. Sipping on warm herbal teas, like chamomile or ginger, can help ease cramps and digestion, while applying essential oils such as lavender or clary sage to your abdomen, temples, feet, or behind your ears can bring a sense of calm and relaxation. Epsom salt baths are another wonderful way to reduce bloating, relax tense muscles, and support detoxification. These small, nurturing acts of self-care can help you feel more grounded and connected to your body during this phase, allowing you to honor the slower pace your body craves.

By aligning your diet and lifestyle with your body's needs during the menstrual phase, you can ease discomfort, restore energy, and nurture yourself from within. In the following recipes, you'll find comforting meals packed with nutrients to help you feel your best during this phase—foods that are easy on digestion, rich in key minerals, and full of flavor. Let's dive into nourishing your body, one delicious meal at a time!

During this three- to seven-day window, your routine might look like:

- TWO DAYS OF REST Let your body fully recharge—think sleep, cozy meals, and saying no to extra obligations.
- TWO TO THREE DAYS OF GENTLE MOVEMENT Try a walk in nature, a light stretch session, or a slow yoga flow. Focus on your breath and connection to your body.
- ONE OPTIONAL DAY OF INTUITIVE MOVEMENT If you're feeling up for it, do something that feels good in the moment—a short Pilates class, a solo dance session, or a mellow swim.

What to Eat

- BREAKFASTS Go for warming, iron-rich meals like cacao oatmeal with chia seeds and almond butter, or sweet potato hash with eggs.
- LUNCHES Try comforting bowls like a lentil soup with spinach, or a chicken and root veggie stew with bone broth.
- DINNERS Focus on mineral-rich, grounding meals like grass-fed ground beef with sautéed kale and rice, or baked salmon with roasted squash and turmeric. Add ginger or cinnamon for warmth and digestion support.

Menstrual Phase Superfoods

- CACAO Contains iron, magnesium, and antioxidants, helping to reduce cravings, improve mood, and alleviate cramps.
- SWEET POTATOES High in complex carbohydrates, potassium, and fiber, helping to stabilize blood sugar levels, boost energy, and reduce water retention.
- BANANAS Excellent source of potassium, which can help reduce bloating and water retention.

- **SALMON** Packed with omega-3 fatty acids that reduce inflammation.
- **GRASS-FED BEEF** High in iron and vitamin B12, essential for energy levels and replenishing red blood cell production.
- **PUMPKIN SEEDS** Rich in magnesium, iron, and zinc, supporting hormone balance and reducing PMS symptoms.
- **SPINACH** High in iron, folate, and magnesium, aiding in energy production and reducing menstrual cramps.
- **QUINOA** A complete protein and high in fiber, helping to keep you full and stabilize blood sugar levels.
- **AVOCADO** Rich in healthy fats, fiber, and potassium, supporting overall hormonal balance.
- **BLUEBERRIES** Packed with antioxidants and vitamin C, helping to reduce inflammation and boost immunity.
- **CHIA SEEDS** High in omega-3 fatty acids and fiber, reducing inflammation and supporting digestion.
- **GINGER** Can help alleviate menstrual cramps and nausea.
- **LENTILS** Great source of plant-based protein, iron, and folate, supporting energy levels and hormonal health.
- **GREEK YOGURT** High in protein and calcium, supporting bone health and satiety.
- **WALNUTS** Rich in omega-3 fatty acids, magnesium, and antioxidants, promoting brain health and reducing inflammation.
- **OATS** High in fiber and complex carbohydrates, stabilizing blood sugar levels and supporting digestion.
- **APPLES** High in fiber and antioxidants, aiding in digestion and reducing inflammation.
- **TURMERIC** Contains curcumin, which has powerful anti-inflammatory properties.

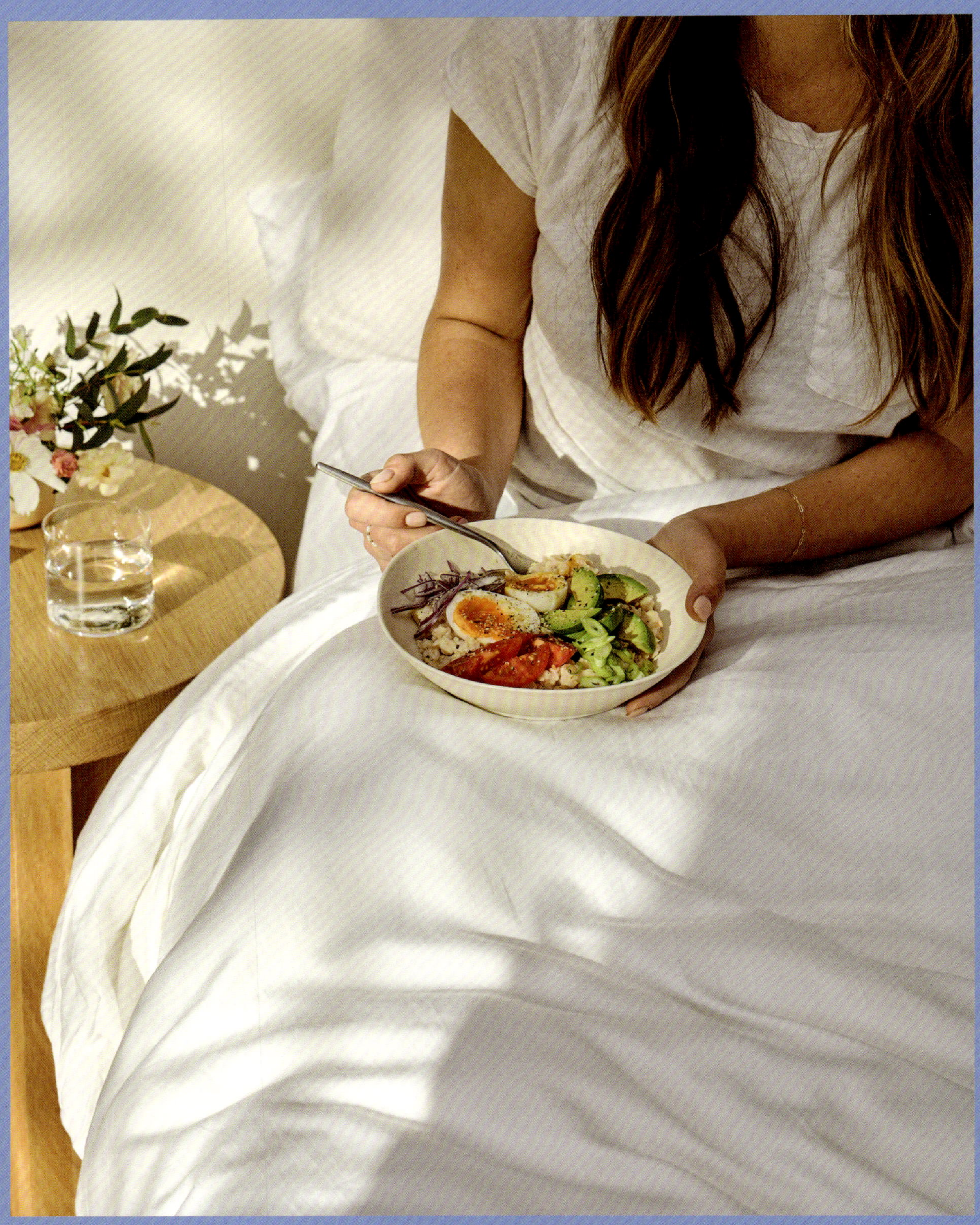

Breakfasts

Rich and Chocolatey Menstrual Phase Cacao Oatmeal

Serves 1
Prep Time: 5 minutes
Cook Time: 10 minutes

I've been relying on this recipe during my menstrual phase for years; it satisfies the chocolate cravings that hit during this time, but offers increased nutritional value and without the extra sugars that most store-bought chocolates contain. Your progesterone and estrogen are still low here in the first few days of your cycle, which can leave you feeling drained and craving comfort. Subbing cacao powder for the cocoa powder or chocolate chips in your oats is a great way to start the day; you'll get the chocolatey flavor without the extra sugar, which can cause blood sugar spikes that lead to energy crashes, water retention, bloating, and irritation. Plus, cacao powder is packed with magnesium and iron to help relax those tight muscles, ease cramps, and give you a much-needed energy boost.

½ cup old-fashioned rolled oats (I suggest looking for sprouted oats)

1 cup unsweetened almond milk (or other milk of choice)

1 tablespoon cacao powder

1 tablespoon pure maple syrup or honey

1 teaspoon vanilla extract

¼ teaspoon ground cinnamon

Pinch of salt

1 scoop protein powder (optional)

Optional toppings: 1 tablespoon almond butter, 2 tablespoons cacao nibs, walnuts and pumpkin seeds, berries (fresh or frozen), plain Greek yogurt

1 — In a small saucepan, combine the oats and almond milk. Bring to a boil over medium heat, then reduce to a simmer.

2 — Stir in the cacao powder, maple syrup, vanilla, cinnamon, and salt. Continue to stir and cook for 5 to 7 minutes, until the oats are tender and the mixture thickens. If using, stir in the protein powder as well.

3 — Remove the pan from the heat and transfer the oatmeal to a bowl. Top with some almond butter, cacao nibs, walnuts and pumpkin seeds, and berries to your liking, and spoon on the Greek yogurt, if using.

Note

You can also make this oatmeal ahead of time, or double- or triple-batch the recipe for easy breakfasts throughout the week. Just follow the instructions through step 2, portion it into individual containers, and store in the fridge for up to 3 days. Simply reheat and add your toppings when you're ready to enjoy!

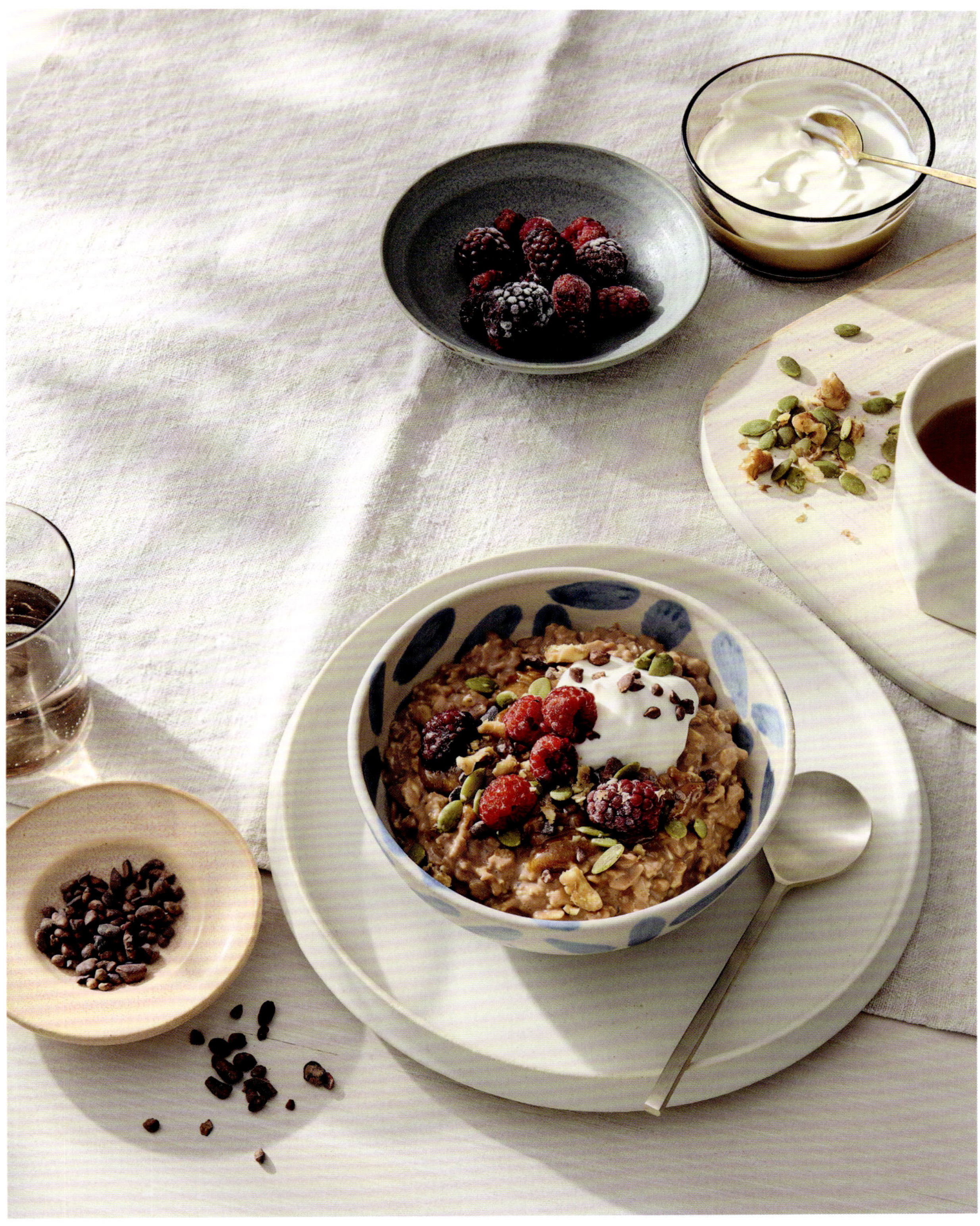

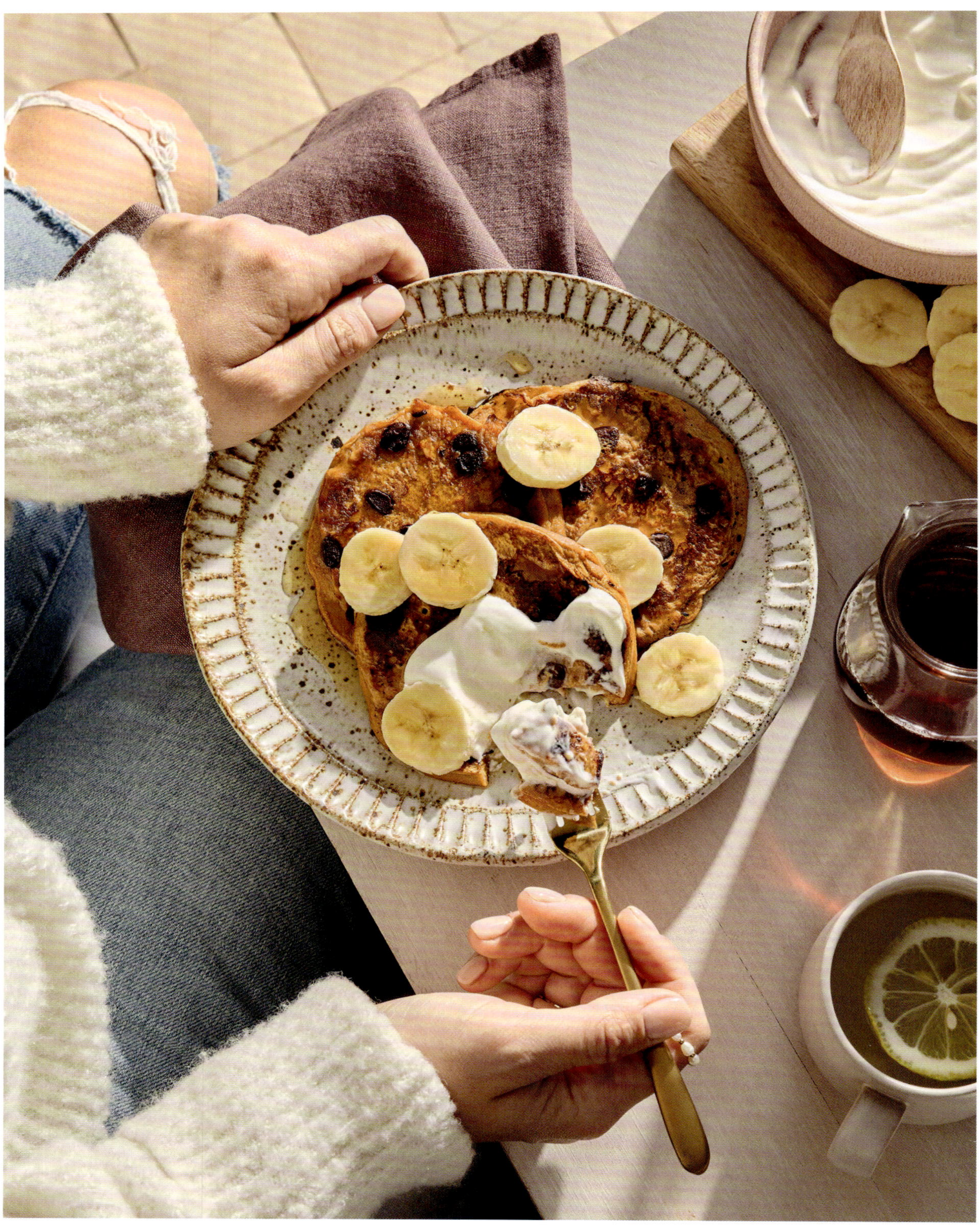

Conquer-Your-Cravings Sweet Potato Pancakes

Serves 2

Prep Time: 10 minutes

Cook Time: 15 minutes

These sweet potato pancakes are a fan favorite among my followers! They're packed with complex carbs and fiber to keep your energy steady and your hormones happy. While simple carbs (think cereals, pastries, white bread) are digested quickly by the body and can leave your stomach grumbling soon after you eat, complex carbs (think whole wheat bread, oatmeal, root vegetables) take much longer to break down and provide much steadier sources of energy—the kind you need while your body is in its menstrual phase. These pancakes are a tasty, wholesome option that will satisfy your cravings and even help with digestion. Sweet potatoes are also loaded with vitamin C and B6, both of which support mood and energy production. To make this a hassle-free breakfast, toss an extra sweet potato into the oven next time you're making some for dinner!

- 1 medium sweet potato, baked, peeled, and mashed
- 2 large eggs
- ¼ cup oat flour or 1:1 gluten-free flour
- 1 teaspoon ground cinnamon
- 1 teaspoon vanilla extract
- 2 to 3 tablespoons dark chocolate chips (optional)
- 1 tablespoon coconut oil or ghee
- Optional toppings: scoop of plain Greek yogurt or coconut yogurt, sliced banana, maple syrup or honey

1 — In a medium bowl, combine the mashed sweet potato, eggs, oat flour, cinnamon, and vanilla. Mix until smooth. Fold in the chocolate chips, if using.

2 — Heat the coconut oil or ghee in a nonstick skillet over medium heat.

3 — Spoon the batter into the skillet, forming 3-inch pancakes. Cook each side for 3 to 4 minutes, until golden brown. Repeat with remaining batter.

4 — Serve the pancakes warm, topped with the yogurt, banana slices, or a drizzle of maple syrup or honey, if desired.

PSL-Vibes Pumpkin Spice Smoothie Bowl

Serves 1
Prep Time: 10 minutes

When the phases of your cycle are related to the seasons of the year, the menstrual phase is considered your body's "winter," so it's no wonder you crave satisfying meals with warming ingredients during this phase. But since you go through the four phases year-round, sometimes you need something cold and refreshing that tastes just as comforting. This pumpkin spice smoothie bowl blends the warming flavors of pumpkin and cinnamon into a smooth, easily digestible breakfast. Blending helps your body absorb the nutrients more efficiently by breaking them down before they even hit your stomach. I love adding a crunchy, low-sugar granola made with nuts and seeds for extra texture and nutrition; I've included a simple recipe here, but feel free to add your favorite hormone-friendly brand!

½ frozen peeled banana
¼ cup pumpkin puree
½ teaspoon pumpkin spice blend
¼ cup unsweetened almond milk
1 scoop vanilla protein powder
1 cup crushed ice
¼ cup low-sugar granola (recipe follows)
2 tablespoons pomegranate seeds

1 — In a blender, combine the banana, pumpkin puree, pumpkin spice, almond milk, protein powder, and ice. Blend on high speed until smooth and creamy.

2 — Pour the smoothie into a bowl and top with the granola and pomegranate seeds.

continued

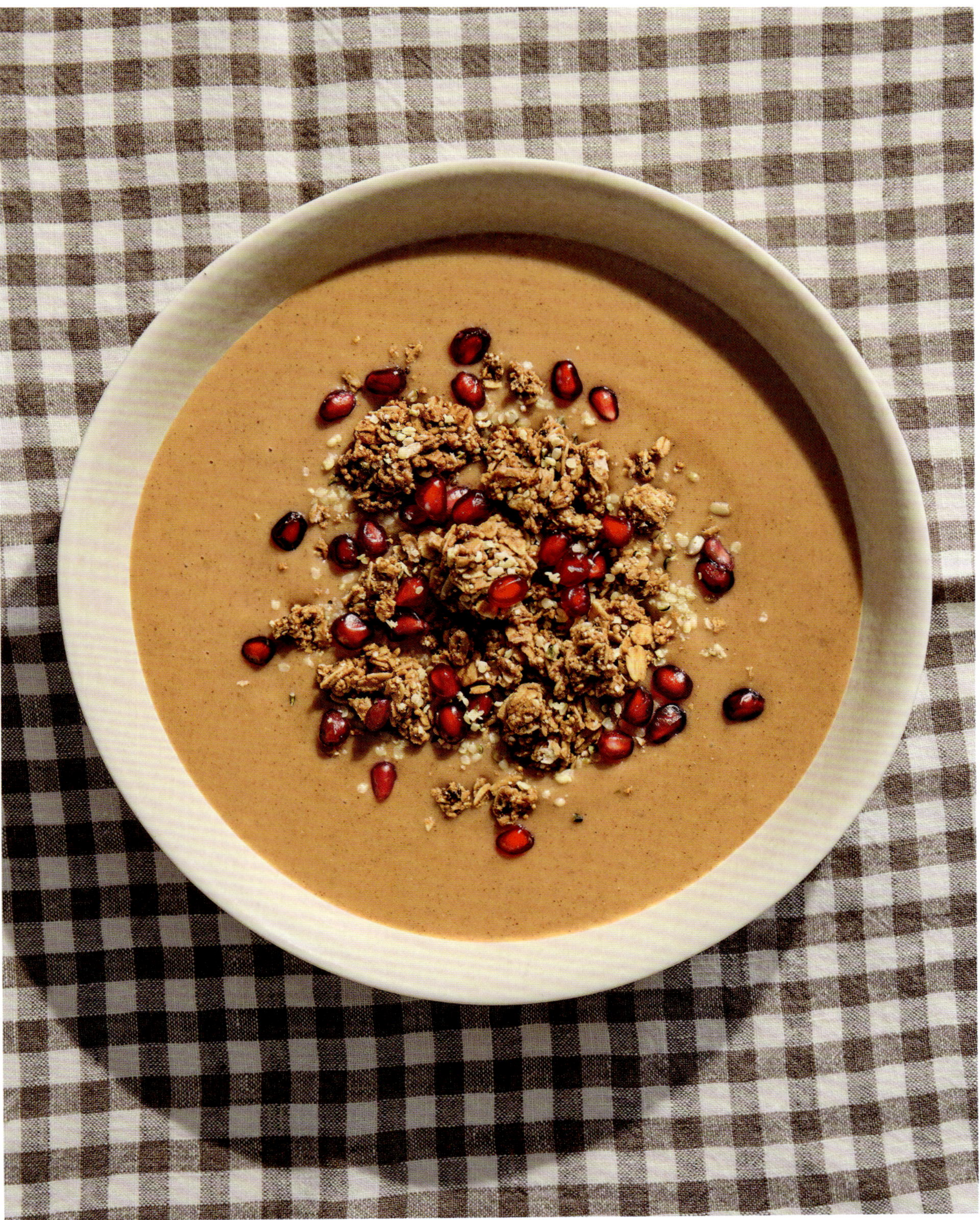

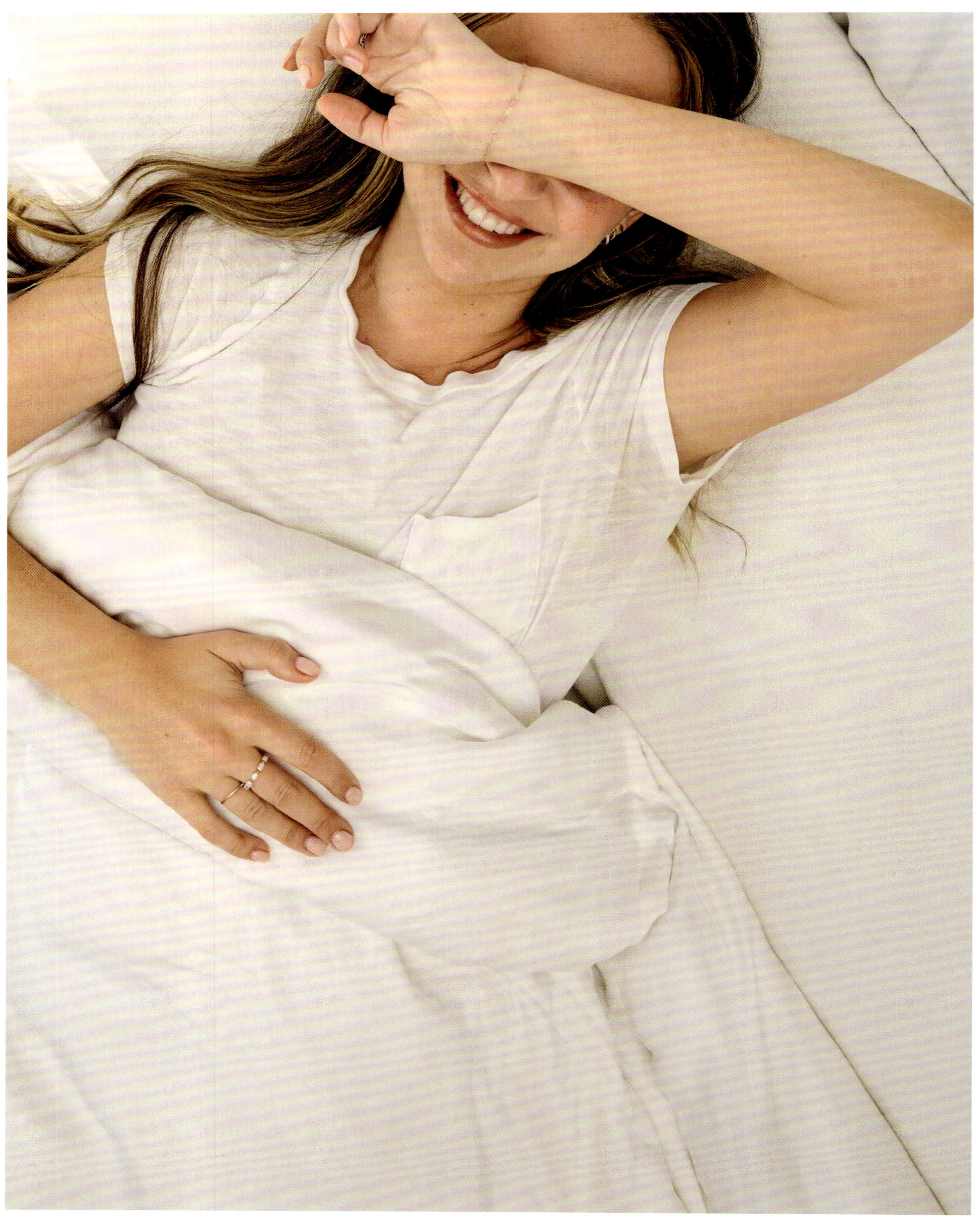

Maple-Walnut Superseed Granola

Makes 3½ cups
Prep Time: 10 minutes
Cook Time: 22 to 25 minutes

Granola

2 cups gluten-free rolled oats
½ cup raw walnuts, chopped
½ cup sunflower seeds
¼ cup unsweetened coconut flakes
2 tablespoons ground flaxseed
1 tablespoon chia seeds
1½ teaspoons ground cinnamon
¼ teaspoon sea salt
¼ cup melted coconut oil
¼ cup pure maple syrup
1 teaspoon vanilla extract

Optional Add-ins (after baking)

2 tablespoons hemp seeds
2 tablespoons dried unsweetened cherries or mulberries
2 tablespoons mini dark chocolate chips

1 — Preheat the oven to 325°F. Line a baking sheet with parchment paper.

2 — Make the granola: In a large bowl, mix the oats, walnuts, sunflower seeds, coconut flakes, flaxseed, chia seeds, cinnamon, and salt.

3 — In a small bowl, whisk together the melted coconut oil, maple syrup, and vanilla. Pour over the dry mix and stir until everything is well coated.

4 — Spread the mixture evenly on the baking sheet and bake for 22 to 25 minutes, stirring halfway through, until golden and crisp.

5 — Remove from the oven and let cool completely, then stir in any optional add-ins. Store the granola in a glass jar or airtight container at room temperature for up to 2 weeks.

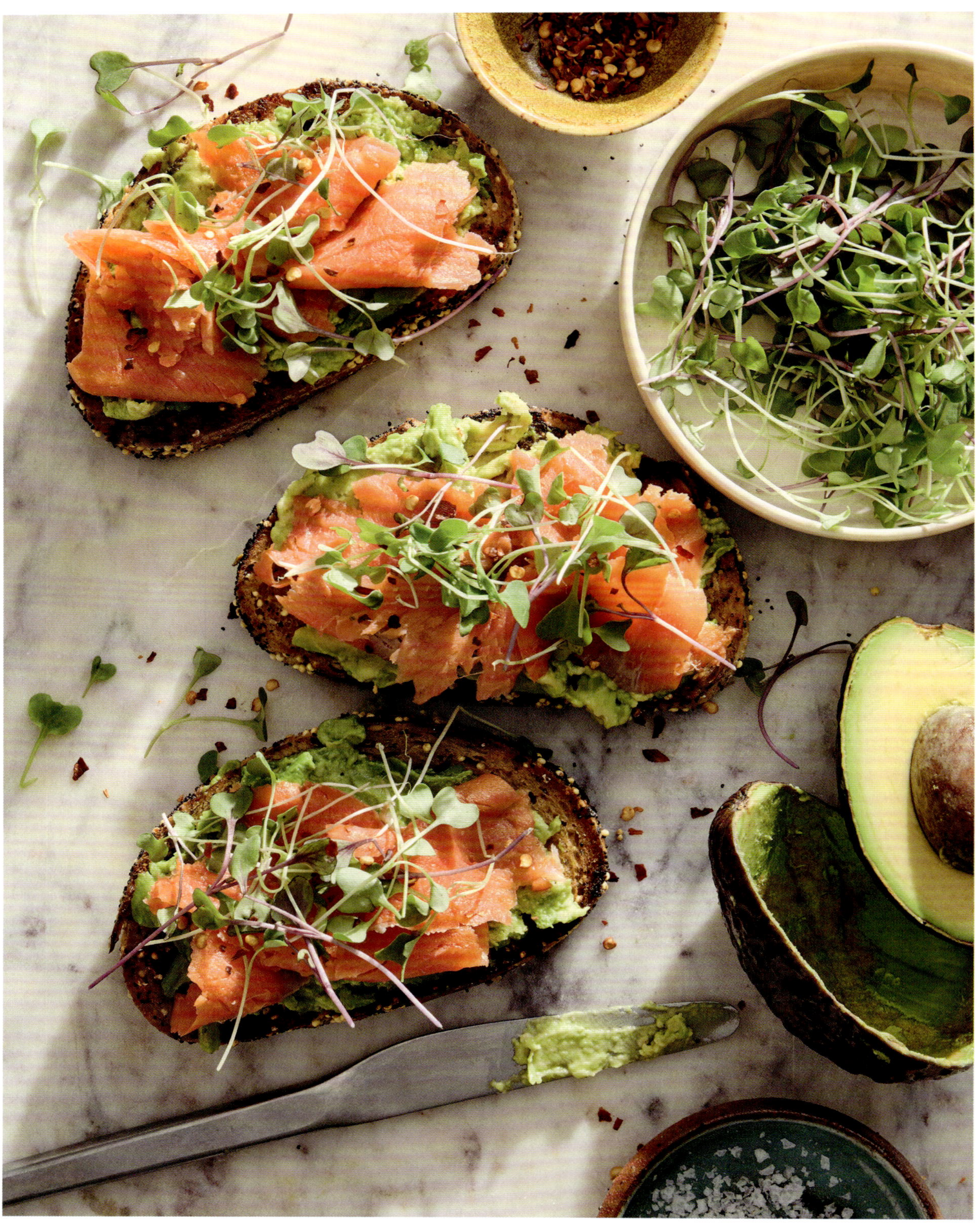

Happy Macros Avocado Toast

Serves 1
Prep Time: 10 minutes

This nutritious toast has become a go-to breakfast for me when I wake up craving something savory. Around your period time, cravings for salty, savory foods can kick in as your body seeks out iodine and omega-3s, which are essential for supporting your thyroid, hormones and mood. The avocado and smoked salmon here deliver an excellent dose of healthy fats, which can help with mood swings, bloating, anxiety, depression, insomnia, and more. You might be tempted to skip the microgreens, but make sure to add them: These vegetable sprouts are incredibly nutrient dense and pack a healthy punch of vitamins C, E, and K, as well as antioxidants and dietary fiber, which can help keep things running smoothly as your digestion tends to slow down during this restful time.

- ½ ripe avocado, peeled and pitted
- 1 teaspoon freshly squeezed lemon juice
- Salt and freshly ground black pepper
- 1 slice sourdough or gluten-free bread, toasted
- 2 ounces smoked salmon (preferably wild-caught)
- ¼ cup fresh microgreens (such as arugula, radish, or broccoli sprouts)
- Red pepper flakes, for garnish

1 — In a small bowl, mash the avocado with a fork. Add the lemon juice, and salt and pepper to taste, then mix until smooth and creamy.

2 — Spread the avocado mixture evenly over the toast. Top with the smoked salmon, arranging it neatly on the slice.

3 — Finish with a sprinkle of the microgreens and, if desired, a pinch of red pepper flakes for a bit of heat.

Happy Gut Breakfast Skillet

Serves 1
Prep Time: 10 minutes
Cook Time: 20 minutes

Research has shown that gut health and hormone health are linked, and that eating a variety of plants is highly beneficial to both—so, when in doubt, fill your plate with color! The mix of sweet potato, red bell pepper, and spinach in this skillet creates a colorful and nutrient-rich base, with plenty of fiber and essential vitamins to fuel your morning. Sweet potatoes offer complex carbs for steady energy, while spinach provides the iron and folate your body needs for optimal hormone function. The eggs add a hit of protein, and the avocado brings in those nourishing fats—keeping you full, focused, and balanced until lunch! This is also a great meal-prep option; simply chop your veggies ahead of time and you'll have a healthy breakfast in under 20 minutes.

1 tablespoon olive oil
¼ red onion, diced
½ small sweet potato, diced
½ red bell pepper, cleaned and diced
1 cup fresh baby spinach, trimmed
2 large eggs
¼ avocado, peeled, pitted, and sliced
Salt and freshly ground black pepper
Hot sauce or salsa, for serving (optional)

1 — Heat the olive oil in a large skillet over medium heat. Add the red onion and sweet potato and cook for 8 to 10 minutes, stirring occasionally, until the sweet potato is tender and slightly crispy.

2 — Add the bell pepper to the skillet and cook for an additional 3 minutes, until softened. Add the spinach and cook just until wilted, about 1 minute.

3 — Make 2 small wells in the vegetable mixture and crack an egg into each. Cover the skillet with a lid and cook until the eggs are set to your liking, 4 to 5 minutes for soft yolks or 5 to 7 minutes for firm.

4 — Transfer the contents of the skillet to a serving plate and top with the avocado slices. Add salt and pepper to taste, then add a dash of hot sauce or salsa, if desired.

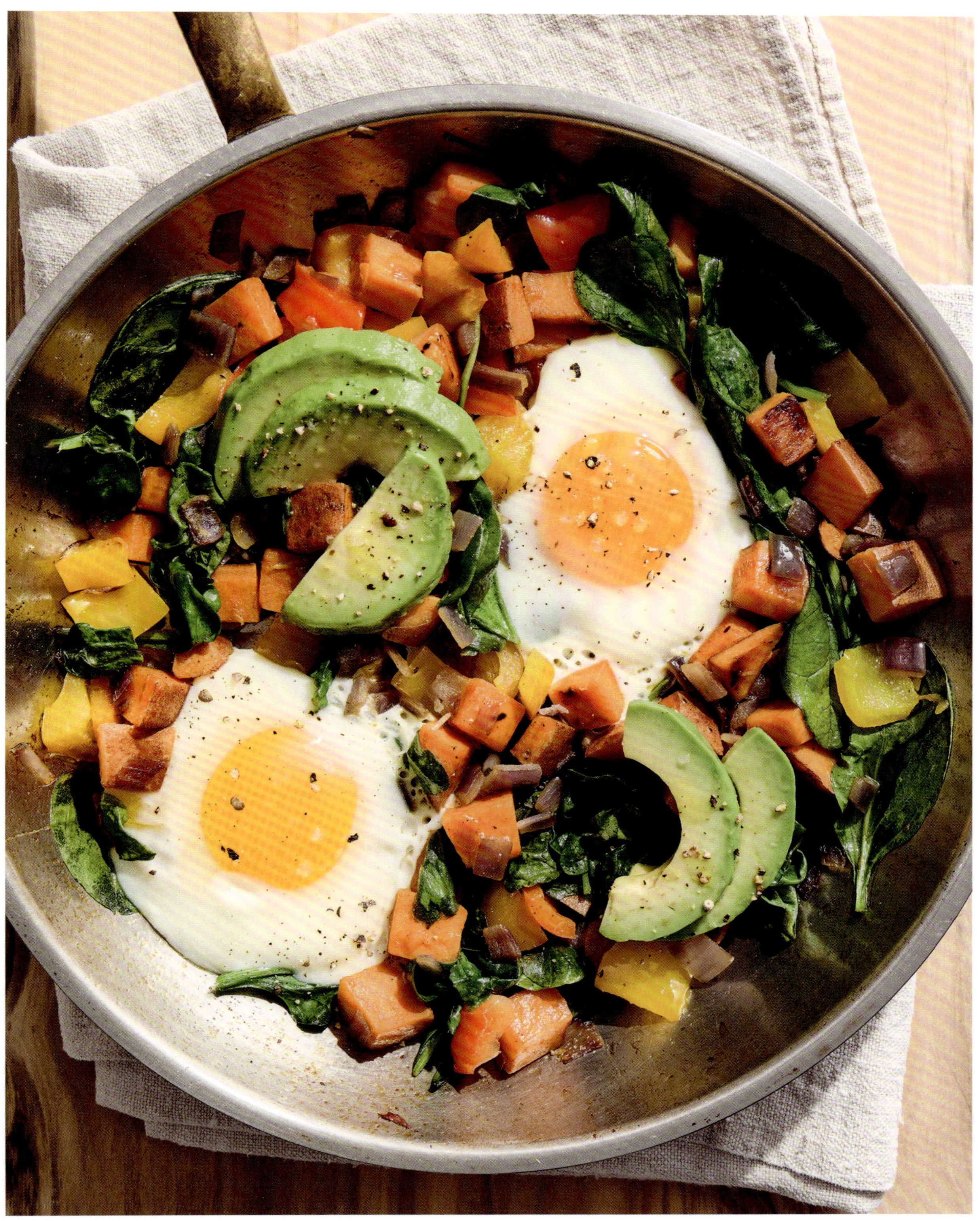

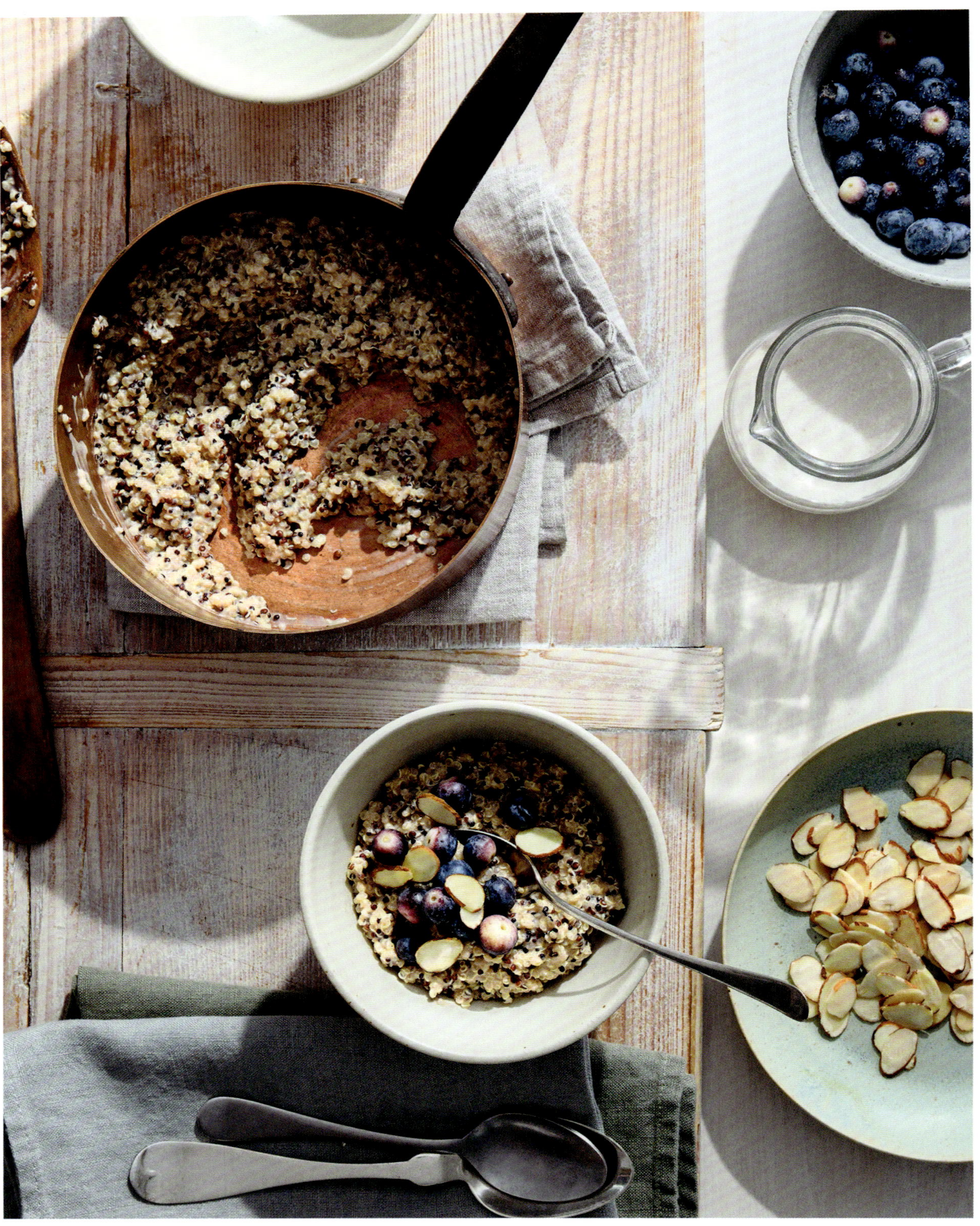

Cozy Quinoa Porridge with Cinnamon and Almond Milk

Serves 1
Prep Time: 5 minutes
Cook Time: 15 minutes

This quinoa porridge is like a warm, comforting blanket for your morning, and it will help you get out of bed even when you're feeling at your worst. Quinoa is a complete protein, making it a perfect addition to your breakfast, as your body craves nourishment during your period. Protein is especially important as well because it helps stabilize your blood sugar, keeps you feeling fuller longer, and supports your body's repair processes that are hard at work during menstruation. Its rich magnesium content also helps soothe muscle cramps and tension. I especially recommend adding some fresh blueberries as a garnish—they contain vitamin K, which can help reduce heavy bleeding—but any berries will be delicious with this. It's the ultimate feel-good breakfast when you need extra care!

¼ cup quinoa, rinsed
½ cup unsweetened almond milk
¼ teaspoon ground cinnamon
1 tablespoon pure maple syrup
¼ teaspoon vanilla extract
Optional toppings: chopped nuts, fresh fruit, or a drizzle of almond butter

1 — In a small saucepan, combine the quinoa, almond milk, and cinnamon.

2 — Bring to a simmer over medium heat, then reduce the heat to low, cover the pan, and cook for 15 minutes, until the quinoa is tender and the liquid is absorbed.

3 — Stir in the maple syrup and vanilla.

4 — Spoon the porridge into a bowl and top with your choice of chopped nuts, fresh fruit, or almond butter for added flavor and texture.

Carrot Cake Breakfast Muffins

Makes 12 muffins
Prep Time: 10 minutes
Cook Time: 20 to 22 minutes

Your menstrual phase can be a great time to slow down, stay home, and do mindful activities like journaling, puzzles, crafts, or, if you like being in the kitchen as much as I do, baking. These carrot cake muffins are a lifesaver for those days when you prioritize sleeping in and you need something quick but nourishing. Carrots are loaded with beta-carotene, which promotes healthy progesterone levels and can also help metabolize estrogen, making them ideal no matter where you are in your cycle. Naturally sweetened, these muffins are gentle on your blood sugar and give you lasting energy while satisfying your sweet tooth. I like to add them to a yogurt bowl in the morning for extra protein!

1¼ cups almond flour
⅔ cup oat flour
¾ teaspoon baking soda
¾ teaspoon ground cinnamon
⅓ teaspoon grated nutmeg
3 large eggs
⅓ cup pure maple syrup
⅓ cup unsweetened applesauce
1¼ cups grated carrots
⅓ cup chopped walnuts or pecans

1 — Preheat the oven to 350°F. Line a 12-cup muffin tin with paper liners.

2 — In a medium bowl, whisk together the almond flour, oat flour, baking soda, cinnamon, and nutmeg.

3 — In another medium bowl, whisk the eggs, maple syrup, and applesauce until smooth.

4 — Gradually add the wet ingredients to the dry ingredients, stirring until just combined. Fold in the grated carrots and chopped nuts.

5 — Divide the batter evenly among the muffin cups and bake for 20 to 22 minutes, or until a toothpick inserted into the center of a muffin comes out clean.

6 — Let the muffins cool slightly before turning out onto a rack to cool completely before serving.

Note

I recommend two muffins as a serving, which then make a great breakfast, especially when they are warmed up with a little nut butter on top. Sometimes, though, I'll just take one muffin and use it as a garnish for another breakfast!

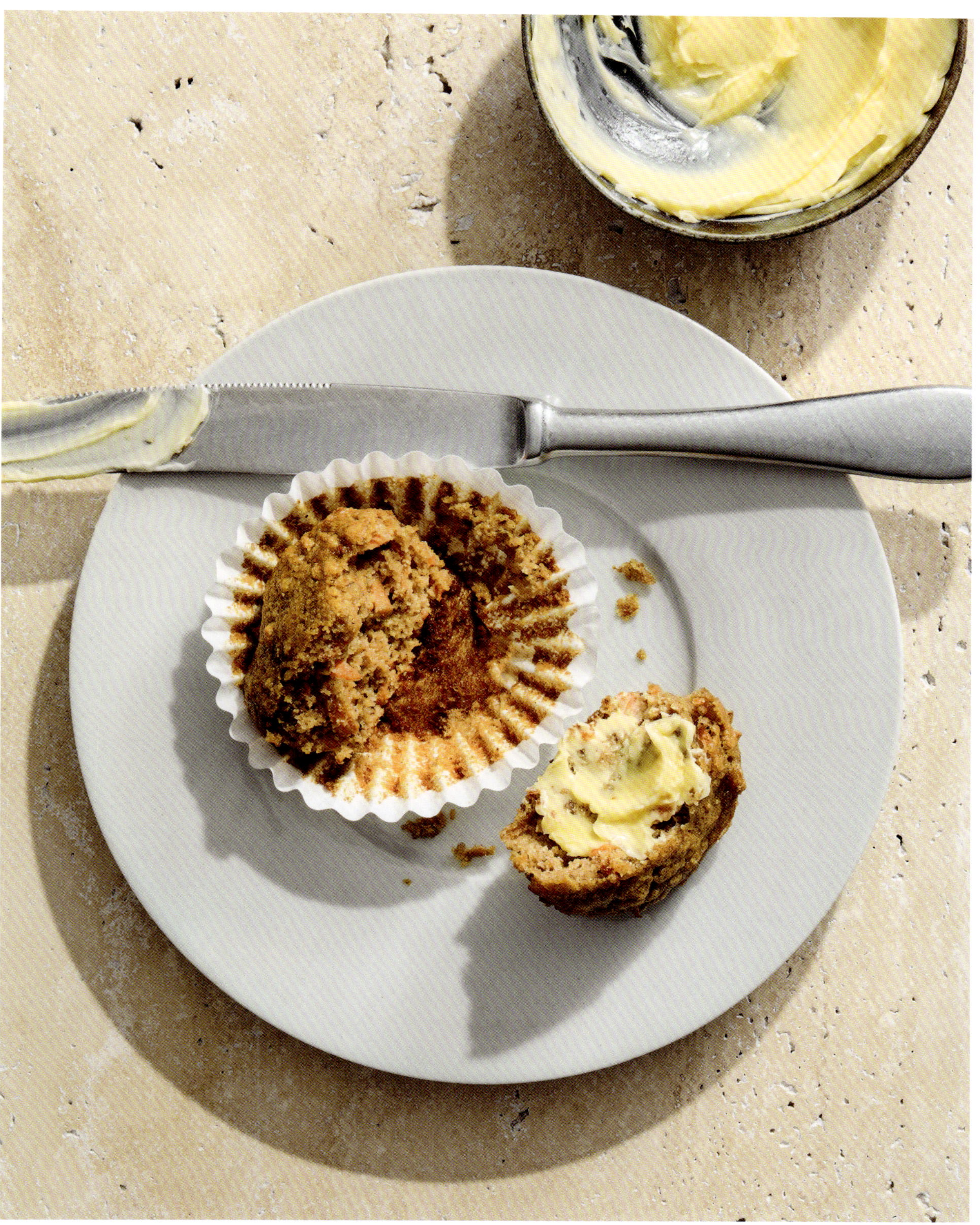

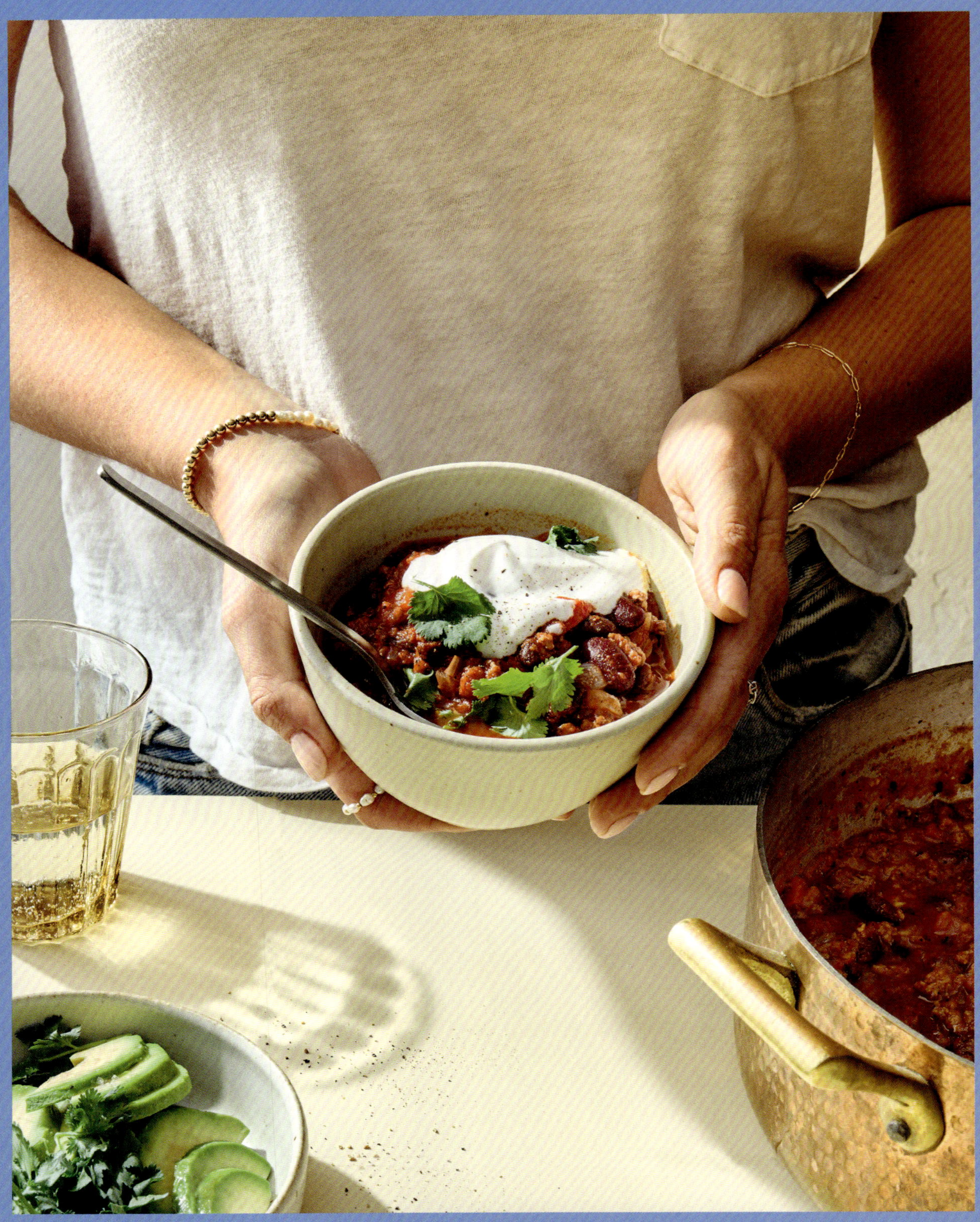

Lunches & Dinners

Soothing Ground Beef and Bean Chili

Serves 4
Prep Time: 15 minutes
Cook Time: 1 hour

Menstruation is all about listening to your body's needs, and this chili has become one of my go-to's when I need something hearty that also feels easy on digestion but still energizes me. Inspired by a classic family recipe, it's loaded with iron-rich ground beef to support your energy when your levels are low, while the fiber from the beans is a great way to keep digestion running smoothly. I love the smoky blend of cumin and chili powder, which doesn't just add flavor; it also promotes circulation, a little secret weapon for easing cramps. This chili reminds me of cozy nights with friends, perfect for batch cooking and freezing leftovers when you want something simple for later. Pro tip: Pair this chili with a side of avocado slices or mix in some fresh cilantro and lime for a bright, fresh contrast!

1 tablespoon olive oil
1 pound ground beef (preferably grass-fed)
1 small onion, chopped
2 garlic cloves, minced
1 red bell pepper, stemmed, seeded, and diced
1 (15-ounce) can kidney beans, drained and rinsed
1 (15-ounce) can black beans, drained and rinsed
1 (28-ounce) can diced tomatoes
2 tablespoons tomato paste
2 teaspoons chili powder
1 teaspoon ground cumin
1 teaspoon paprika
Salt and freshly ground black pepper
Optional toppings: chopped cilantro, avocado slices, and a dollop of plain Greek yogurt

1 — In a large pot, heat the olive oil over medium heat. Add the ground beef and cook for about 5 minutes, until browned, breaking it apart with a wooden spoon.

2 — Add the onion, garlic, and bell pepper. Cook for 5 minutes, until softened.

3 — Stir in the beans, tomatoes, tomato paste, chili powder, cumin, and paprika. Season to taste with salt and pepper.

4 — Bring the chili to a simmer, then reduce the heat to low and cook for 45 minutes, stirring occasionally.

5 — Serve the chili with your favorite toppings, like cilantro, avocado, and Greek yogurt.

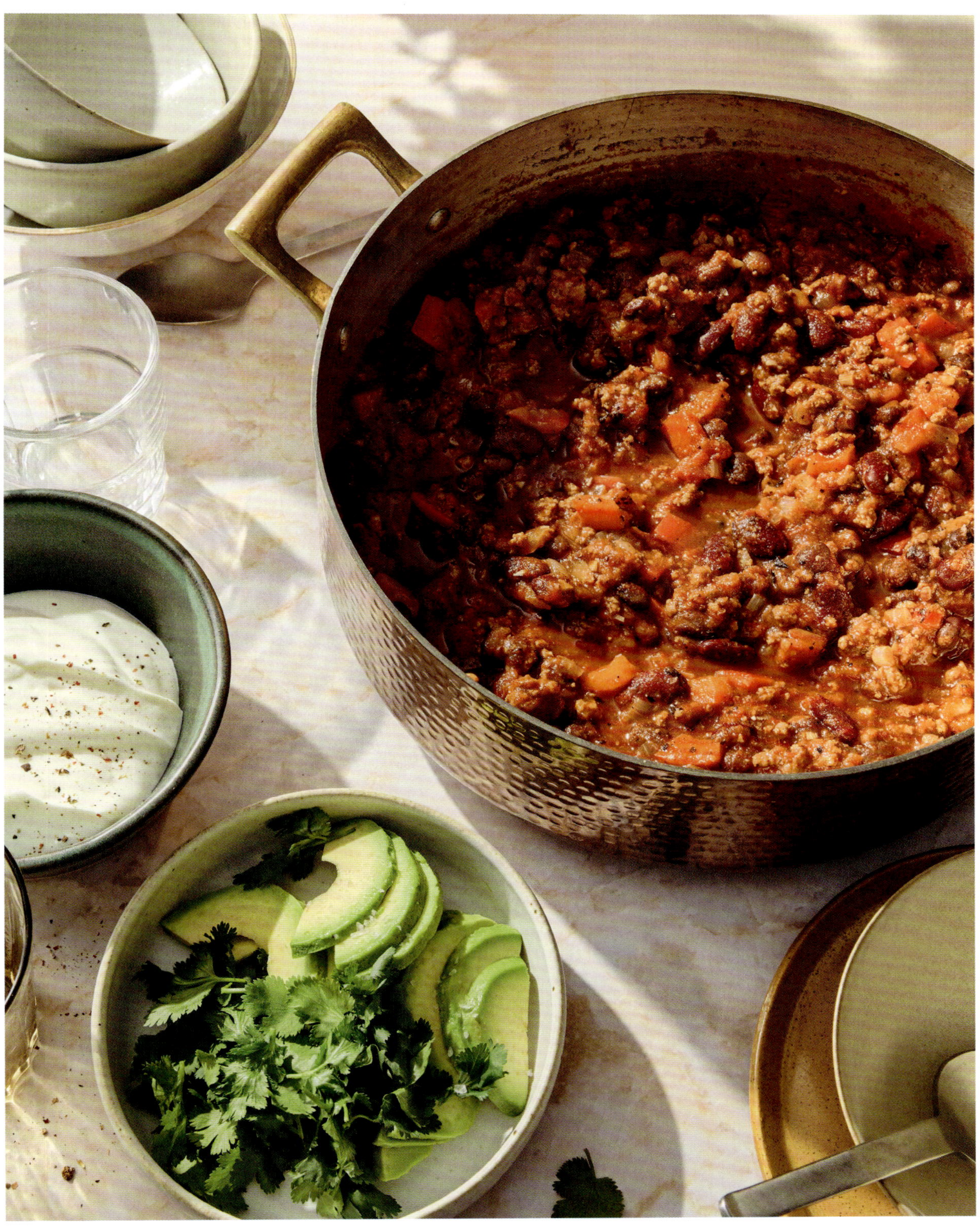

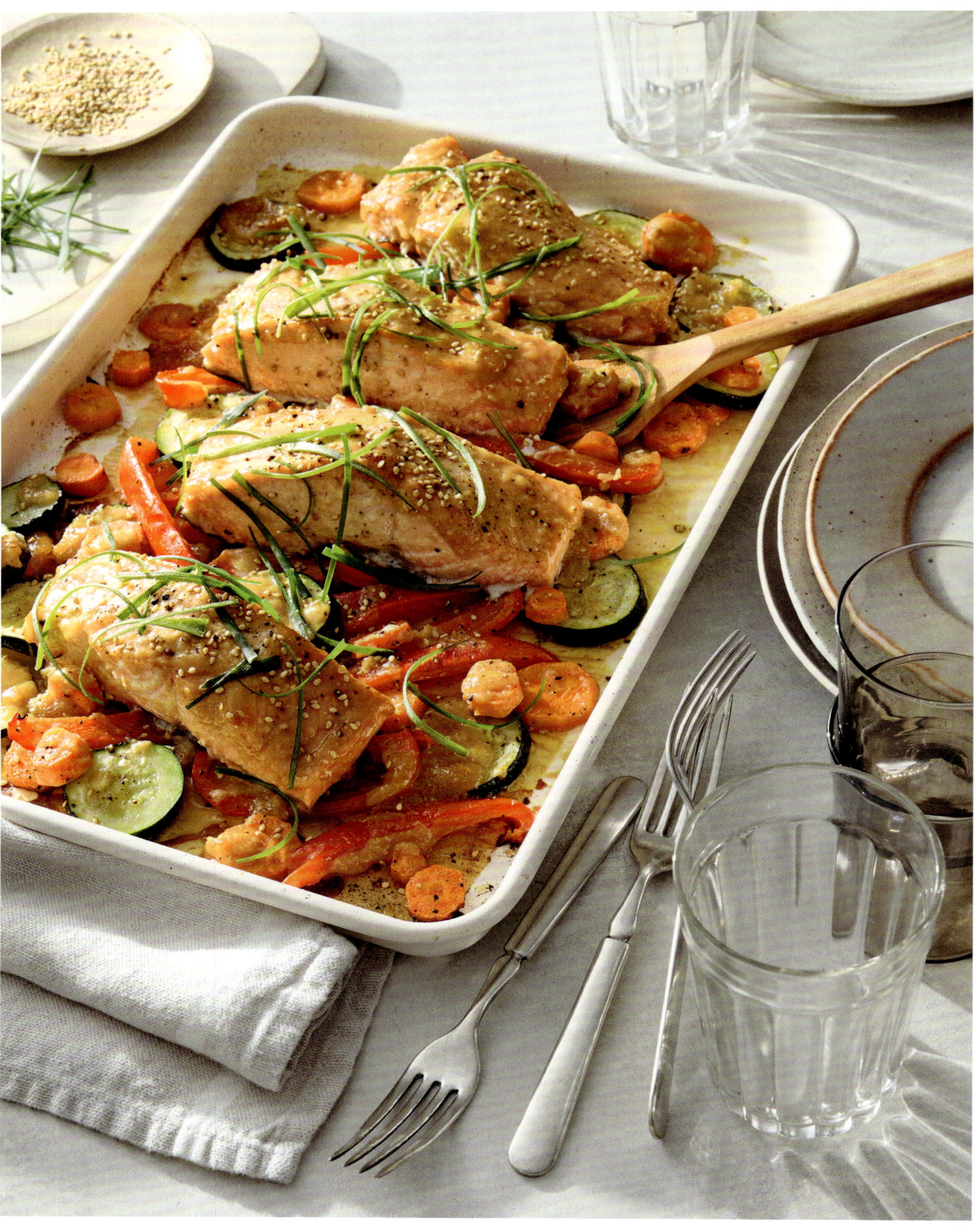

Miso-Glazed Salmon Veggie Sheet Pan

Serves 4
Prep Time: 15 minutes
Cook Time: 20 minutes

This is a dinner I turn to time and time again when I need a meal that feels effortless but still fuels me. The miso glaze brings a perfect umami punch that pairs beautifully with tender roasted veggies, while the salmon's omega-3s work behind the scenes to reduce inflammation, ease cramps, and support both your skin and mood during your period. Everything cooks in one sheet pan, leaving you with minimal cleanup, which—let's be honest—is always a win (especially when you're low on energy). I recommend serving this with some rice or quinoa. I like to cook mine in bone broth for extra flavor and protein; simply follow the cooking instructions on the label and replace the called-for amount of water with the broth.

4 salmon fillets, about 6 ounces each
2 tablespoons miso paste
1 tablespoon pure maple syrup
1 tablespoon rice vinegar
1 teaspoon toasted sesame oil
1 red bell pepper, stemmed, seeded, and sliced
1 medium zucchini, sliced
1 medium carrot, sliced
1 tablespoon olive oil
Salt and freshly ground black pepper
Sesame seeds and chopped green onions, for garnish

1 — Preheat the oven to 400°F. Line a sheet pan with parchment paper.

2 — In a small bowl, whisk together the miso paste, maple syrup, rice vinegar, and sesame oil. Place the salmon fillets on a cutting board and brush each with the marinade.

3 — Toss the bell pepper, zucchini, and carrot slices with the olive oil and salt and pepper to taste. Spread the vegetables on the sheet pan and place the salmon fillets on top. Drizzle any remaining marinade over the vegetables and salmon.

4 — Roast for 20 minutes, until the salmon is cooked through and the veggies are tender.

5 — Garnish with some sesame seeds and green onions before serving.

Baked Beef Tacos with Cauliflower Spanish Rice

Serves 4
Prep Time: 20 minutes
Cook Time: 25 minutes

As the menstrual phase encourages you to slow down, these baked beef tacos provide a satisfying way to fuel your body without requiring too much effort. Packed with grass-fed ground beef, they offer a protein-rich iron boost to help replenish what your body loses during your period. The cauliflower Spanish rice adds a light, nutrient-dense base while providing fiber to support blood sugar balance and keep your digestion smooth. The bold spices spark your digestive fire, keeping you warm from the inside out while creating a comforting flavor profile. I love to top mine with fresh avocado and a squeeze of lime for added creaminess and a burst of freshness that enhances each bite. You can usually find riced cauliflower in the frozen-food section of your grocery store; if not, simply cut a head of cauliflower into florets, place them in a blender or food processor, and pulse until you achieve small grains.

Tacos

2 tablespoons avocado oil
1 pound ground beef (preferably grass-fed)
1 cup chopped fresh mushrooms
1 teaspoon chili powder
1 teaspoon ground cumin
1 teaspoon paprika
½ teaspoon garlic powder
½ teaspoon onion powder
8 taco shells
1 cup shredded Cheddar cheese (or dairy-free alternative)

Cauliflower Spanish Rice

1 tablespoon avocado oil
½ medium onion, chopped
1 garlic clove, minced
1 cup frozen cauliflower rice (see Headnote)
½ cup tomato sauce
½ teaspoon ground cumin
Salt and freshly ground black pepper

Optional toppings: shredded lettuce, diced tomatoes, sliced avocado

1 — Preheat the oven to 375°F.

2 — Make the tacos: In a large skillet, add the avocado oil and beef and cook over medium heat for 5 minutes, browning it lightly and breaking up any clumps. Add the mushrooms, chili powder, cumin, paprika, garlic powder, and onion powder. Cook for 8 to 10 minutes, until the meat is browned and cooked through.

3 — Fill the taco shells with the beef mixture and arrange into an 8 x 8-inch baking dish, folded and lined up so they can bake into a hard-shell taco shape. Sprinkle with the cheese and bake in the oven for 10 minutes, until the cheese is melted.

4 — While the tacos bake, make the cauliflower rice: Heat the avocado oil in a skillet over medium heat. Add the onion and garlic, cooking about 2 minutes, until softened. Stir in the cauliflower rice, tomato sauce, cumin, and salt and pepper to taste. Cook for 5 minutes, until heated through.

5 — Serve the tacos with the cauliflower Spanish rice and toppings of choice.

Anti-Inflammatory Ginger and Turmeric Chicken Stir-Fry

Serves 4
Prep Time: 15 minutes
Cook Time: 15 minutes

Ginger and turmeric have been used for centuries for their anti-inflammatory and digestion-supporting benefits, and they bring a vibrant, flavorful twist to this easy stir-fry. The zing of ginger pairs perfectly with the earthiness of the turmeric, creating layers of flavor that make this dish anything but ordinary. Lean chicken adds a solid dose of protein to keep your energy stable, while the spices help ease the bloating and discomfort that can come with your period. Serve it over brown rice for a hearty, filling meal that leaves you feeling balanced and satisfied without the fuss.

2 tablespoons olive oil
1 pound boneless, skinless chicken breasts, thinly sliced into strips
Salt and freshly ground black pepper
1 tablespoon grated fresh ginger
1 tablespoon grated fresh turmeric (or 1 teaspoon ground)
2 cups mixed sliced bell peppers
1 cup broccoli florets
2 medium carrots, julienned
3 tablespoons coconut aminos
2 tablespoons sesame oil
2 cups cooked brown rice, warmed
Sesame seeds and minced green onions, for garnish (optional)

1 — Heat 1 tablespoon of the olive oil in a large skillet or wok over medium-high heat. Add the chicken and season to taste with salt and pepper. Cook for 5 to 7 minutes, stirring and flipping until the chicken pieces are cooked through and lightly browned. Remove from the skillet and set aside.

2 — In the same skillet, add the remaining tablespoon olive oil, then add the ginger, turmeric, bell peppers, broccoli, and carrots. Stir-fry for about 5 minutes, until the vegetables are tender-crisp.

3 — Return the chicken to the skillet. Add the coconut aminos and sesame oil, stirring to combine. Cook for an additional 2 to 3 minutes, allowing the flavors to meld.

4 — Serve the stir-fry over a bed of the warm brown rice. Garnish with the sesame seeds and green onions, if desired.

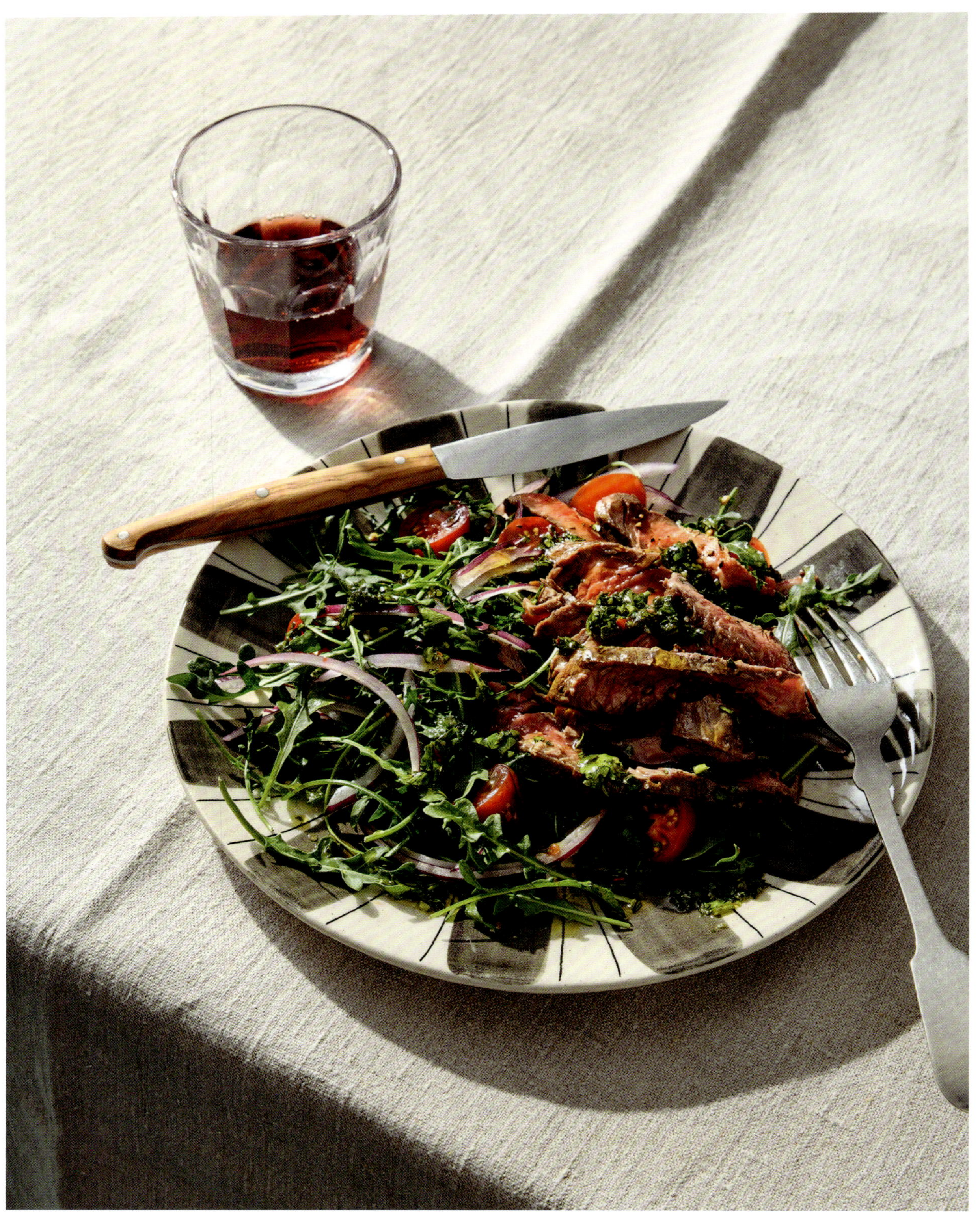

Zesty Chimichurri Steak and Arugula Salad

Serves 1

Prep Time: 15 minutes

Cook Time: 10 minutes

A lot of people tend to avoid cooking steak at home; it can seem hard to get it just right. The key, though, is to focus on quality; ideally you want organic, grass-fed beef, from a cut that looks bright, bright red when you pick it up from the store. In general, when cooking for hormone health, you want to prioritize organic produce and proteins; other options tend to have been sprayed with pesticides or contain added hormones that can act as disruptors.

Apart from being delicious, this chimichurri steak provides plenty of iron, which helps replenish what your body loses during menstruation. The vitamin C in the tomatoes actually boosts your body's ability to absorb that iron more effectively. The peppery arugula aids digestion, while the vibrant flavors of the chimichurri sauce bring a bright, uplifting element to the meal, ideal for when you need an energy and mood lift.

Steak and Salad

1 (8-ounce) flank steak (preferably grass-fed)

Salt and freshly ground black pepper

2 cups fresh arugula

¼ cup cherry tomatoes, halved

¼ medium red onion, thinly sliced

1 tablespoon olive oil

Juice of ½ lemon

Chimichurri

½ cup chopped fresh parsley

2 garlic cloves, minced

¼ cup olive oil

2 tablespoons red wine vinegar

¼ teaspoon red pepper flakes

Salt and freshly ground black pepper

1 — Prepare the steak and salad: Heat a large skillet over medium-high heat. Season the steak with salt and pepper, add to the skillet, and cook for 3 to 4 minutes per side for medium-rare, or until cooked to your desired doneness. Set aside to rest.

2 — Toss the arugula, cherry tomatoes, and red onion in a large bowl with the olive oil, lemon juice, and salt and pepper to taste.

4 — Prepare the chimichurri: In a small bowl, stir together the parsley, garlic, olive oil, vinegar, red pepper flakes, and salt and pepper to taste.

5 — Slice the steak, cutting against the grain. Place the arugula salad on plates, add some steak slices, and drizzle with the chimichurri sauce.

Almond Flour–Crusted Chicken and Roasted Veg Buddha Bowl with Maple-Tahini Dressing

Serves 4
Prep Time: 20 minutes
Cook Time: 50 minutes

We all know that low-energy days during your period can make preparing even the simplest meal feel like a chore. When you're tired but craving something nourishing, having a meal prepped and ready to go is a lifesaver. Here, you can roast the veggies, cook the quinoa, and prepare the tahini dressing in advance, so when it's time to eat, all you have to do is cook the chicken and assemble. Or, if you are in a pinch for time, you can swap out the almond flour–crusted chicken for store-bought rotisserie chicken! The healthy fats in the tahini dressing bring a rich and creamy element to the mix, while also helping calm inflammation and support balanced hormones, which can ease cramps and bloating!

Chicken and Veg Bowl

1 medium sweet potato, diced
1 medium zucchini, sliced
1 red bell pepper, stemmed, seeded, and chopped
1½ tablespoons olive oil
Salt and freshly ground black pepper
1 large egg
¾ cup almond flour
1 teaspoon paprika
½ teaspoon garlic powder
1 pound boneless, skinless chicken breasts, sliced

Maple-Tahini Dressing

¼ cup tahini
1 tablespoon freshly squeezed lemon juice
1 teaspoon cider vinegar
1½ tablespoons pure maple syrup
1 garlic clove, minced
Salt

For Serving

2 cups cooked quinoa
1 (15-ounce) can chickpeas, drained and rinsed

1 — Preheat the oven to 400°F. Line a baking sheet with parchment paper.

2 — Toss the sweet potato, zucchini, and bell pepper in a medium bowl with the olive oil and salt and pepper to taste. Spread the mix on the parchment-lined baking sheet and roast for 20 minutes, until the vegetables are tender. Transfer to a plate to cool. Retain the baking sheet and keep the oven turned on.

3 — In a small shallow bowl, lightly beat the egg. In another shallow dish, mix the almond flour, paprika, garlic powder, and salt and pepper to taste. Dip each piece of chicken into the beaten egg, then dust with the seasoned flour. Place the chicken on the same baking sheet and bake for 20 to 25 minutes, flipping halfway through, until golden and cooked through.

4 — While the chicken bakes, make the dressing: In a small bowl, whisk together the tahini, lemon juice, vinegar, maple syrup, garlic, and a pinch of salt. Add a little water, about ½ tablespoon at a time, until the dressing reaches your desired consistency.

5 — Divide the cooked quinoa, roasted veggies, chickpeas, and cooked chicken among serving bowls. Drizzle the bowls with some of the tahini dressing and serve.

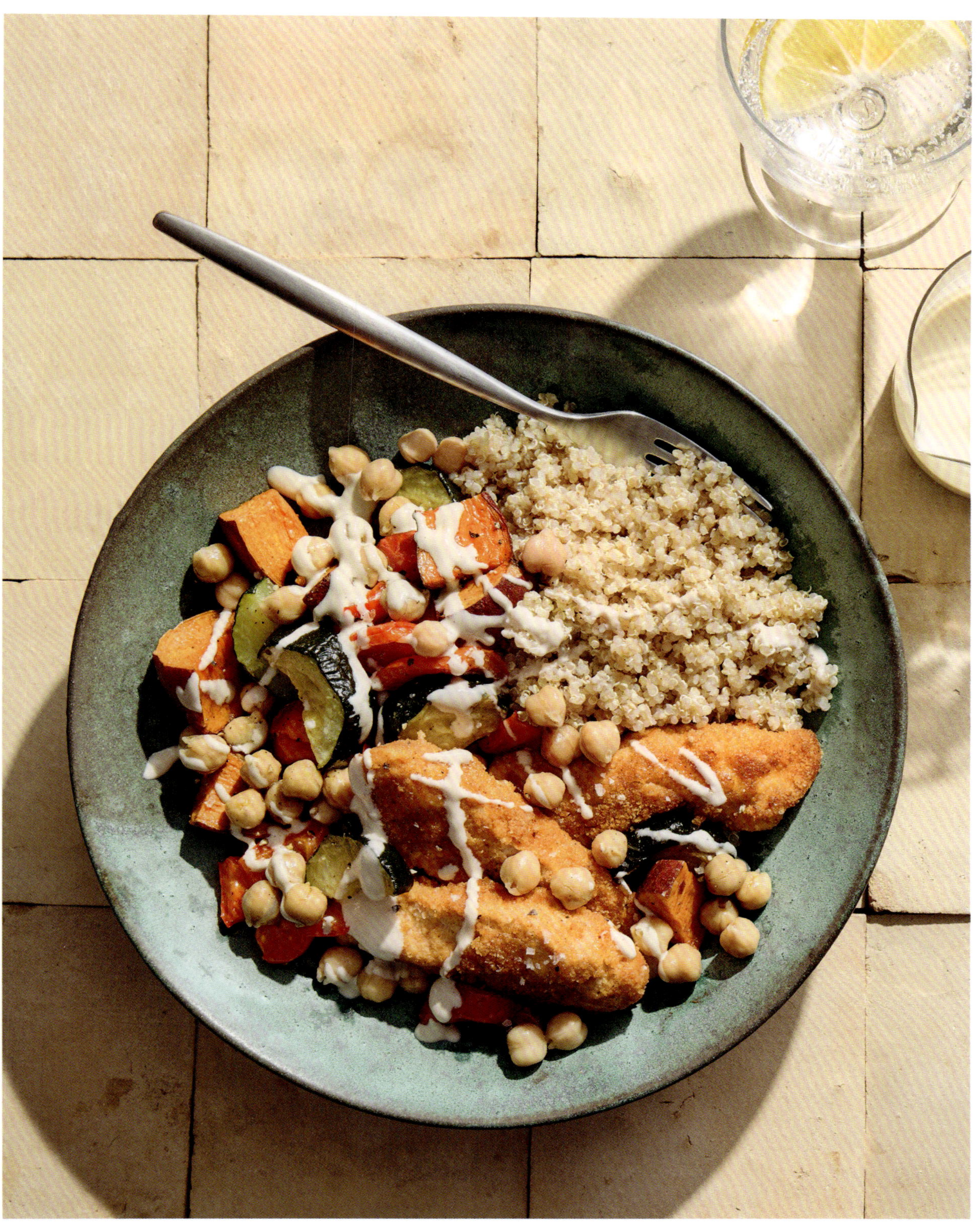

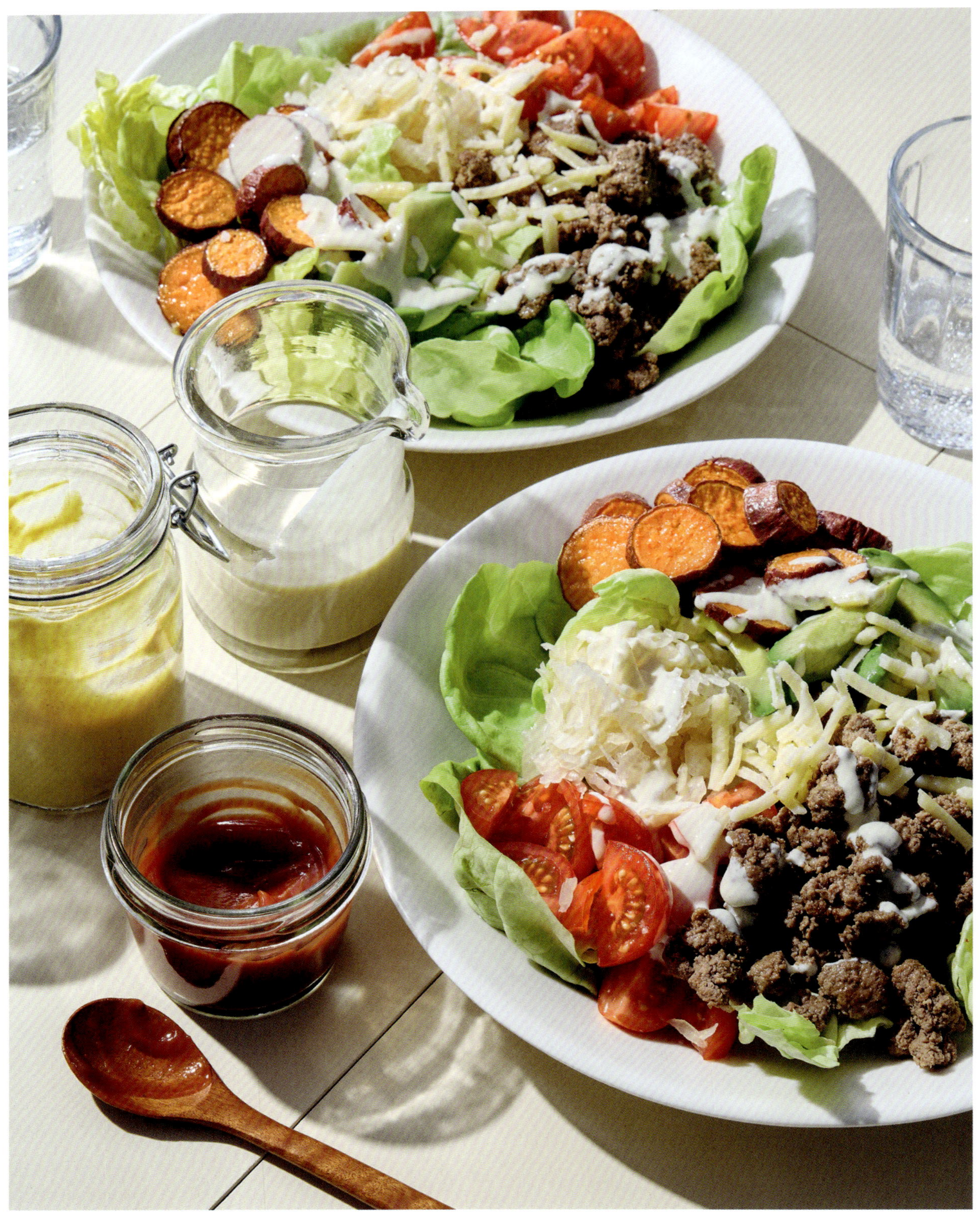

Low-Effort Burger Bowls with Sweet Potato Coins and "Secret Sauce"

Serves 4

Prep Time: 20 minutes

Cook Time: 25 minutes

When period cravings hit, nothing beats the comfort of a burger! I love burger bowls because they ditch the processed carbs and load up on nutrient-dense, hormone-supportive ingredients. Grass-fed beef provides a rich source of heme iron, which is crucial for replenishing your iron stores during menstruation and for combating fatigue. The healthy fats from avocado help reduce inflammation, support hormone production, and soothe menstrual cramps. Instead of adding raw onion, which can be tough to digest during this phase, you swap in sauerkraut for the same satisfying crunch and tang. The probiotics in sauerkraut help promote gut health, improve digestion, and reduce bloating—perfect for a bloated belly during your period. Add in roasted sweet potato coins, which are rich in vitamin A and fiber to keep you feeling satisfied. This is comfort food that works with your body, not against it!

Sweet Potatoes and Beef

2 medium sweet potatoes, sliced into ½-inch rounds

1 tablespoon olive oil

Salt and freshly ground black pepper

1 pound ground beef (preferably grass-fed)

1 teaspoon garlic powder

1 teaspoon onion powder

½ teaspoon smoked paprika

Secret Sauce

¼ cup plain Greek yogurt (or dairy-free yogurt)

1 tablespoon Dijon mustard

1 tablespoon cider vinegar

1 teaspoon honey (optional, for a touch of sweetness)

Salt and freshly ground black pepper

Assembly

4 cups torn butter lettuce

1 avocado, halved, pitted, and sliced

1 cup cherry tomatoes, halved

¼ cup sauerkraut

¼ cup shredded Cheddar cheese (or dairy-free alternative)

¼ cup ketchup or mustard (optional)

1 — Preheat the oven to 400°F and lightly grease a baking sheet.

2 — Prepare the sweet potatoes and beef: Toss the sweet potato rounds in the olive oil, and season to taste with salt and pepper. Spread the coins evenly in one layer on the greased baking sheet and roast for 20 to 25 minutes, flipping halfway through, until golden and tender.

3 — While the sweet potatoes roast, heat a large skillet over medium-high heat. In a large bowl, mix the ground beef with the garlic powder, onion powder, smoked paprika, and salt and pepper to taste. Add the beef to the hot skillet and cook for 5 to 6 minutes, breaking it up into small pieces as it cooks, until browned and fully cooked.

4 — Prepare the sauce: In a small bowl, whisk together the yogurt, mustard, vinegar, honey (if using), and salt and pepper to taste. Taste and adjust seasoning as needed.

5 — Assemble the bowls: Divide the lettuce, avocado slices, cherry tomatoes, and sauerkraut among 4 serving bowls. Add a handful of sweet potato coins to each bowl, then spoon some of the cooked beef over each bowl. Top each with some of the shredded cheese and drizzle with the sauce. Serve with your choice of ketchup or mustard on the side.

Dinner-on-the-Couch Creamy Mushroom, Spinach, and Chicken Pasta

Serves 4

Prep Time: 10 minutes

Cook Time: 25 minutes

A creamy bowl of pasta is my ultimate comfort meal, so I wanted to find a way to make a pasta dish that will love my body back. The result was this creamy mushroom, spinach, and chicken pasta. The rotisserie chicken adds protein with minimal effort, while the mushrooms and spinach deliver iron and magnesium to help ease cramps and fatigue. The coconut milk creates that rich, creamy texture we all love but without the dairy, so it's gentle on digestion. This pasta is sure to become your cozy, nourishing go-to when your body needs a little extra love!

4 cups brown rice pasta (such as Jovial brand from Whole Foods or brown rice quinoa pasta from Trader Joe's)

1 tablespoon olive oil

2 garlic cloves, minced

1 medium onion, diced

3 cups sliced cremini mushrooms

3 cups (packed) fresh baby spinach

½ cup full-fat coconut milk

¼ cup nutritional yeast

Salt and freshly ground black pepper

2 cups shredded rotisserie chicken

Chopped fresh parsley, for garnish

1 — Bring a large pot of salted water to a boil. Add the pasta and cook according to the package instructions, until al dente. Drain and set aside.

2 — In a large skillet, heat the olive oil over medium heat. Add the garlic and onion and sauté until soft and translucent, about 3 minutes.

3 — Add the mushrooms and cook, stirring occasionally, until browned, about 5 minutes.

4 — Stir in the spinach and cook just until wilted, about 2 minutes.

5 — Pour in the coconut milk and stir to combine. Let the sauce simmer for 2 to 3 minutes, until slightly thickened. Stir in the nutritional yeast, and season to taste with salt and pepper.

6 — Add the chicken and pasta to the skillet. Toss everything together until well coated and heated through, about 2 minutes.

7 — Garnish with the parsley and serve.

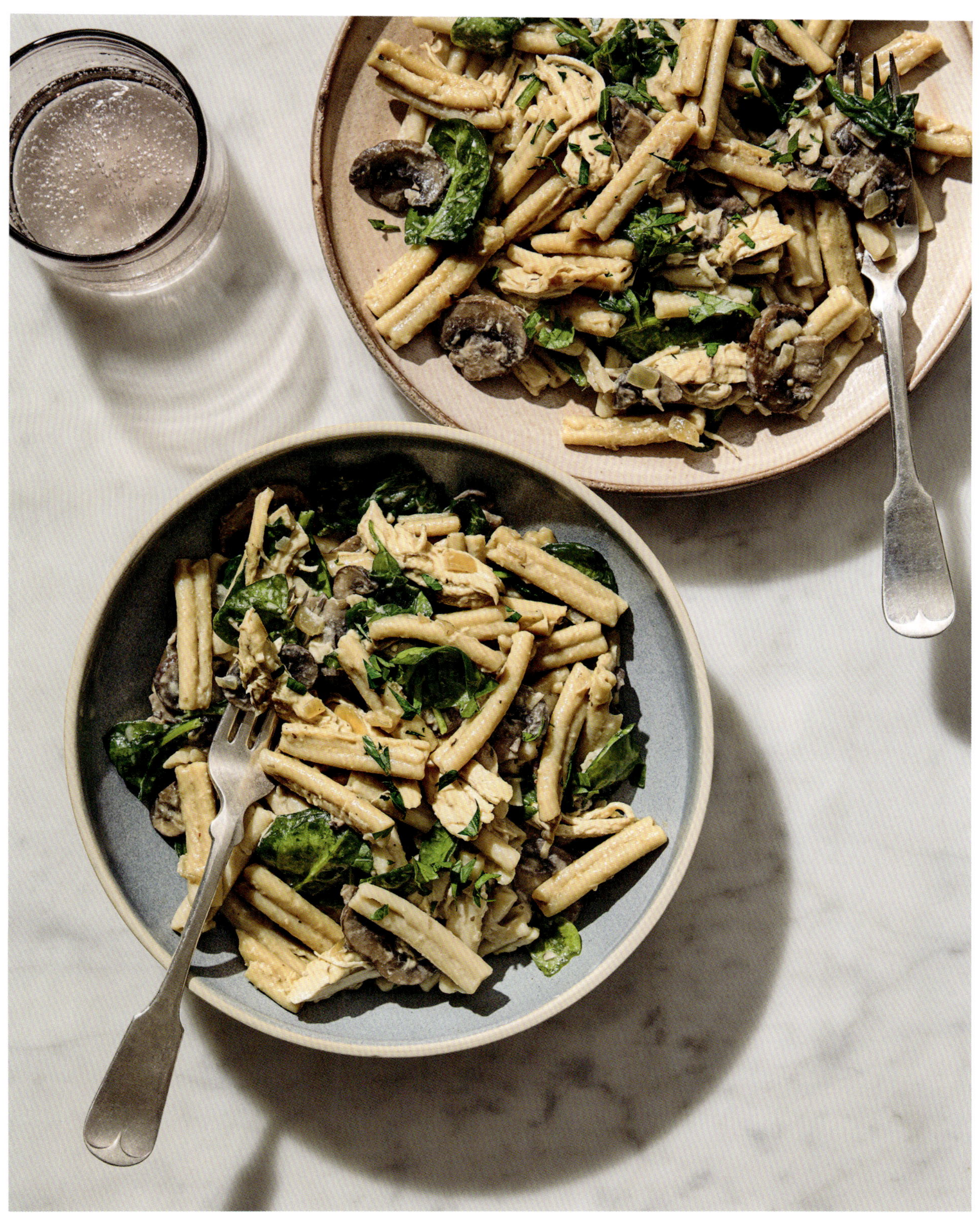

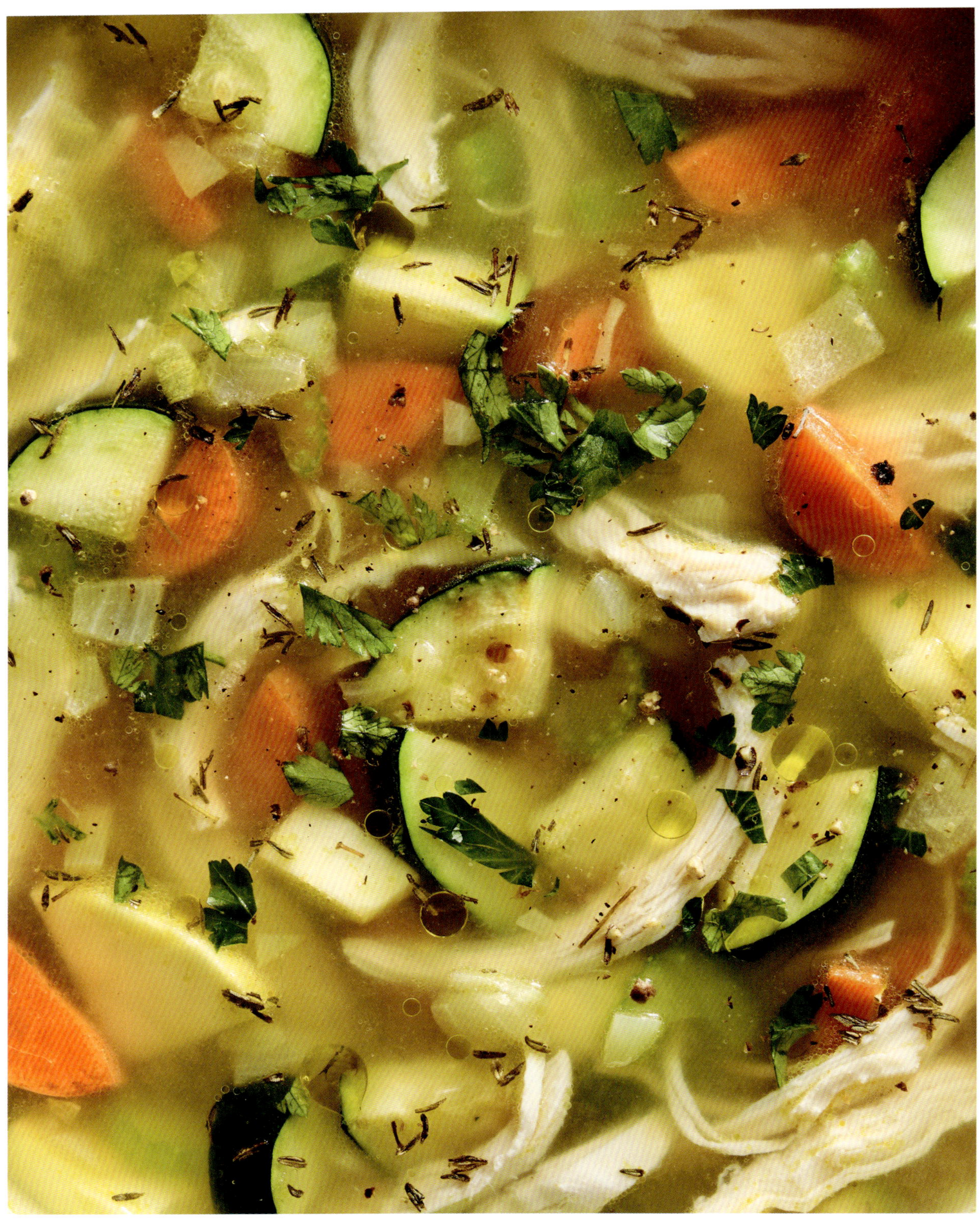

It's Okay to Cry into Your (Chicken Bone Broth) Soup

Serves 6
Prep Time: 15 minutes
Cook Time: 35 minutes

There's nothing like a bowl of chicken soup when you're feeling off, but this isn't your average recipe—it's your go-to for menstrual phase recovery. This version features grounding root vegetables like carrots and parsnips, packed with slow-digesting carbs that help stabilize blood sugar and provide sustained energy. Chicken bone broth takes it to the next level, delivering collagen and minerals to support your gut and immune system—both of which can feel a little more delicate during your bleed. With anti-inflammatory herbs like thyme and a finishing touch of fresh parsley for an extra nutrient boost, this soup is designed to nourish deeply while being gentle on your digestion. The best part? Making this soup is just as healing as eating it. So put on some music, get into the kitchen, and relax as the healing begins.

---

1 tablespoon olive oil
1 medium onion, chopped
2 garlic cloves, minced
3 medium carrots, sliced
2 celery stalks, sliced
1 medium parsnip, chopped
1 medium zucchini, chopped
2 cups shredded rotisserie chicken
8 cups chicken bone broth
1 teaspoon dried thyme
1 dried bay leaf
Salt and freshly ground black pepper
Chopped fresh parsley, for garnish

1 — Heat the olive oil in a large pot over medium heat. Add the onion and garlic, and cook for 5 minutes, until softened.

2 — Stir in the carrots, celery, parsnip, zucchini, chicken, bone broth, thyme, and bay leaf. Season to taste with salt and pepper.

3 — Bring the soup to a boil, then reduce the heat and simmer for 25 to 30 minutes, until the vegetables are tender.

4 — Remove the bay leaf, then pour into bowls and garnish with the parsley before serving.

Pro tip

Make a big batch and freeze individual portions to have on hand for next month. It's the meal prep you'll thank yourself for later!

The Instant Classic Lentil and Sweet Potato Shepherd's Pie

Serves 6
Prep Time: 20 minutes
Cook Time: 40 minutes

One of the things I like to focus on when I know I'm about to hit my time of the month is self-care. It's easy to get down on yourself when you have a harder time making it through the workout you smashed just two weeks ago, or when you can't concentrate during that 2 p.m. meeting because you need a nap so badly. Just remember your body is asking you to slow down during this time; that's because it's doing really important things behind the scenes, and the more you can do to listen to it, the better you are in setting yourself up for success for the rest of the month. Personally, I love to turn on some music (maybe for you it's an audiobook or your favorite comfort show!) and make a self-care activity out of cooking this special shepherd's pie. It's a vegetarian dinner packed with iron-rich lentils and sweet potatoes, loaded with fiber and vitamin C to boost iron absorption! This might not be your mama's traditional shepherd's pie, but it's pretty dang close!

1 cup dried green or brown lentils, rinsed and drained
2 cups vegetable broth
2 large sweet potatoes, peeled and cubed
2 tablespoons olive oil
Salt and freshly ground black pepper
1 medium onion, diced
2 garlic cloves, minced
2 medium carrots, diced
2 celery stalks, diced
1 tablespoon tomato paste
1 teaspoon dried thyme
1 teaspoon smoked paprika
1 cup frozen peas
Chopped fresh parsley, for garnish (optional)

1 — In a medium saucepan, combine the lentils and broth. Bring to a boil, then reduce the heat and simmer for about 20 minutes, or until the lentils are tender. Drain excess liquid, if necessary. (Make sure to finish cooking the lentils before you move on to the next step.)

2 — While the lentils are cooking, bring a medium pot of salted water to a boil, then add the sweet potato cubes. Cook until tender, about 15 minutes. Drain and return the sweet potato cubes to the pot. Mash them with 1 tablespoon of the olive oil and some salt and pepper to taste.

3 — In a large skillet, heat the remaining tablespoon olive oil over medium heat. Add the onion, garlic, carrots, and celery. Sauté for 5 to 7 minutes, until softened. Add the lentils, then stir in the tomato paste, thyme, smoked paprika, peas, and some salt and pepper to taste. Stir to combine well and cook for an additional 5 minutes.

4 — Preheat the oven to 375°F. Lightly grease a 1 quart baking dish.

5 — Transfer the mixture from the skillet to the baking dish, spreading it in an even layer with a spatula. Spread the sweet potato mash over the lentil filling, smoothing it out evenly. Put the dish in the oven and bake for 20 minutes, or until the top is slightly golden. Let it cool slightly before serving. Garnish with fresh parsley, if desired.

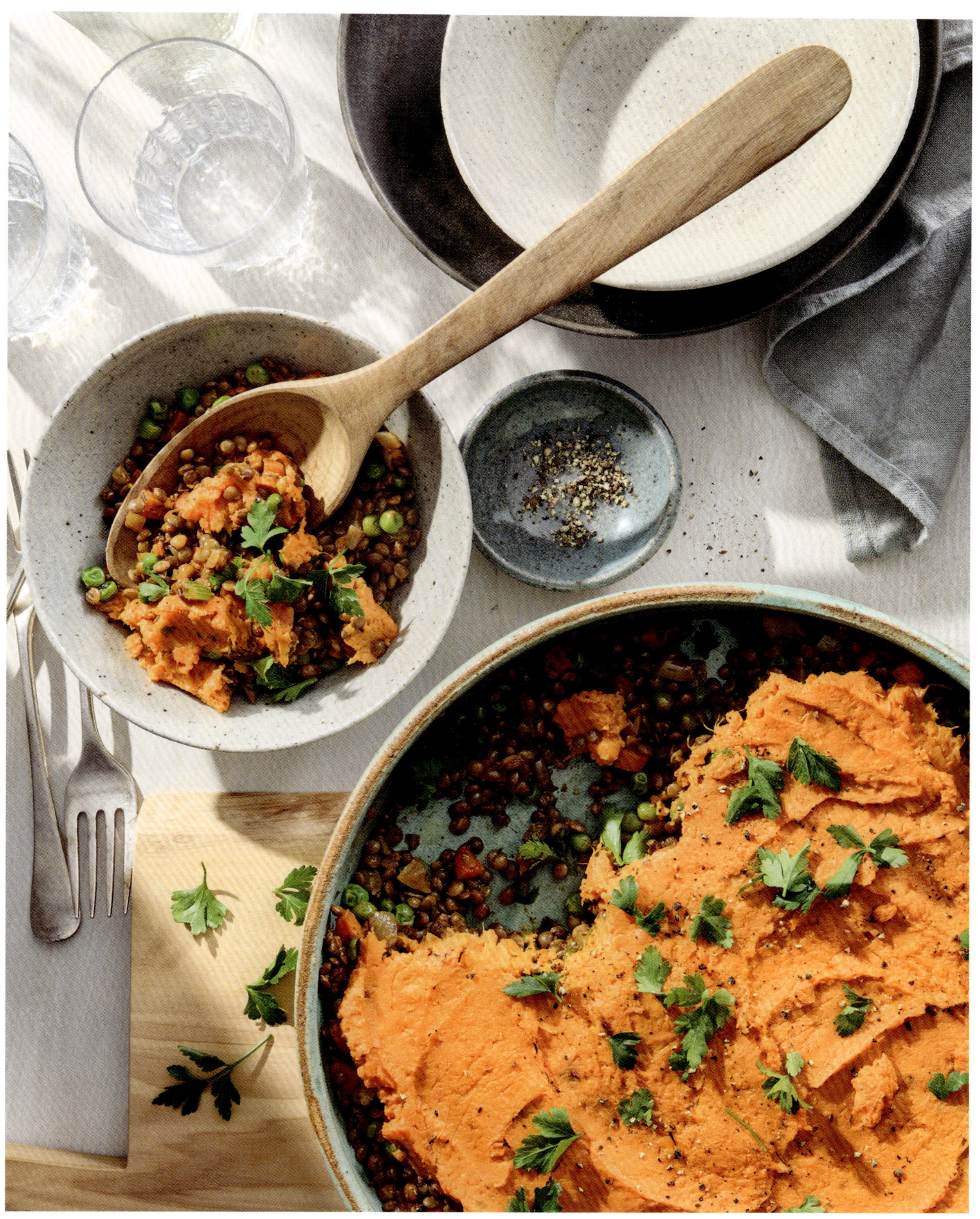

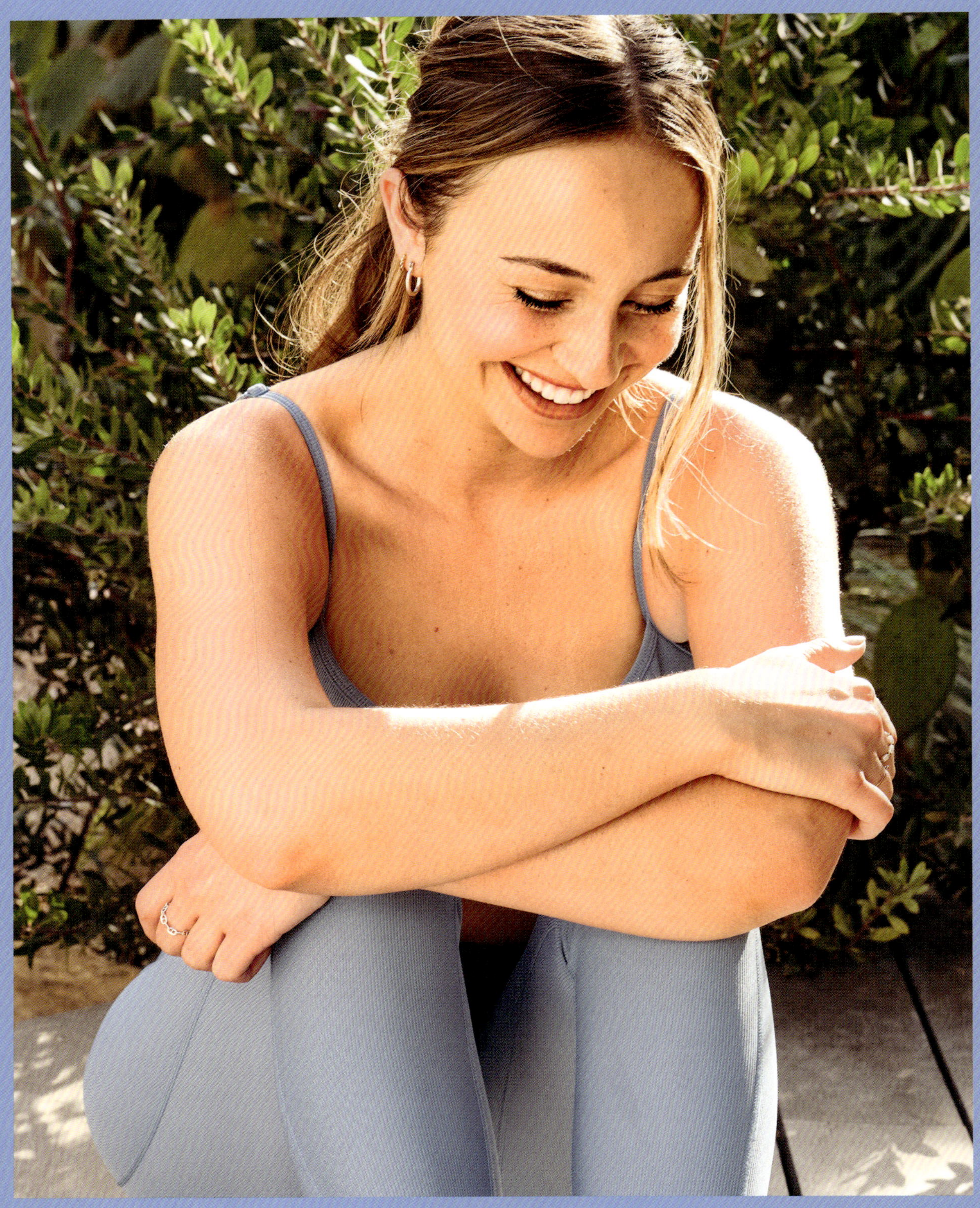

Snacks & Desserts

Cacao Dreams Chocolate Protein Pudding

Serves 2

Prep Time: 10 minutes, plus 1 hour chilling

When those chocolate cravings strike during my period (thank your dipping progesterone levels for that), this is one of my favorite desserts to make! As progesterone levels continue to flatline during the menstrual phase, your body often craves quick energy and comfort foods like chocolate. This happens because lower progesterone can decrease serotonin, the "feel good" hormone, making your body reach for serotonin-boosting foods like chocolate. The cacao powder here is packed with magnesium, which supports serotonin production, helping to lift your mood and soothe tension. Bananas bring in potassium to reduce bloating and water retention, while the avocado provides healthy fats and fiber to keep your blood sugar stable and prevent energy crashes. Almond butter adds a subtle nuttiness and a boost of healthy fats, and the chocolate protein powder makes it a satisfying snack that tackles both cravings and nutritional needs!

1 ripe avocado, halved, pitted, and sliced

1 banana, sliced

2 tablespoons cacao powder

1 tablespoon almond butter

1 tablespoon honey or pure maple syrup (optional)

1 scoop chocolate protein powder

1 teaspoon vanilla extract

¼ cup unsweetened almond milk (or other plant-based milk)

Cacao nibs or sliced almonds, for topping (optional)

1 — Scoop the avocado into a blender or food processor, then add the banana, cacao powder, almond butter, honey (if using), protein powder, vanilla, and almond milk. Blend on high speed until smooth and creamy, scraping down the sides of the container as needed.

2 — Transfer the pudding to individual serving bowls and refrigerate for at least 1 hour to allow it to set.

3 — Before serving, top the puddings with the cacao nibs or almonds for added crunch and flavor, if desired.

Note

This is a great option for preparing ahead so you have a healthy sweet treat to reach for throughout the week! This pudding will last in the fridge for up to 4 days.

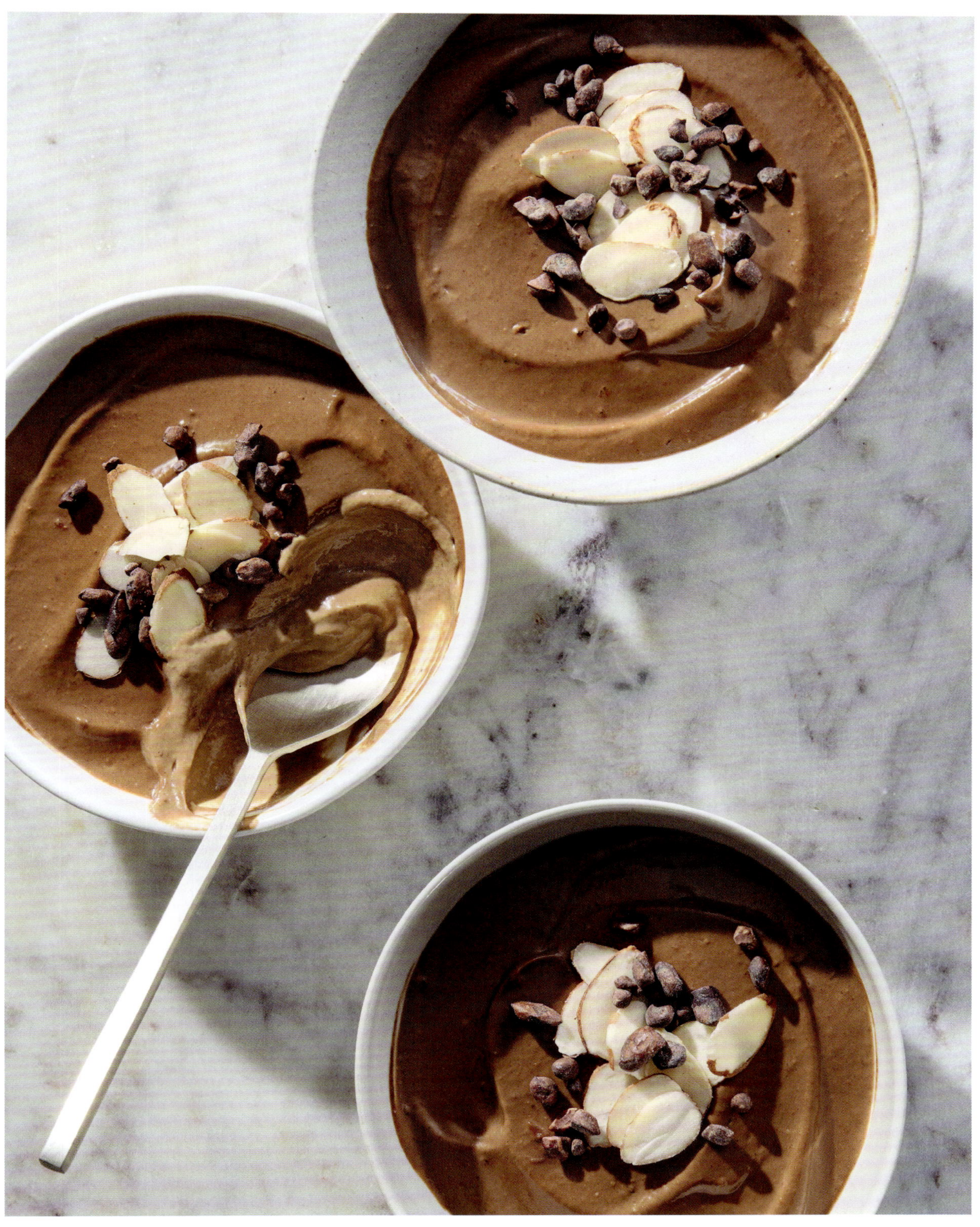

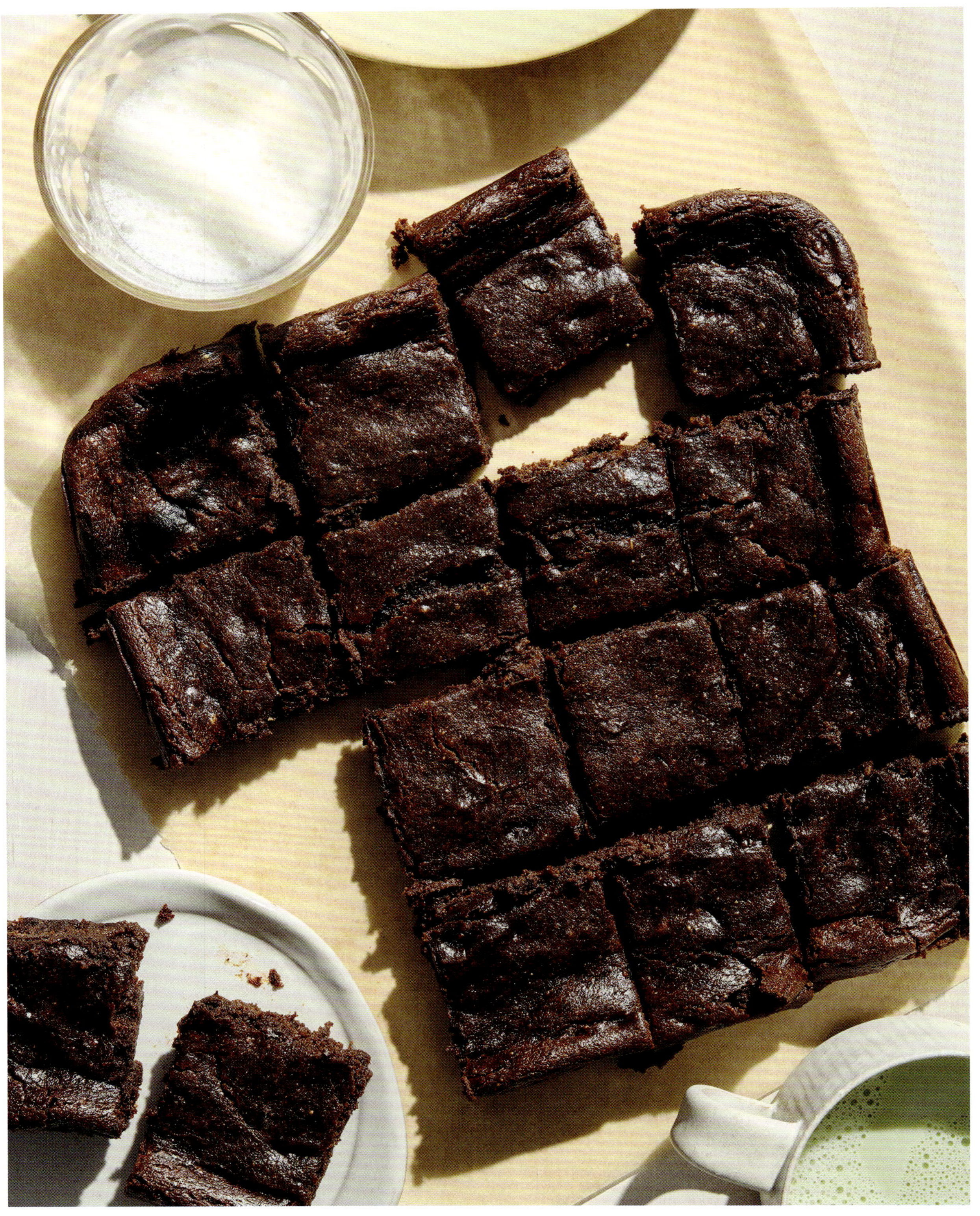

My Famous Sweet Potato Brownies

Makes 12 brownies
Prep Time: 15 minutes
Cook Time: 25 minutes

When I was 22, I lost my period, and when I finally got it back about a year and a half later, I wanted to celebrate in a way that also supported my body and my cycle. That's when these sweet potato brownies were born! Sweet potatoes are loaded with complex carbs and beta-carotene, which help keep your energy steady; the cinnamon works to stabilize blood sugar levels, and the almond butter provides those healthy fats that fuel our hormones, fight inflammation, and keep us feeling satisfied. When I have it on hand, I like to add two scoops of collagen (you can fold it in with the cinnamon and nutmeg) for an extra protein boost and that deliciously gooey texture!

½ cup canned sweet potato puree
½ cup almond butter
½ cup pure maple syrup
⅓ cup cacao powder
1 teaspoon ground cinnamon
¼ teaspoon grated nutmeg
½ teaspoon baking soda
¼ teaspoon sea salt
⅓ cup dark chocolate chips

1 — Preheat the oven to 350°F. Line an 8 × 8-inch baking dish with parchment paper.

2 — In a large bowl, whisk together the sweet potato puree, almond butter, and maple syrup until smooth.

3 — Add the cacao powder, cinnamon, nutmeg, baking soda, and sea salt. Stir until well combined. Fold in the chocolate chips.

4 — Pour the batter into the baking dish and spread evenly into the corners. Bake for 25 to 30 minutes, or until a toothpick inserted in the center comes out clean.

5 — Let the brownies cool completely before slicing. Enjoy as a snack or dessert!

Afternoon Pick-Me-Up Brownie Batter Protein Bites

Makes 12 bites

Prep Time: 10 minutes, plus 30 minutes chilling

When the mid-afternoon slump hits, these brownie batter bites come to the rescue every time. Each bite is loaded with protein, healthy fats, and fiber from the combination of nuts, seeds, and cacao, helping to keep blood sugar stable—super important for maintaining steady energy during the ups and downs of your cycle. Ground flaxseed is a true powerhouse in this recipe; it's packed with omega-3 fatty acids, which are known to help reduce inflammation and support overall hormone health. Plus, it contains lignans, which can help balance estrogen levels and may alleviate some PMS symptoms. Flaxseed also provides a good dose of fiber, aiding digestion and keeping you feeling full longer. I love pairing these bites with my morning matcha, enjoying them as a midday snack, or treating myself to one as a sweet finish to a meal!

½ cup almond butter
¼ cup cacao powder
¼ cup chocolate protein powder
2 tablespoons honey or pure maple syrup
¼ cup ground flaxseed
½ teaspoon vanilla extract
Pinch of sea salt
¼ cup dark chocolate chips

1 — In a medium bowl, mix the almond butter, cacao powder, protein powder, honey, flaxseed, vanilla, and sea salt until well combined.

2 — Fold in the chocolate chips.

3 — Using a spoon or scoop, shape and roll portions of the mixture into 12 bite-size balls, then place them on a baking sheet.

4 — Chill in the refrigerator for 30 minutes to firm up.

5 — Store the protein bites in an airtight container in the fridge for up to 1 week. Grab one whenever you need a quick, satisfying snack!

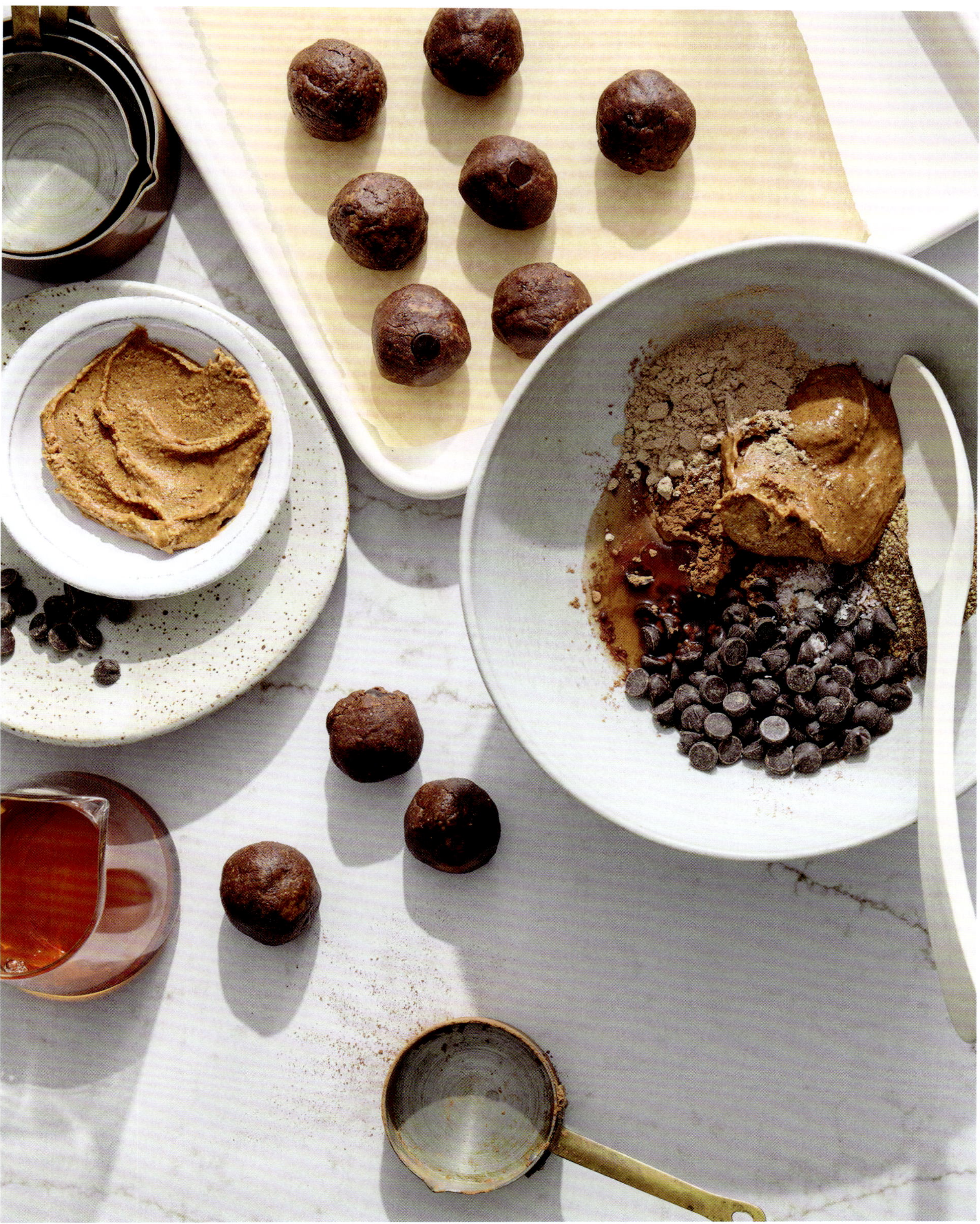

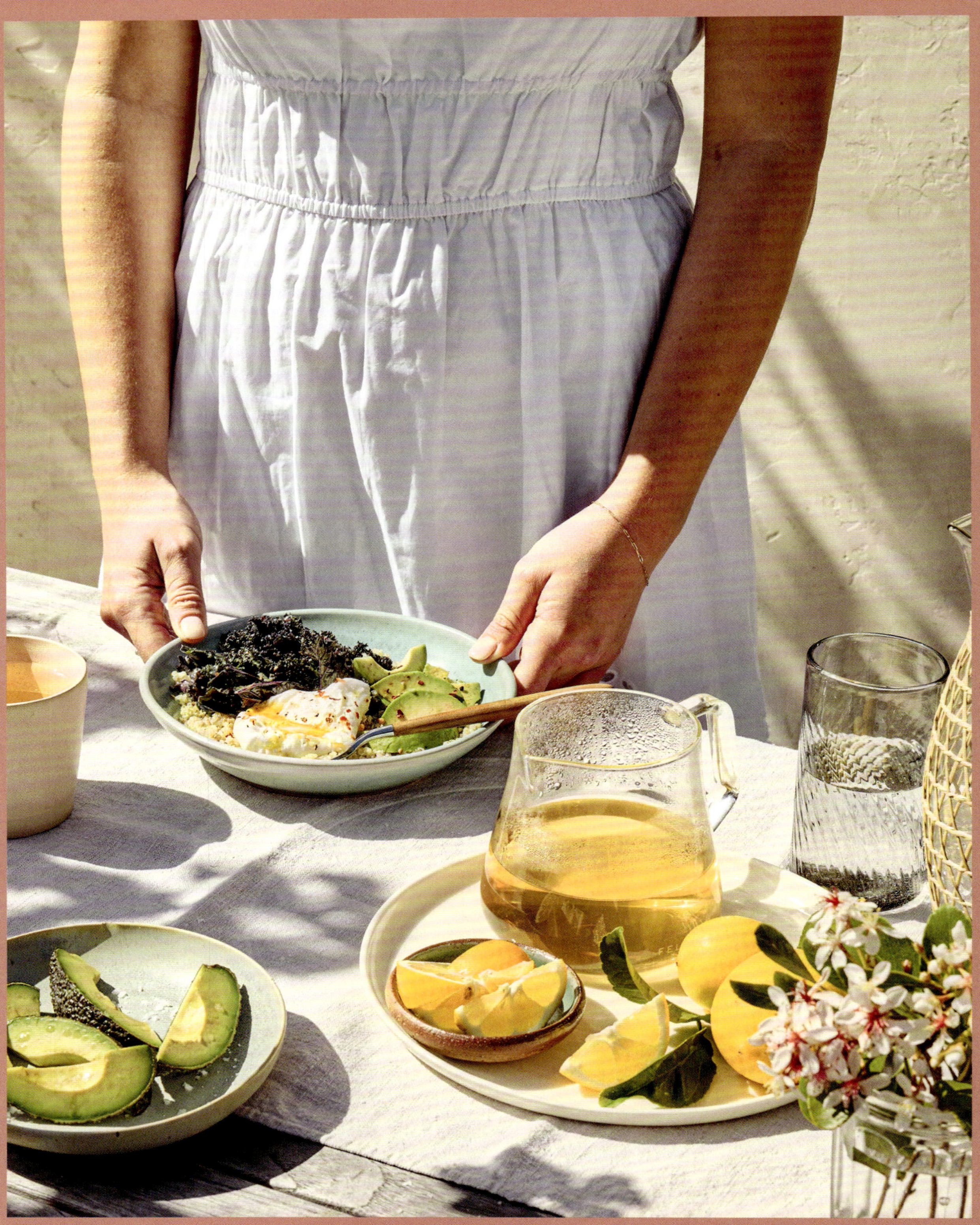

Follicular Phase

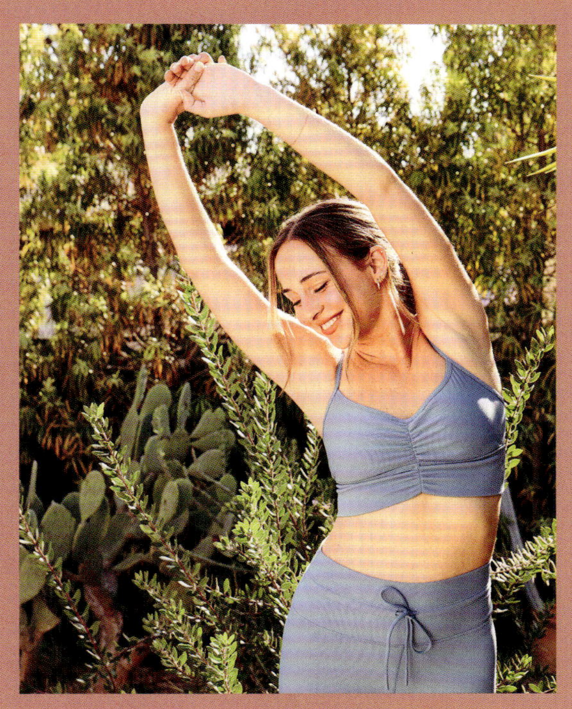

Energizing Your Body

The follicular phase begins the moment your period ends, typically lasts seven to ten days, and is a time of renewal! During menstruation, the uterine lining is shed, and your body is essentially in a recovery phase. During the follicular phase, your body focuses on rebuilding that uterine lining (endometrium). This rebuilding is essential because a healthy, thickened uterine lining is necessary to support a fertilized egg if conception occurs. As this process happens, the body also works to restore nutrient levels that were depleted during the shedding process, while also supporting rising estrogen levels. Estrogen is the key hormone that helps the follicles in the ovaries grow and mature.

On the cellular level, the body is working on the regeneration of tissues, particularly in the uterus, but also in other areas like the skin, hair, and muscles. The liver, which plays a vital role in detoxifying the body and processing excess hormones, is working overtime to help balance and metabolize the hormones circulating during this phase.

Hormonal Breakdown: What's Happening?

Let's talk hormones:

- ESTROGEN is your follicular phase MVP. It starts to climb steadily, preparing your body for ovulation. Estrogen is a powerhouse: It boosts your energy, sharpens your mind, and even helps your skin glow. It also enhances your body's ability to tolerate physical stress, making this a good time to step up your fitness game.
- TESTOSTERONE also rises but more gradually. This hormone gives you an extra edge, supporting muscle strength, libido, and motivation. It's one of the reasons why you might feel more bold and confident during this phase.

Together, these hormones create the perfect environment for growth, both physical and mental. They also make your body more efficient in using carbohydrates, so let's use that to our advantage!

How Food Can Support You

During the follicular phase, the body is in a state of rebuilding, so it requires a variety of nutrients to support the processes.

1 — Protein and Amino Acids

The body is repairing and regenerating tissues, so adequate protein intake is essential. Protein is needed to create the building blocks for muscle, skin, and hormone production.

2 — Healthy Fats

Estrogen production relies on healthy fats, so omega-3 fatty acids (found in foods like flaxseed, walnuts, and fatty fish) are especially important. These fats not only support hormone production but also help reduce inflammation, which can be a concern in the follicular phase as the body is recovering from the inflammatory effects of menstruation.

3 — Fiber-Rich Foods

Dr. Amersi notes that as the body starts metabolizing and eliminating excess hormones, fiber plays a key role in supporting digestion and helping the liver detoxify. Fiber from vegetables, fruits, legumes, and whole grains supports gut health and hormone metabolism, ensuring that any excess estrogen or toxins are efficiently eliminated.

4 — B Vitamins

The B vitamins, particularly B6 and B12, are vital during the follicular phase, as they help regulate hormonal balance, boost energy, and support the production of red blood cells. Foods like leafy greens, beans, and eggs can provide these nutrients.

5 — Magnesium

Dr. Amersi explains that magnesium levels tend to be lowest during the follicular phase, so consuming magnesium-rich foods now can help prevent period pain later in the cycle. This mineral helps the body maintain balance, particularly as estrogen rises. It also helps with muscle relaxation, supports healthy blood flow, and relieves tension in muscles (including those in the pelvic area). Magnesium is also important for maintaining stable blood sugar levels and preventing irritability or fatigue. Sources of magnesium include leafy greens, nuts, seeds, and whole grains.

6 — Antioxidants

Your body is repairing tissues, so antioxidants are essential to combat oxidative stress. Berries, nuts, seeds, and leafy greens are great sources of antioxidants, which help protect your cells from damage as the body rebuilds.

Top Nutrition Tips for the Follicular Phase

1 — Support Rising Estrogen

As estrogen begins to rise during the follicular phase, it's important to support its production and metabolism. Cruciferous veggies like broccoli, cauliflower, Brussels sprouts, and kale contain compounds that help the liver process and eliminate excess estrogen. These foods also provide fiber, which supports healthy digestion and hormone balance by promoting regular detoxification through the gut.

2 — Focus on Fresh, Light, and Energizing Foods

Your body is naturally more insulin sensitive during this time, meaning it handles carbohydrates more efficiently. This is a great phase to enjoy lighter meals with plenty of fresh fruits, lean proteins, legumes, and whole grains like quinoa, oats, and brown rice. These foods provide steady energy and help fuel the boost in physical and mental activity that often comes with this phase.

3 — Incorporate Fermented Foods

With your digestive system functioning more optimally, this is a great time to support your gut health. Fermented foods like sauerkraut, kimchi, kefir, and unsweetened yogurt introduce beneficial bacteria that can support hormone metabolism, immune function, and overall mood—especially as estrogen levels continue to climb.

4 — Include Omega-3s for Brain and Mood Support

Estrogen has a natural mood-boosting effect, and omega-3 fatty acids can enhance that outcome even more. Foods like wild salmon, chia seeds, flax seeds, and walnuts support brain health, reduce inflammation, and keep your mood elevated. They're also great for keeping your skin glowing as estrogen enhances collagen production.

5 — Power Up with Protein

You might notice an increase in motivation and activity during this time, so be sure to fuel your body properly with high-quality protein. Options like eggs, pasture-raised chicken, lentils, and tofu help build lean muscle and keep you feeling satisfied. Pairing protein with complex carbs also helps maintain blood sugar balance and sustain energy throughout the day.

Exercise and Lifestyle Tips

With your hormones working in your favor, this phase is perfect for embracing activities that get your heart pumping and your mind inspired.

Embrace Vigorous Movement

Rising estrogen improves your endurance and recovery, so don't be afraid to push yourself. Try jogging, cycling, crossfit, or a fun dance class.

Why Strength Training Shines

The rise in hormones in this phase enhances muscle recovery, increases strength, and improves your body's tolerance for physical stress. This makes it the perfect time to lift weights! Not only does this build lean muscle and support bone density, but it also improves insulin sensitivity, helping stabilize blood sugar levels. Strength training during this phase lays the foundation for long-term metabolic and hormonal health, all the while making you feel strong and empowered.

Get Creative with Your Energy

The follicular phase is a time of heightened creativity. Try something new! Whether it's experimenting with recipes from this book, starting a creative project, or diving into a hobby like painting or writing, this phase is all about exploration and growth!

During this follicular phase, your seven to ten days might look like a balance of movement and nourishment designed to match your rising energy:

- TWO DAYS OF CARDIO Enjoy a light jog, an energizing run, or a fun cycling session to boost endurance.
- THREE DAYS OF STRENGTH TRAINING Focus on full-body workouts with squats, dead lifts, and push-ups, alternating with upper- and lower-body sessions to build lean muscle.
- TWO DAYS OF ACTIVE RECOVERY Try a restorative yoga class or a playful dance session to stay loose, flexible, and centered.

Self-Care Practices to Support Your Follicular Phase

While your energy is high, it's important to keep some grounding practices in your routine:

- OUTDOOR TIME Exposure to morning sunlight supports your circadian rhythm, boosts serotonin, and regulates cortisol. Walking, hiking, or grounding barefoot can nourish your nervous system, which is important to keep in mind during all phases.
- GENTLE YOGA OR MEDITATION These practices help balance energy, which is important in preventing burnout while also keeping your body and mind in sync.
- SLEEP AS A NON-NEGOTIABLE Sleep is one of the most underrated pillars of hormone health. Even with the energy boost in this phase, aiming for seven to nine hours of quality rest each night is essential. Sleep plays a critical role in regulating hormones, supporting muscle recovery, maintaining healthy cortisol levels, and so much more. Don't "sleep" on the importance of quality rest—it's the foundation for feeling your best throughout your cycle!

What to Eat

- BREAKFASTS Energize with a berry chia pudding, avocado toast with eggs, or a maca smoothie for hormone support and steady energy.
- LUNCHES Build Buddha bowls with fiber-rich veggies like roasted sweet potatoes, leafy greens, and quinoa, and with lean proteins like chicken or turkey.
- DINNERS Lean into poultry-heavy dishes like grilled chicken with roasted vegetables or turkey stir-fry over cauliflower rice. Include healthy fats like avocado or olive oil for hormone support.

Note

You'll be using a lot of pre-cooked quinoa this week! Go ahead and meal-prep a batch on Sunday night; you can even use bone broth instead of water to add extra protein and nutrients.

Follicular Phase Superfoods

- FLAX SEEDS Rich in lignans and omega-3s, they help modulate estrogen levels and support hormone balance during this phase.
- PUMPKIN SEEDS A great source of zinc, they support follicle development and promote healthy ovulation as your body prepares for the next phase.
- CHIA SEEDS High in omega-3 fatty acids and fiber, they support blood sugar balance and promote healthy hormone metabolism as estrogen begins to rise.
- QUINOA A complete protein and rich in fiber, it provides sustained energy and stabilizes blood sugar during this naturally higher-energy phase.
- KALE Packed with vitamins A, C, and K, as well as calcium, it supports detoxification pathways and overall hormone balance.
- WHITE BEANS High in protein, fiber, and iron, they help to boost energy levels and replenish iron stores post-menstruation.
- CHICKPEAS A great source of plant-based protein and fiber, they support digestion and provide key nutrients like folate for cellular growth.
- LENTILS High in protein, iron, and folate, they are essential for supporting energy production and healthy cell development as your body gears up for ovulation.
- SPINACH Rich in iron, magnesium, and vitamins A and C, it promotes energy production and reduces inflammation, which is particularly helpful after menstruation.
- AVOCADO Loaded with healthy fats and potassium, it helps stabilize blood sugar and supports estrogen production during this phase.
- BROCCOLI A cruciferous vegetable, it aids in liver detoxification and supports healthy estrogen metabolism.
- BERRIES High in antioxidants and fiber, they help combat oxidative stress and support healthy digestion as hormone levels rise.
- HEMP SEEDS They provide a balanced ratio of omega-3 and omega-6 fatty acids along with plant-based protein, supporting hormonal health and energy.
- TURMERIC Contains curcumin, a powerful anti-inflammatory compound that can help combat any residual inflammation from menstruation.

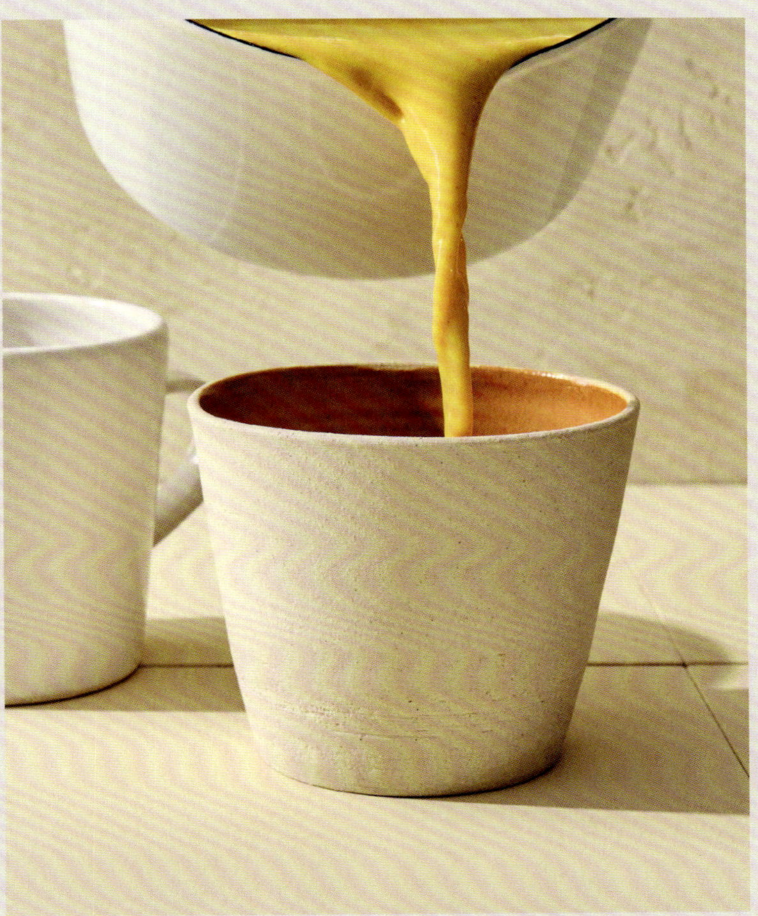

- **BRUSSELS SPROUTS** High in fiber, vitamins C and K, and folate, they aid in liver detoxification and hormonal balance.
- **PINEAPPLE** Contains bromelain and vitamin C, which support digestion and help reduce inflammation as your energy increases.
- **ASPARAGUS** High in folate, fiber, and vitamins A, C, and K, it promotes healthy cell growth and detoxification.
- **GREEN TEA** Packed with antioxidants and catechins, it helps reduce inflammation and boosts metabolism during this energized phase.
- **COCONUT OIL** Provides medium-chain triglycerides (MCTs) that offer quick, sustained energy and support hormone production.

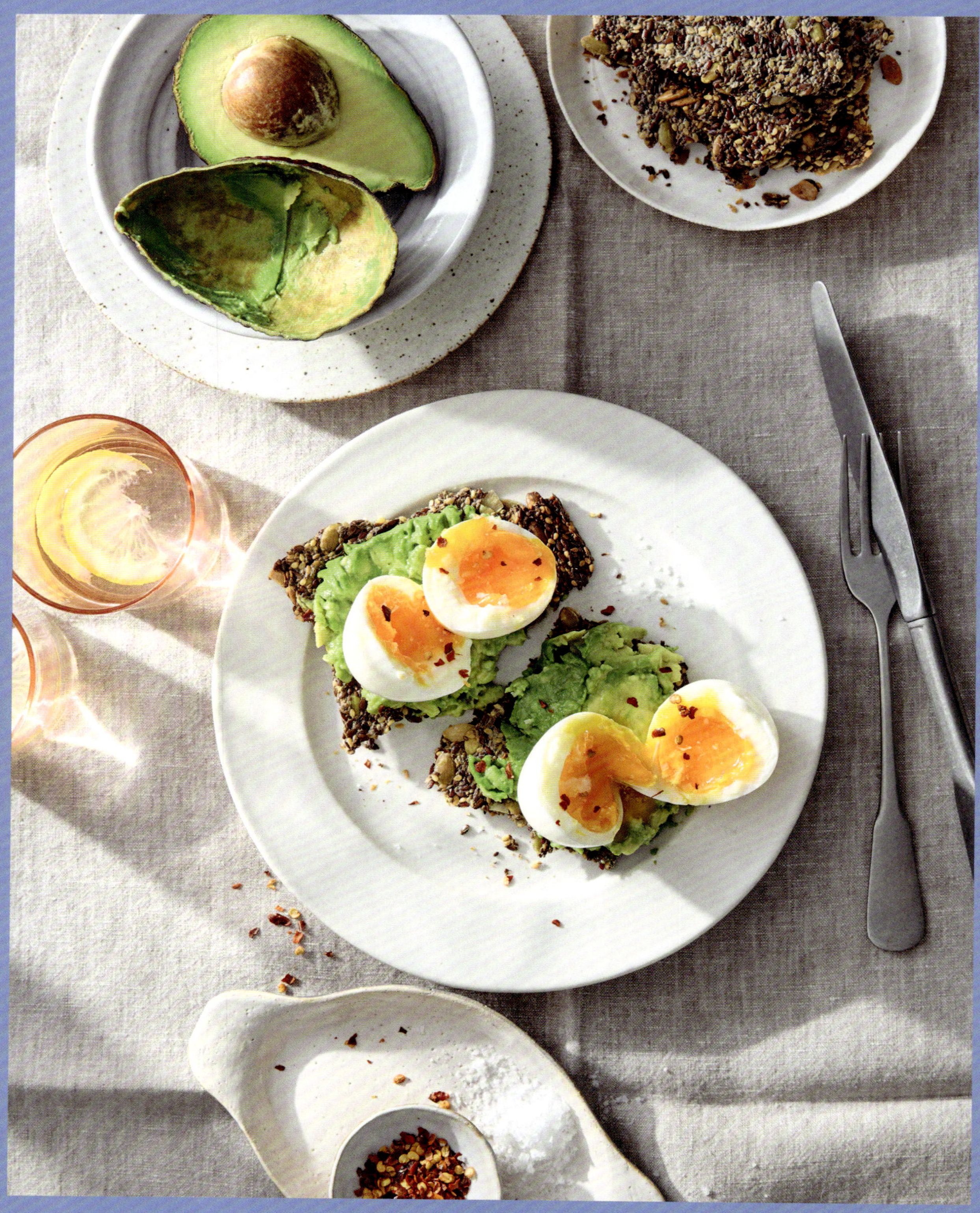

Breakfasts

Cha-Cha Chia Pudding (3 Ways)

Serves 2

Prep Time: 10 minutes, plus 4 hours or overnight to set

Chia pudding has been one of my go-to breakfasts for years because it's like a blank canvas, ready to take on whatever flavors I'm in the mood for. Chia seeds are rich in omega-3s and fiber, which help support steady energy levels—just what you need during the follicular phase as your body gears up for ovulation, when energy demands increase, hormone production ramps up, and balanced blood sugar becomes essential to support your rising estrogen levels. Chia seeds absorb liquid to create a creamy, pudding-like texture that's endlessly customizable. If the texture bothers you, you can even blend it! Whether you're craving earthy matcha (my favorite), sweet berries, or a spiced turmeric kick, these three variations give you options to keep things fresh!

Basic Mix

¼ cup chia seeds

1 cup almond milk (or any milk of choice)

1 teaspoon vanilla extract

1 tablespoon pure maple syrup or honey

Matcha Chia Pudding

1 teaspoon matcha powder

Berry Chia Pudding

¼ cup fresh or frozen berries (blueberries, raspberries, or strawberries)

Turmeric Chia Pudding

½ teaspoon ground turmeric

¼ teaspoon ground cinnamon

Optional Toppings

Greek yogurt, granola, berries, nuts, seeds, honey, or coconut flakes

1 — Make the basic mix (for Matcha or Turmeric Chia. See below for Berry): Combine the chia seeds, almond milk, vanilla, and maple syrup in a small bowl.

2 — Choose your variation:

FOR MATCHA Whisk the matcha powder into the bowl along with the other ingredients.

FOR BERRY First add the milk and the berries to a blender, and blend to combine, then mix with the chia seeds, vanilla, and maple syrup in the bowl.

FOR TURMERIC Stir the turmeric and cinnamon into the bowl with the other ingredients.

3 — Refrigerate for 30 minutes, then remove and stir to avoid clumping. Cover the bowl and return to the refrigerator to chill for 4 hours or overnight.

4 — Serve chilled, topped with your choice of Greek yogurt, granola, berries, nuts, seeds, honey, or coconut flakes.

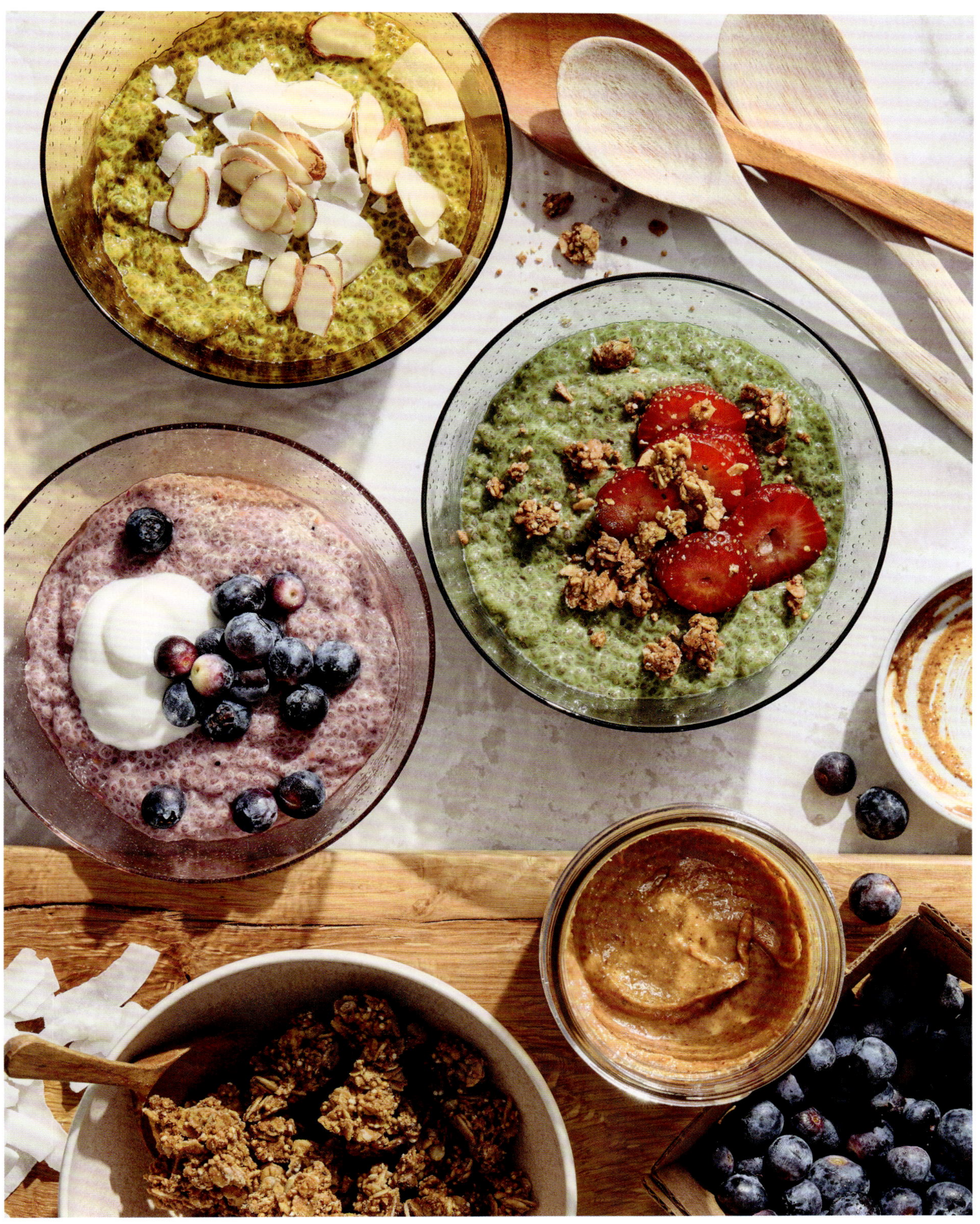

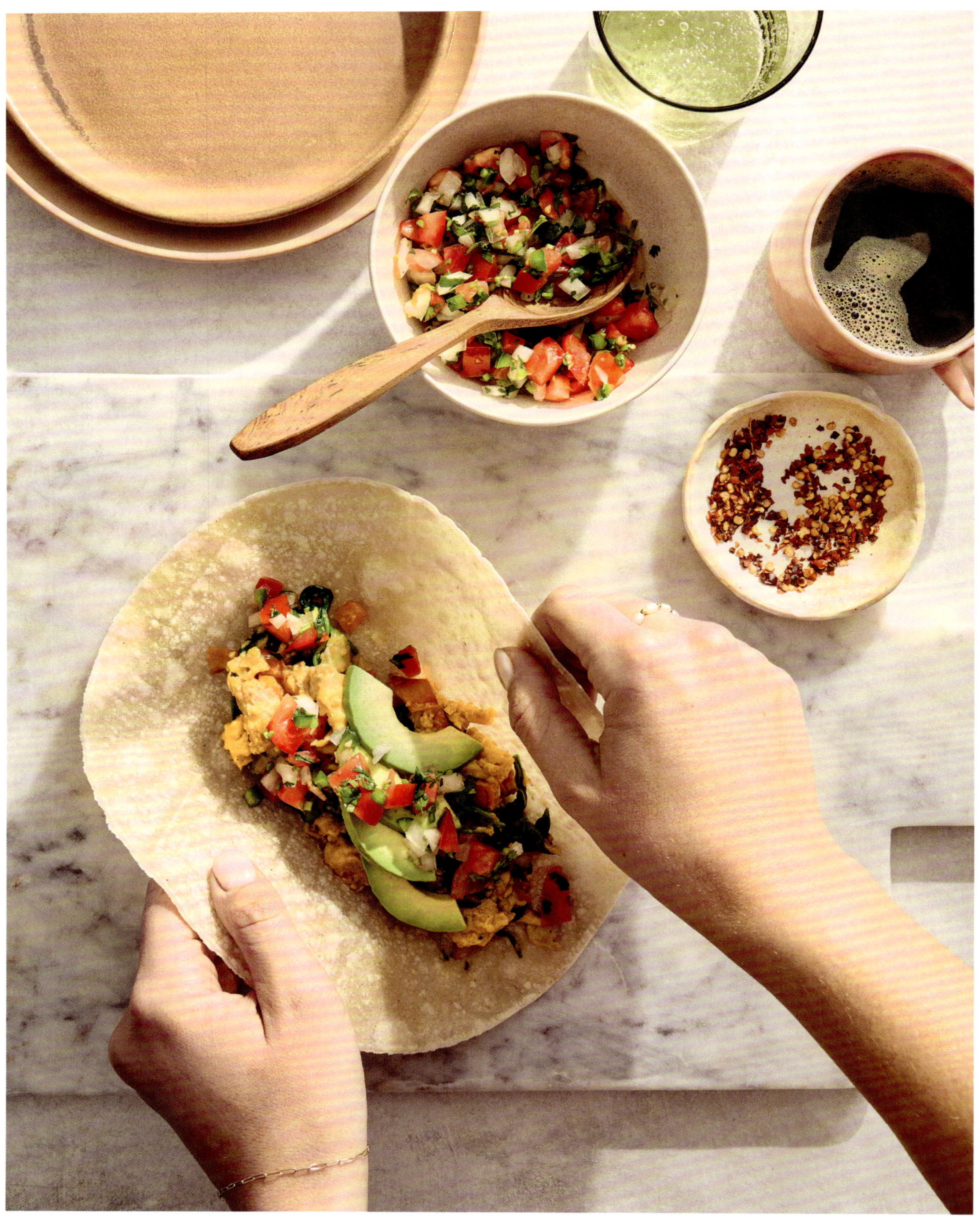

Make-It-Yours Veggie and Egg Breakfast Burrito

Serves 1
Prep Time: 10 minutes
Cook Time: 10 minutes

This breakfast burrito is my go-to when the follicular phase energy surge kicks in, and I'm ready to fuel up for a productive day. The eggs provide a solid protein and choline boost, while the sautéed veggies and creamy avocado offer healthy fats, fiber, and antioxidants to keep energy steady and focused. It's quick, filling, and adaptable to whatever veggies are on hand, like cooked broccoli, tomato, or zucchini. It also makes for a great meal-prep option; just wrap the prepared burrito in foil, store it in the freezer, unwrap, and reheat it when you wake up craving flavor and fuel!

1 tablespoon olive oil
¼ cup diced bell pepper
¼ cup fresh baby spinach
2 large eggs
1 whole wheat or gluten-free burrito-size tortilla
¼ avocado, pitted and sliced
1 tablespoon salsa of choice
Salt and freshly ground black pepper

1 — Place a large skillet over medium heat and add the olive oil. Add the bell pepper and sauté until softened, about 3 minutes.

2 — Add the spinach and cook just until wilted.

3 — Lightly whisk the eggs in a small bowl, then pour into the pan and scramble and cook with the veggies for 3 minutes, until firm.

4 — Spoon the egg-and-veggie mixture into the tortilla and top with the avocado slices. Spoon the salsa over the top and season to taste with salt and pepper.

5 — Fold in the sides of the tortilla and roll the burrito up snugly. Enjoy warm.

Quinoa Breakfast Bowl with Sautéed Kale, Avocado, and Poached Egg

Serves 1

Prep Time: 5 minutes

Cook Time: 10 minutes

Quinoa is a complete protein that is also packed with fiber, which is why I love using it as a base for breakfast bowls! The sautéed kale and avocado deliver healthy fats and folate to support hormone production and they complement the gradual rise in energy and focus you'll feel as estrogen begins to increase. I like to top this bowl with a poached egg for extra protein and richness, while a sprinkle of red pepper flakes adds a bit of heat!

Vinegar, for poaching (optional)
1 teaspoon olive oil
1 cup chopped fresh kale
1 large egg
½ cup cooked quinoa, warmed
¼ avocado, pitted and sliced
Salt and freshly ground black pepper
Red pepper flakes (optional)

1 — Fill a small saucepan with about 3 inches of water and bring it to a gentle simmer over medium heat. Add a splash of vinegar, if desired, to help the egg whites set more easily.

2 — While the water is heating, warm the olive oil in a large skillet over medium heat. Add the kale and sauté about 4 minutes, until just wilted. Remove from the heat, cover, and set aside to stay warm.

3 — Crack the egg into a small bowl or ramekin. When the water is simmering (not boiling), stir it gently to create a slight whirlpool, then carefully slide the egg into the center. Let it cook for 3 to 4 minutes, until the egg white is set but the yolk remains runny. Use a slotted spoon to carefully remove the egg and place it on a paper towel to briefly drain.

4 — In a serving bowl, layer the quinoa, sautéed kale, and avocado slices. Top with the poached egg. Season to taste with salt and pepper, then add a sprinkle of red pepper flakes, if desired. Serve immediately.

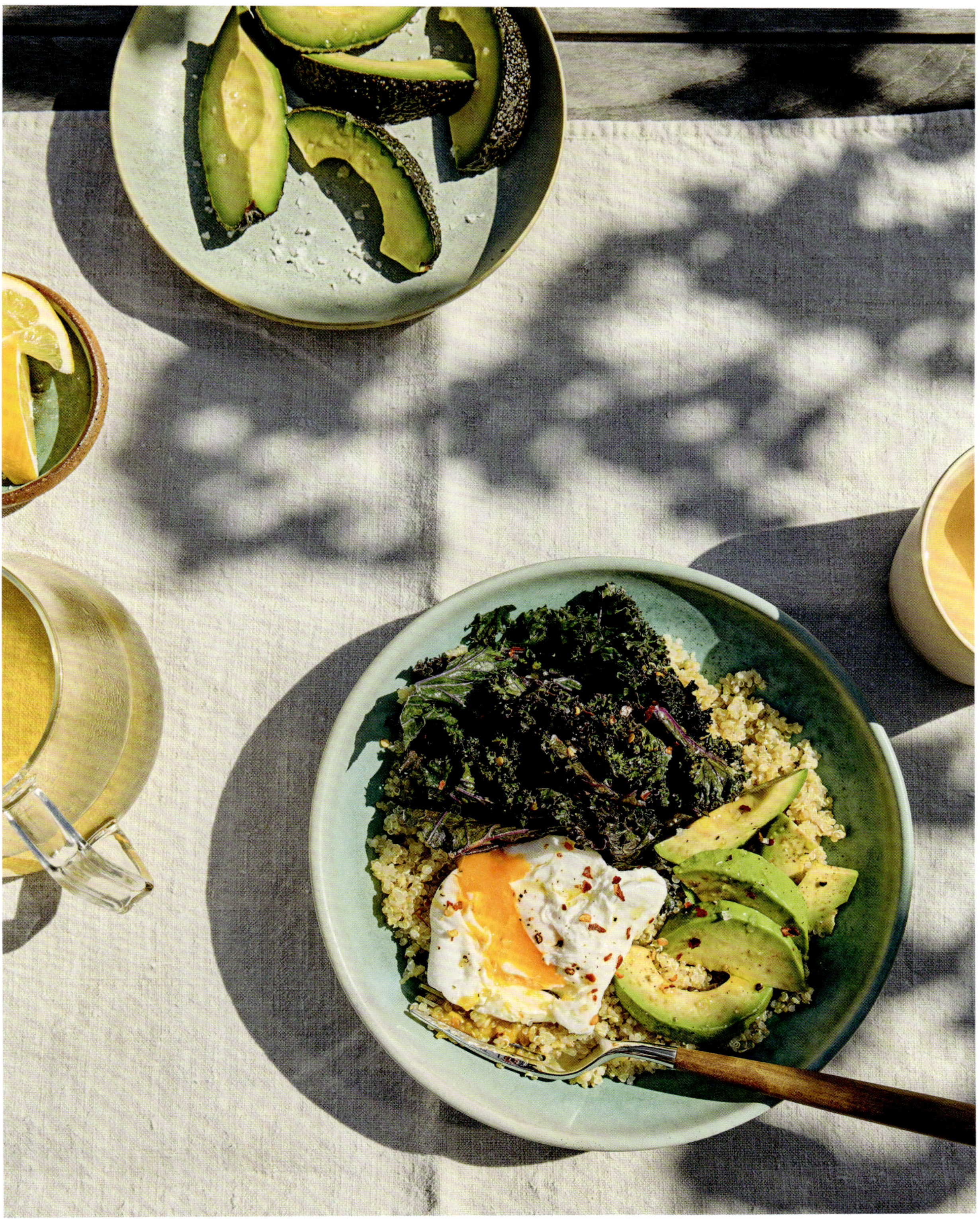

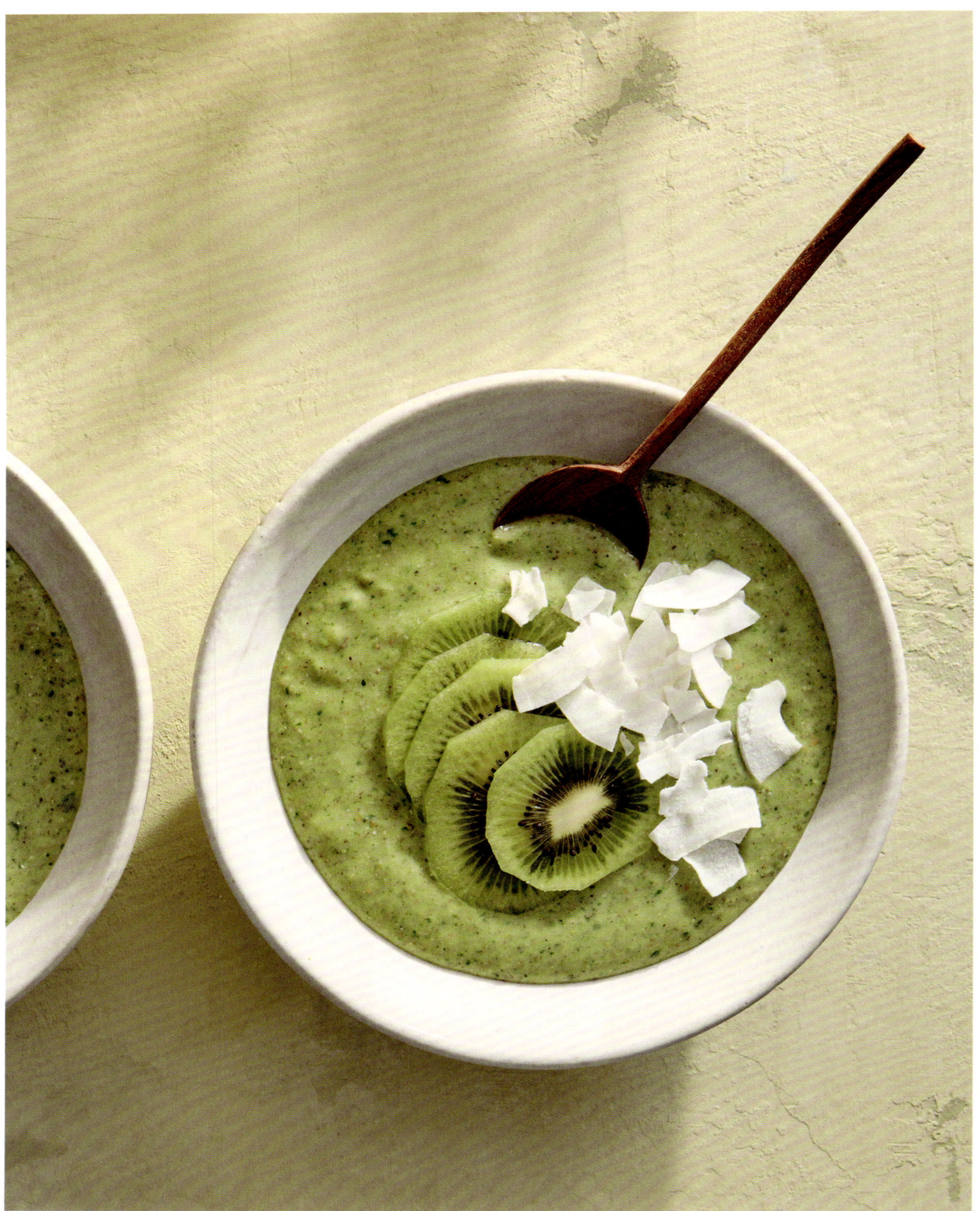

Green Dreams Smoothie Bowl with Kiwi and Coconut

Serves 1

Prep Time: 5 minutes

Years ago, my doctor taught me about the power that kiwi fruit has for digestion, and it's become my go-to when things need a little help to get moving along. The follicular phase is an ideal time to support your body's natural detoxification process because, as estrogen begins to rise, it's crucial to help the liver and gut efficiently metabolize and clear out any excess hormones lingering from the previous cycle. Kiwi plays a key role here: Its fiber and enzymes aid digestion, promoting regular bowel movements that are essential for hormone clearance.

For an extra nutrient boost, keep the peel on the kiwi! The peel contains even more fiber and nutrients, further enhancing its detoxifying power and supporting optimal gut health. By keeping things "moving," you're ensuring that estrogen levels stay balanced as they rise, preventing sluggish digestion or hormone build-up. Topped with shredded coconut for healthy fats, this bowl provides a gentle yet energizing nutrient boost!

---

1 frozen peeled banana

½ cup fresh baby spinach

1½ kiwis (peel on), 1 whole and ½ sliced, for topping

½ cup almond milk

½ cup plain Greek yogurt (or 1 scoop vanilla protein powder)

1 cup crushed ice

1 tablespoon chia seeds

2 tablespoons shredded unsweetened coconut

1 tablespoon almond butter (optional)

1 — Place the frozen banana, spinach, whole kiwi, almond milk, yogurt, crushed ice, and chia seeds in a blender and blend on high power until smooth.

2 — Pour the mixture into a serving bowl and top with the kiwi slices, coconut, and almond butter (if using). Enjoy.

Crunchy Seed Crackers with Avocado and Soft-Boiled Eggs

Serves 4 to 6

Prep Time: 10 minutes, plus 10 minutes soaking

Cook Time: 50 to 65 minutes

Seed cycling has become one of my favorite hormone-supportive practices, and these seed crackers make it easy. The idea is simple: During the follicular phase, flax and pumpkin seeds help support natural estrogen production, while in the luteal phase, sunflower and sesame seeds help maintain steady progesterone levels (see page 20 for more). Here, flax and pumpkin seeds supply the phytoestrogens and omega-3s that keep your hormones balanced and your body's rhythm on track. I love piling on the creamy avocado and soft-boiled eggs for a protein- and fiber-packed breakfast that's as nourishing as it is delicious!

Crackers

½ cup flax seeds

½ cup pumpkin seeds (or sunflower seeds, if you're in the luteal phase)

¼ cup sesame seeds

¼ cup chia seeds

1 cup water

½ teaspoon sea salt

½ teaspoon garlic powder (or dried herbs like rosemary or thyme; optional)

Toppings

½ avocado, pitted and mashed

2 large eggs, soft-boiled and kept warm

½ teaspoon red pepper flakes (optional)

1 — Preheat the oven to 300°F. Line a baking sheet with parchment paper.

2 — Make the crackers: In a medium bowl, combine all the seeds, the water, sea salt, and garlic powder. Let the mixture sit for about 10 minutes, until it thickens, as the seeds absorb the water and bind together.

3 — Pour the mixture onto the baking sheet and spread it into a thin, even layer using a spatula (aim for about ⅛ inch thick).

4 — Bake for 40 to 50 minutes, checking halfway through. When the edges start to turn golden, remove the baking sheet from the oven and cut the mixture into squares or desired shapes with a knife, being careful not to touch the hot surface of the baking sheet. If the crackers are not fully crisp at this point, carefully flip them over and bake for another 10 to 15 minutes, or until fully dry and crisp.

5 — Allow the crackers to cool completely on the baking sheet. Store them in an airtight container for up to 1 week.

6 — Add the toppings: When ready to enjoy, top some of the crackers with avocado, soft-boiled eggs (I like to just smash mine on top of the crackers, but you can slice and layer if you prefer), and red pepper flakes, if desired.

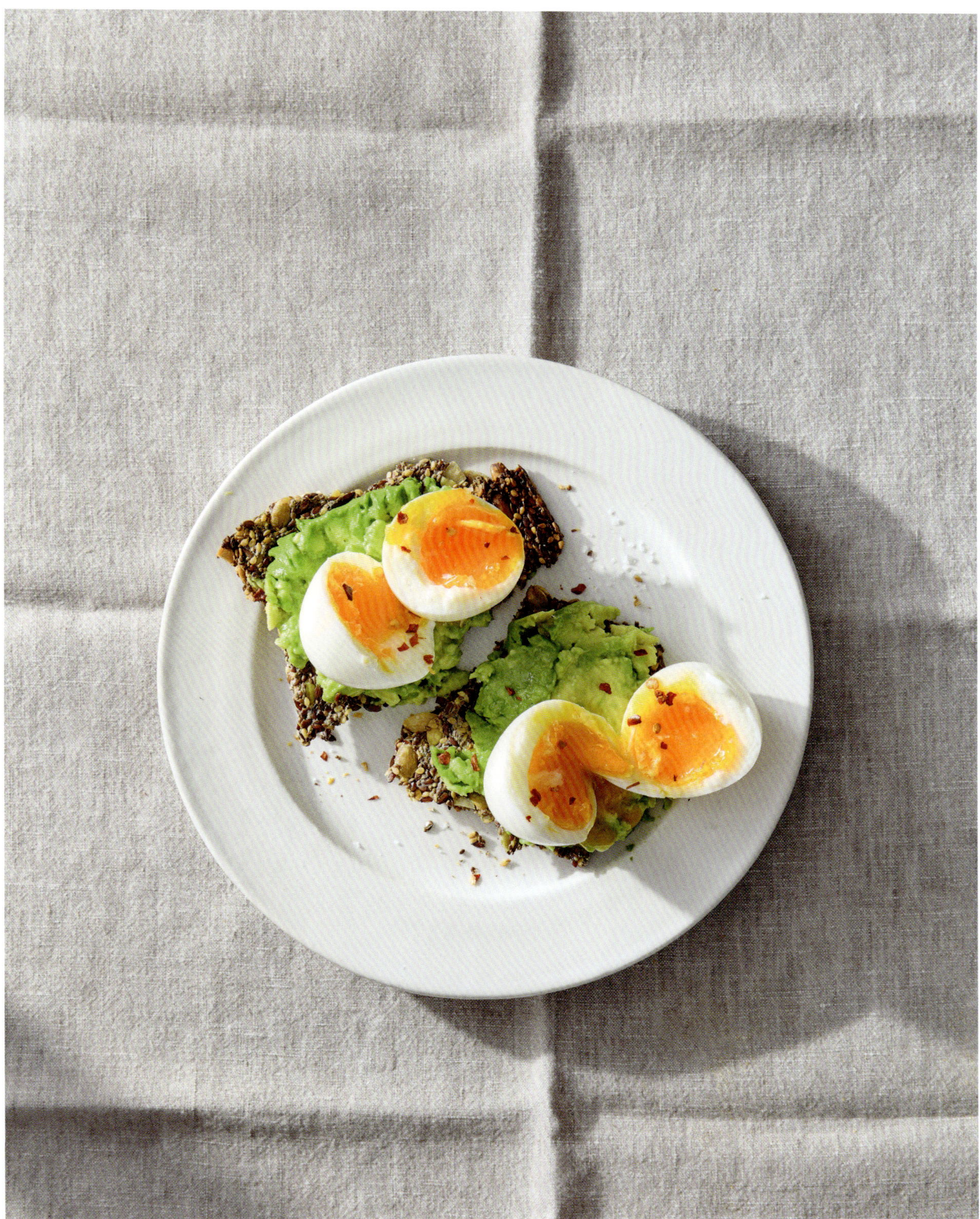

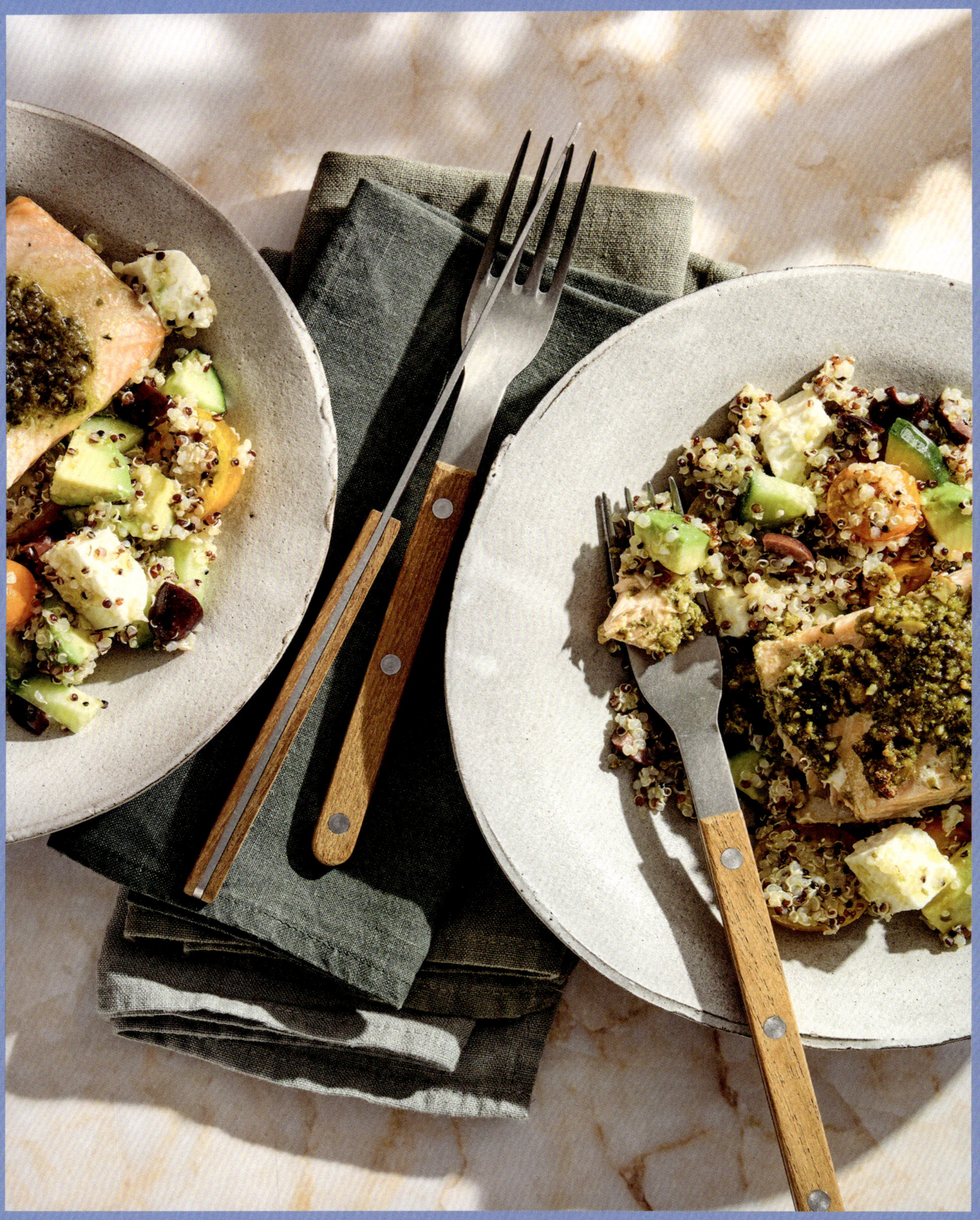

Lunches & Dinners

LA-Dreaming Kale and White Bean Salad

Serves 3

Prep Time: 10 minutes

This was inspired by a salad I love that's available at my favorite health food store in LA. Kale and white beans are both loaded with fiber, which as you've probably gathered is the name of the game in this follicular phase! That's because fiber plays a key role in helping your body clear out excess hormones—particularly the estrogen left from the menstrual phase—by promoting healthy digestion and regular elimination. I toss in pumpkin seeds here for a boost of magnesium, iron, and zinc, which supports energy and hormone balance. I like to pair this salad with grilled salmon or chicken when I'm wanting some extra protein. The salad is fresh, filling, and the perfect way to keep your hormone levels steady while enjoying a little taste of LA wellness in every bite!

---

4 cups chopped fresh kale

2 tablespoons olive oil

½ (15-ounce) can white beans, drained and rinsed

¼ cup pumpkin seeds

¼ avocado, pitted and diced

1 medium grapefruit, peeled and segmented

Juice of 1 lemon

1 teaspoon Dijon mustard

Salt and freshly ground black pepper

1 — In a large bowl, massage the kale with 1 tablespoon of the olive oil for 1 to 2 minutes, until softened.

2 — Toss in the beans, pumpkin seeds, avocado, and grapefruit segments.

3 — In a small bowl, whisk together the remaining tablespoon olive oil, the lemon juice, mustard, and salt and pepper to taste.

4 — Pour the dressing over the mixture in the bowl and toss until everything is evenly coated. Serve chilled or at room temperature.

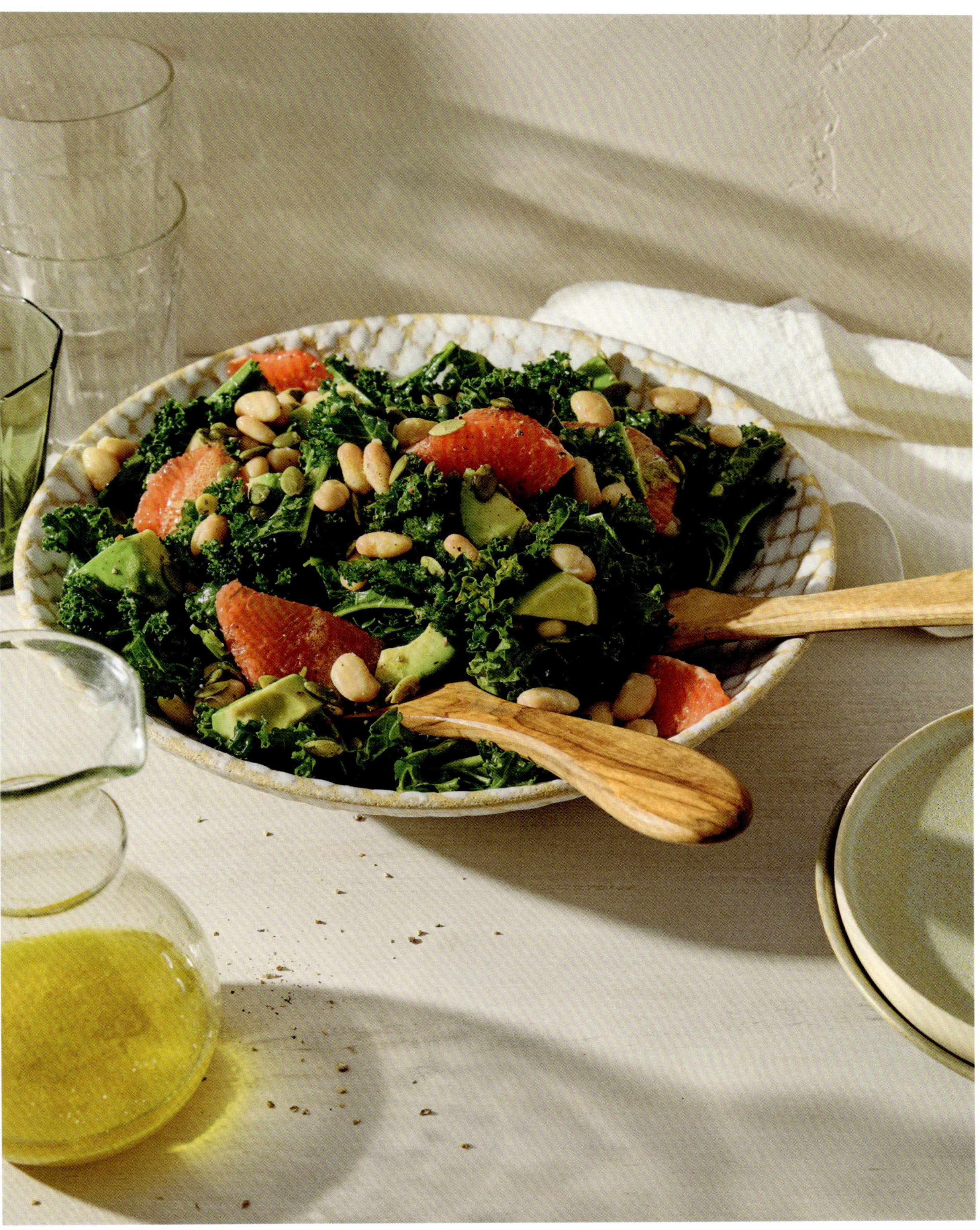

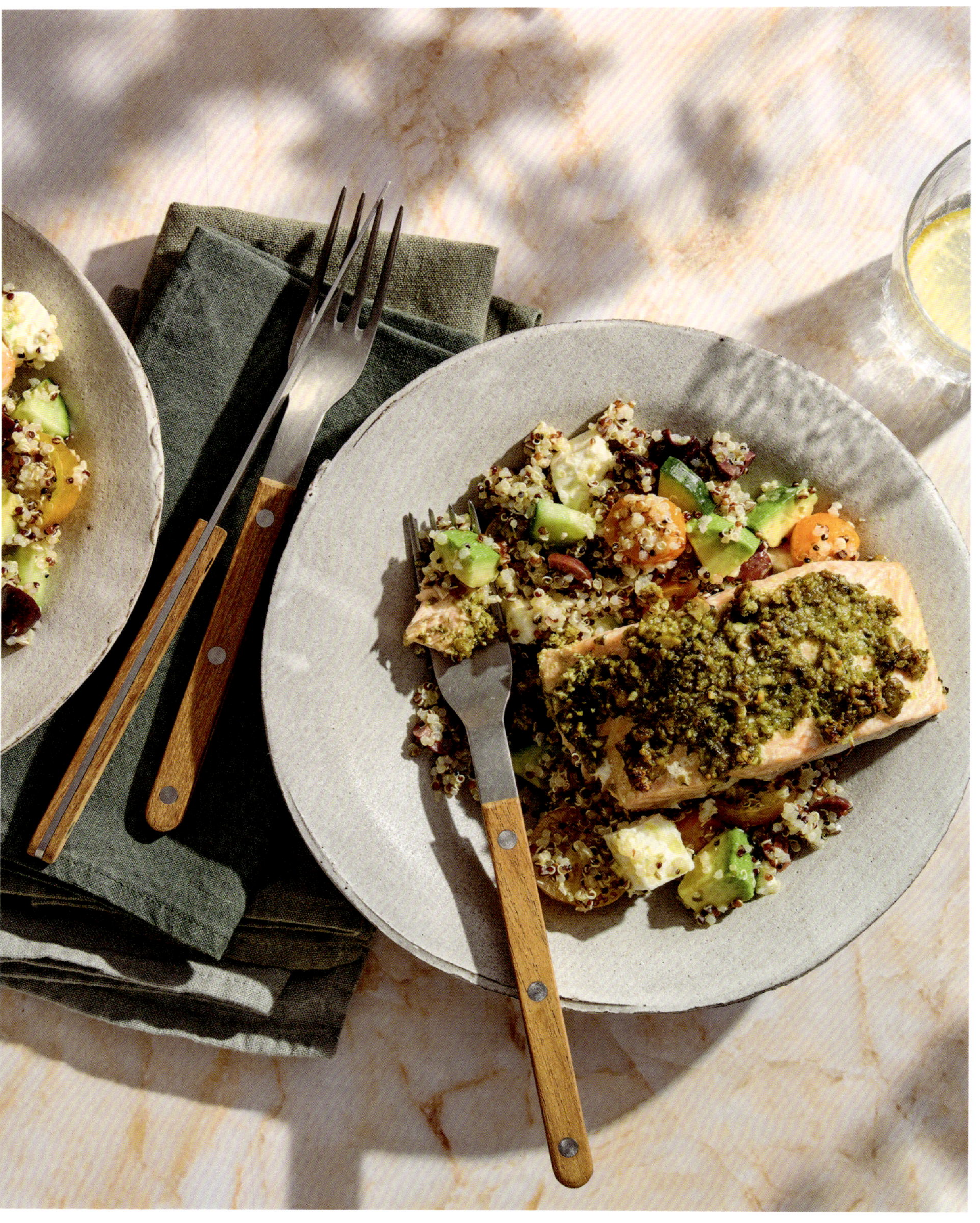

Zippy Greek Quinoa Salad with Pesto Salmon

Serves 2
Prep Time: 20 minutes
Cook Time: 15 minutes

The follicular phase is like your body's springtime—a period of renewal and fresh energy. You're likely feeling lighter, more optimistic, and ready to take on the world. After menstruation, your estrogen levels begin to rise, giving you an energy boost and leaving you craving vibrant, refreshing meals that feel as uplifting as your mood. This salad fits the bill perfectly. It's inspired by the nutrient-rich Mediterranean diet, which is well known for its amazing health benefits, especially when it comes to reducing inflammation! This salad is all about fiber from whole grains and pumpkin seeds; the healthy fats from salmon, olives, olive oil, and avocado; and the fresh veggies!

Pesto

½ cup raw pumpkin seeds
½ cup pine nuts (pignoli)
2 cups fresh basil leaves
2 garlic cloves
Juice of 1 lemon
¼ cup nutritional yeast (for that cheesy flavor)
½ teaspoon sea salt
¼ teaspoon freshly ground black pepper
¼ cup extra-virgin olive oil

Salmon

2 salmon fillets (about 4 ounces each)
1 tablespoon olive oil
Salt and freshly ground black pepper

Salad

½ cup quinoa, cooked and cooled
½ medium cucumber, diced
½ cup cherry tomatoes, halved
¼ cup chopped, pitted Kalamata olives
¼ cup crumbled Greek feta cheese (or dairy-free feta; optional)
1 avocado, halved, pitted, and cubed
1 tablespoon olive oil, plus more for drizzling (optional)
Juice of 1 lemon, plus more for drizzling (optional)
1 teaspoon dried oregano
Salt and freshly ground black pepper

1 — Make the pesto: Toast the pumpkin seeds and pine nuts in a small dry skillet over medium heat for 3 to 4 minutes, until lightly golden and fragrant.

2 — Add the toasted seeds to a food processor along with the basil, garlic, lemon juice, nutritional yeast, salt, and pepper. Pulse a few times to combine. Then slowly drizzle in the olive oil while processing, until the mixture is smooth and creamy.

3 — Taste and adjust seasoning as needed. Set ¼ cup of the pesto aside for the salmon and save the remainder for another use. Makes about 1 cup. (The pesto can be stored in an airtight glass container in the fridge for up to 5 days.)

4 — Preheat the oven to 400°F. Line a baking sheet with parchment paper.

5 — Bake the salmon: Place the fillets on the baking sheet, then drizzle with the olive oil and season to taste with salt and pepper. Spread 2 tablespoons of the pesto on top of each fillet.

6 — Bake the salmon for 12 to 15 minutes, until cooked through and it flakes easily with a fork.

7 — While the salmon bakes, make the salad: In a large bowl, combine the quinoa, cucumber, cherry tomatoes, olives, feta, and avocado. Drizzle on the olive oil and lemon juice, then sprinkle with the oregano and salt and pepper to taste. Toss well to coat everything.

8 — Assemble the meal: Divide the quinoa salad between 2 plates. Top each with a salmon fillet. Drizzle with additional lemon juice or olive oil, if desired, and serve.

Lemon-Herb Chicken with Roasted Brussels Sprouts and Quinoa Pilaf

Serves 4

Prep Time: 15 minutes

Cook Time: 30 minutes

After the restful menstrual phase, your body is primed for a nutrient boost as it ramps up energy and activity during the follicular phase. The lean protein from the chicken aids muscle recovery, while the quinoa provides fiber and essential amino acids to keep your energy steady. The Brussels sprouts bring a rich dose of antioxidants to support liver health, which is key for estrogen detoxification. For added protein and flavor, I love cooking the quinoa in bone broth, but feel free to use vegetable broth or water if you prefer!

Brussels Sprouts

4 cups trimmed and halved Brussels sprouts

2 tablespoons olive oil

Salt and freshly ground black pepper

Chicken

Juice of 1 lemon

4 tablespoons olive oil

2 teaspoons dried oregano

2 teaspoons garlic powder

½ teaspoon salt

½ teaspoon freshly ground black pepper

4 boneless, skinless chicken breasts (about 1 pound)

Quinoa Pilaf

1 cup quinoa, rinsed

2 cups bone broth

1 teaspoon ground cumin

½ teaspoon ground turmeric

½ teaspoon freshly ground black pepper

1 — Preheat the oven to 400°F. Line a baking sheet with parchment paper.

2 — Roast the sprouts: Toss the sprouts with the olive oil and salt and pepper to taste. Spread the sprouts on the baking sheet and roast for 20 to 25 minutes, until lightly charred and crisp. Cover and keep warm.

3 — Meanwhile, marinate the chicken: Combine the lemon juice, 2 tablespoons of the olive oil, the oregano, garlic powder, salt, and pepper in a medium bowl. Add the chicken and marinate for 10 minutes.

4 — Make the quinoa: In a small pot, combine the quinoa, bone broth, cumin, turmeric, and pepper. Bring to a boil over medium-high heat, then reduce to a simmer and cook for 15 minutes.

5 — Cook the chicken: Heat the remaining 2 tablespoons olive oil in a large skillet over medium. When the oil is shimmering, add the chicken, allowing any extra marinade to drip off, and sauté for 6 to 7 minutes per side, until cooked through to an internal temperature of 165°F.

6 — Serve the chicken with the hot quinoa pilaf and the roasted Brussels sprouts.

Springtime-Vibes Chicken and Pumpkin-Seed Salad with Lemon-Tahini Dressing

Serves 2

Prep Time: 10 minutes

Cook Time: 10 minutes

The follicular phase is the spring of your cycle! Your body is waking up, shedding the hibernation of menstrual phase, and craving fresh, vibrant foods that match your rising energy. Raw veggies are light on your digestive system during this phase, helping your body absorb all the nutrients without feeling bogged down. Unlike the luteal phase, where your body craves warming, heartier meals to support your metabolism, the follicular phase thrives on these refreshing, nutrient-dense foods. The grilled chicken and quinoa give you the steady fuel you need, and the lemon-tahini dressing adds just the zesty kick to support your body's natural rejuvenation!

Chicken

2 boneless, skinless chicken breasts, sliced into cutlets

1 tablespoon olive oil

Salt and freshly ground black pepper

Lemon-Tahini Dressing

3 tablespoons tahini

1 tablespoon freshly squeezed lemon juice

1 tablespoon olive oil

1 teaspoon pure maple syrup

1 teaspoon Dijon mustard

Salt and freshly ground black pepper

Salad

4 cups mixed greens (arugula, spinach, kale, etc.)

1 cup cooked quinoa

1 avocado, halved, pitted, and sliced

¼ cup pumpkin seeds

1 — Preheat a grill or place a grill pan over medium heat.

2 — Prepare the chicken: Rub the chicken pieces with the olive oil and salt and and pepper to taste. Grill the chicken for 4 to 5 minutes per side, or until the internal temperature reaches 165°F and the chicken is nicely charred on the outside. Let rest for a few minutes, then slice into strips.

3 — Make the dressing: In a small bowl, whisk together the tahini, lemon juice, olive oil, maple syrup, mustard, and salt and pepper to taste until smooth. Add a splash of water to thin the dressing, if needed.

4 — Assemble the salad: In a large salad bowl, combine the greens, quinoa, and avocado slices. Drizzle the dressing over the salad and toss gently to combine. Top with the grilled chicken strips and sprinkle with the pumpkin seeds. Serve immediately.

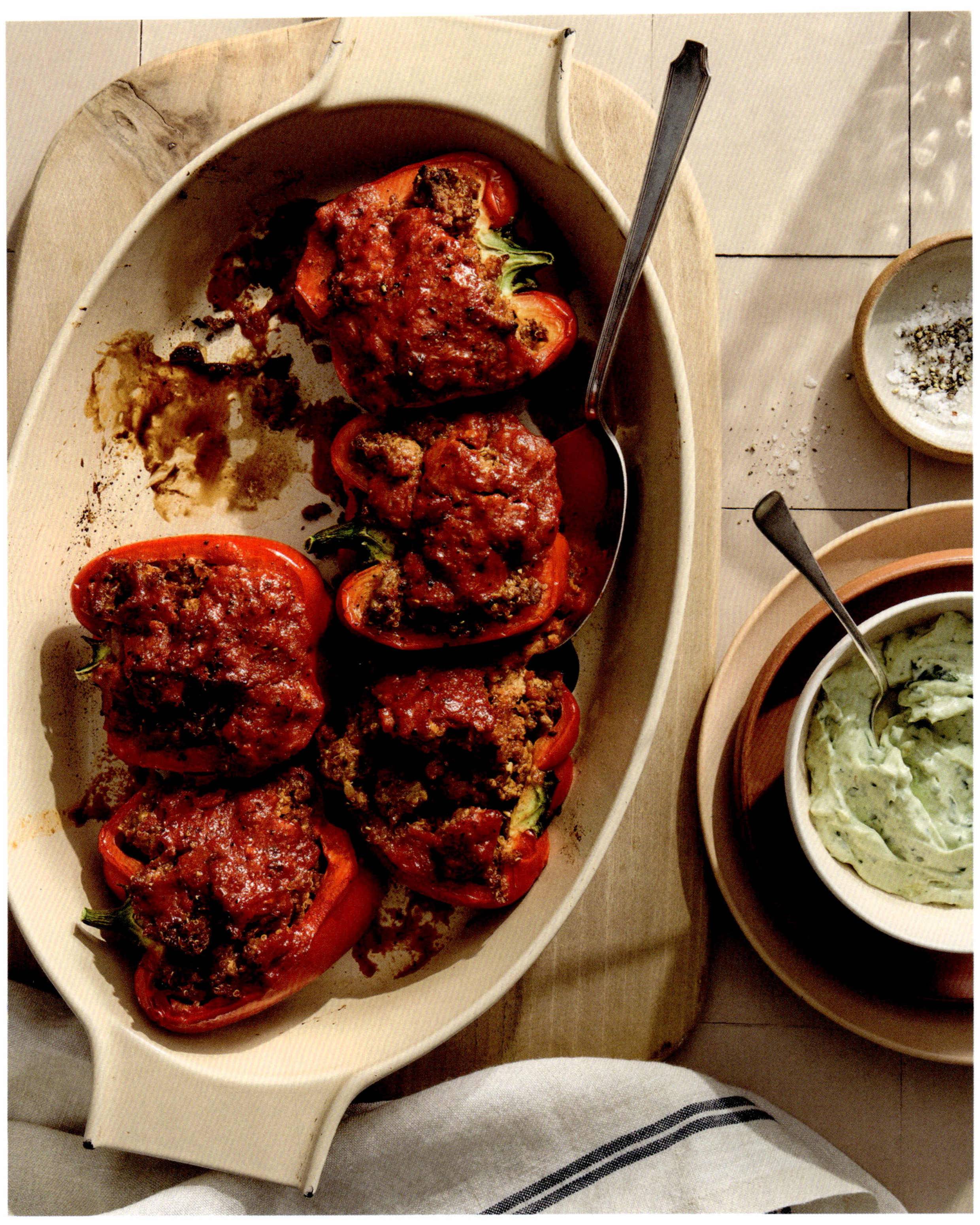

Turkey and Quinoa–Stuffed Bell Peppers with Avocado and Cilantro Yogurt Sauce

Serves 4
Prep Time: 15 minutes
Cook Time: 40 minutes

When I was growing up, stuffed bell peppers were a weekly staple in my household, and they're still one of my favorite comfort meals. I've taken my mom's classic recipe and added a modern twist by swapping out the white rice for quinoa, thereby boosting the dish with extra protein and fiber. This is the perfect meal for the follicular phase, when your body is thriving on nutrient-dense foods to fuel your rising energy and activity. The combination of lean turkey, quinoa, and healthy fats from the avocado helps keep your blood sugar balanced throughout the day. Plus, the zesty cilantro yogurt sauce adds a refreshing, creamy finish. These peppers are filling, energizing, and just as good the next day!

Stuffed Peppers

4 large bell peppers
1 tablespoon olive oil
8 ounces ground turkey
¼ medium onion, finely diced
1 teaspoon ground cumin
1 teaspoon chili powder (optional, for extra flavor)
¼ teaspoon salt
¼ teaspoon freshly ground black pepper
1 cup cooked quinoa
1 cup marinara sauce

Yogurt Sauce

1 ripe avocado
½ cup plain Greek yogurt (or dairy-free alternative)
¼ cup chopped cilantro, plus more for garnish (optional)
Juice of 1 lime, or more as desired
Large pinch of salt and sprinkle of black pepper

1 — Preheat the oven to 375°F.

2 — Prepare the stuffed peppers: Cut the tops off the bell peppers and remove the seeds. Set them aside.

3 — In a large skillet, heat the olive oil over medium heat. Add the turkey, onion, cumin, chili powder (if using), salt, and pepper. Cook for 5 to 7 minutes, breaking up the turkey as it cooks, until it is browned and cooked through.

4 — Stir in the quinoa and add half of the marinara sauce. Continue to cook for another 2 to 3 minutes, until the mixture is well combined and heated through.

5 — Stuff each bell pepper with some of the turkey and quinoa mixture, pressing gently to pack the filling into the peppers all the way down. Place the stuffed peppers in a baking dish large enough to hold them firmly. Top the peppers with the remaining marinara sauce.

6 — Cover the baking dish with foil and bake for 25 to 30 minutes, until the peppers are tender and the filling is heated through.

7 — While the peppers bake, prepare the sauce: In a blender or food processor, combine the avocado, yogurt, cilantro, lime juice, salt, and pepper. Blend until smooth and creamy.

8 — Remove the peppers from the oven and carefully transfer to serving plates. Top each with a generous dollop of the sauce. Garnish with extra cilantro or lime wedges, if desired.

Light and Bright Lentil Soup

Serves 4
Prep Time: 10 minutes
Cook Time: 35 minutes

Making soup feels like self-care to me. There's something especially comforting about a big bowl of lentil soup. It's hearty, it's full of fiber, and it provides plant-based protein to keep you going. Lentils are also a great source of plant-based iron, which is important for energy production—and you produce a lot of energy during the follicular phase. I love whipping up a big batch to enjoy throughout the week; it's a meal that tastes even better as the flavors deepen. I like to serve this with a slice of crusty gluten-free sourdough for an easy, nourishing meal.

1 tablespoon olive oil
½ medium onion, chopped
1 medium carrot, diced
1 celery stalk, diced
2 garlic cloves, minced
1 teaspoon ground cumin
½ teaspoon paprika
½ teaspoon ground turmeric
1 cup dried lentils, rinsed
4 cups vegetable broth
Salt and freshly ground black pepper

1 — Heat the olive oil in a large pot over medium heat. Add the onion, carrot, and celery and sauté about 5 minutes, until softened. Add the garlic, cumin, paprika, and turmeric, and cook for another minute.

2 — Stir the lentils into the pot and add the broth, then bring to a boil, reduce to a simmer, and cook for 25 to 30 minutes, until the lentils are tender.

3 — Season the soup to taste with salt and pepper, and serve hot.

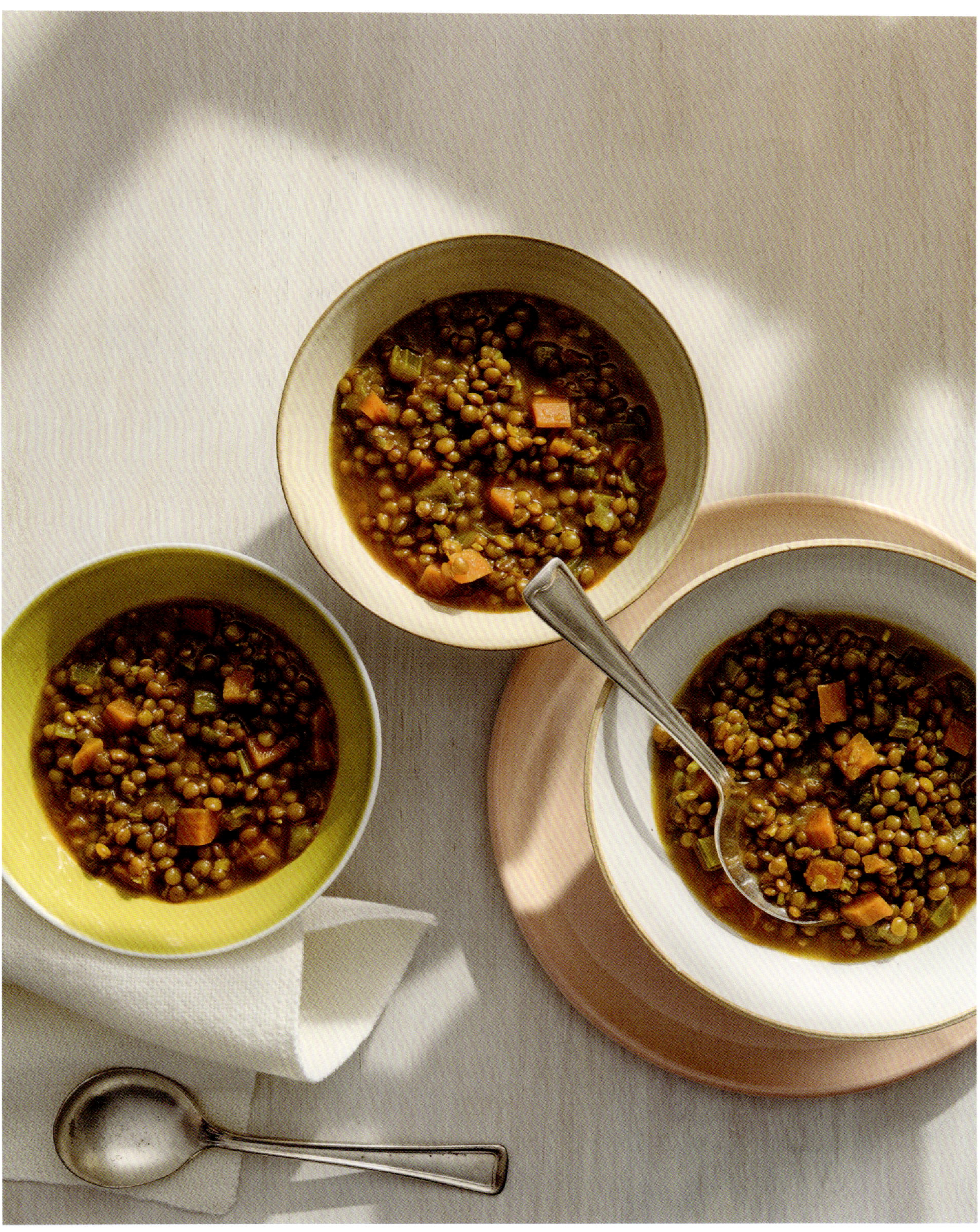

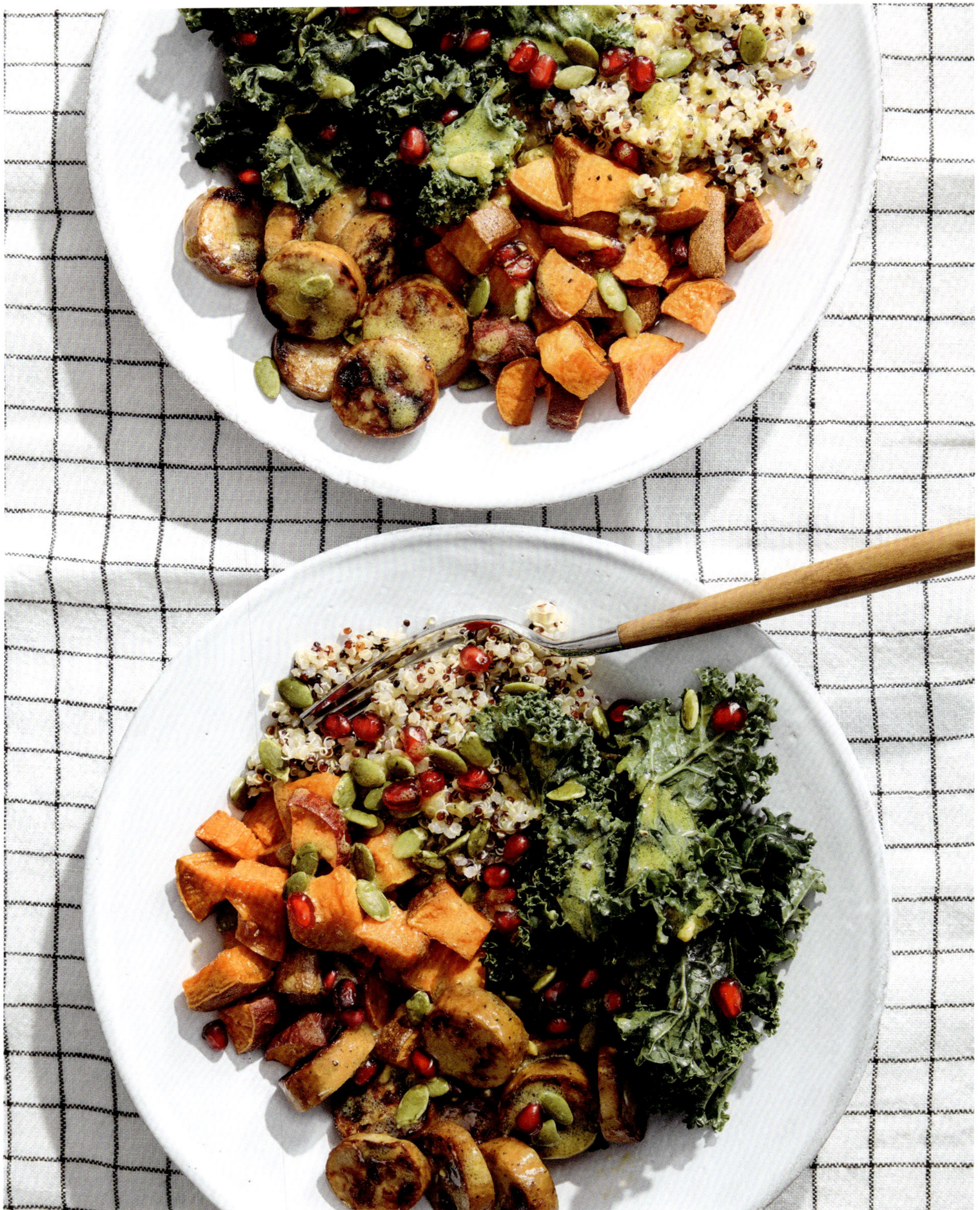

Roasted Harvest Bowl with Creamy Honey Mustard

Serves 2
Prep Time: 10 minutes
Cook Time: 25 minutes

The follicular phase is all about renewal—your energy is rising, your mood is lifting, and your body is craving fresh, vibrant foods to match. This bowl is a perfect way to fuel those feel-good days. Roasted sweet potatoes provide slow-digesting carbs to keep you energized, while kale delivers key nutrients like calcium and antioxidants to support hormone balance. Chicken and apple sausage adds a savory, protein-packed twist (feel free to replace with sprouted tofu, if you are in the mood to keep it veggie focused), and the honey mustard dressing ties everything together with the perfect mix of sweet and tangy. Light and satisfying, this meal is just what your body needs as you step into this new phase feeling refreshed and ready to take on the world.

Harvest Bowl

1 large sweet potato, diced
1 tablespoon olive oil
Salt and freshly ground black pepper
2 cups chopped fresh kale
1 tablespoon balsamic vinegar

Honey-Mustard Dressing

2 tablespoons Dijon mustard
1 tablespoon raw honey or pure maple syrup
1 tablespoon cider vinegar
1 tablespoon olive oil
Salt and freshly ground black pepper

For Serving

½ cup cooked quinoa
¼ cup pumpkin seeds
¼ cup pomegranate seeds

1 — Preheat the oven to 400°F. Line a baking sheet with parchment paper.

2 — Prepare the bowls: In a small bowl, toss the sweet potato dice with the olive oil and salt and pepper to taste. Spread the cubes on the baking sheet and roast for 20 to 25 minutes, flipping halfway through, until they're golden and tender.

3 — While the sweet potatoes roast, place the kale in a large bowl. Drizzle with the vinegar and massage the kale with your hands for 1 to 2 minutes, until it softens and darkens in color. (This will make the kale more tender and less bitter.)

4 — Make the dressing: In a small bowl, whisk together the mustard, honey, vinegar, olive oil, and salt and pepper to taste. Add a small amount of water to thin the dressing to your desired consistency, if needed—about a teaspoon at a time.

5 — Assemble the bowls: Layer the quinoa, the sweet potato cubes, and the massaged kale in serving bowls. Drizzle on the dressing, then sprinkle with the pumpkin seeds and pomegranate seeds for a pop of color and antioxidants.

World-Is-Your-Lentil and Chicken Pesto Pasta

Serves 2 to 3
Prep Time: 10 minutes
Cook Time: 20 minutes

You know those days when your energy starts to return, and you feel lighter, clearer, and ready to take on the world? That's the magic of the follicular phase. As estrogen rises, so does your motivation. Maybe you're signing up for a new workout class, tackling a creative project, or making plans with friends. This dish is the perfect complement to that fresh-start feeling. The lentil pasta provides steady energy without the crash, while roasted veggies and lemon zest brighten each bite, mirroring the vibrancy you're feeling. Protein from the chicken and healthy fats from the pesto help support stable blood sugar, keeping you fueled for whatever the day holds. If I could eat a pasta dish every night, this would be the one!

1 cup diced zucchini
½ cup diced bell pepper
2 tablespoons olive oil
½ teaspoon smoked paprika
Salt and freshly ground black pepper
1 (1-pound) box lentil pasta
1 cup shredded rotisserie chicken
¼ cup pesto (store-bought or homemade; see page 109), plus more if desired
¼ cup halved cherry tomatoes
1 teaspoon grated lemon zest
Fresh basil or arugula, for garnish (optional)

1 — Preheat the oven to 400°F. Line a baking sheet with parchment paper.

2 — In a small bowl, toss the diced zucchini and bell pepper with 1 tablespoon of the olive oil, the smoked paprika, and salt and pepper to taste. Spread evenly on the baking sheet and roast for 20 minutes, until vegetables are tender and slightly caramelized.

3 — While the veggies roast, cook the lentil pasta according to the package instructions. Drain.

4 — In a large saucepan, heat the remaining tablespoon olive oil over medium heat. Add the chicken and sauté for about 3 minutes, just to warm through and slightly brown.

5 — Add the pasta to the pan, then toss with the ¼ cup pesto until everything is evenly coated. Stir in the roasted veggies, then add the cherry tomatoes. Sprinkle on the lemon zest for a burst of freshness.

6 — If desired, season with additional salt and pepper and garnish with the fresh basil for extra flavor. Serve warm, with extra pesto on the side, if desired.

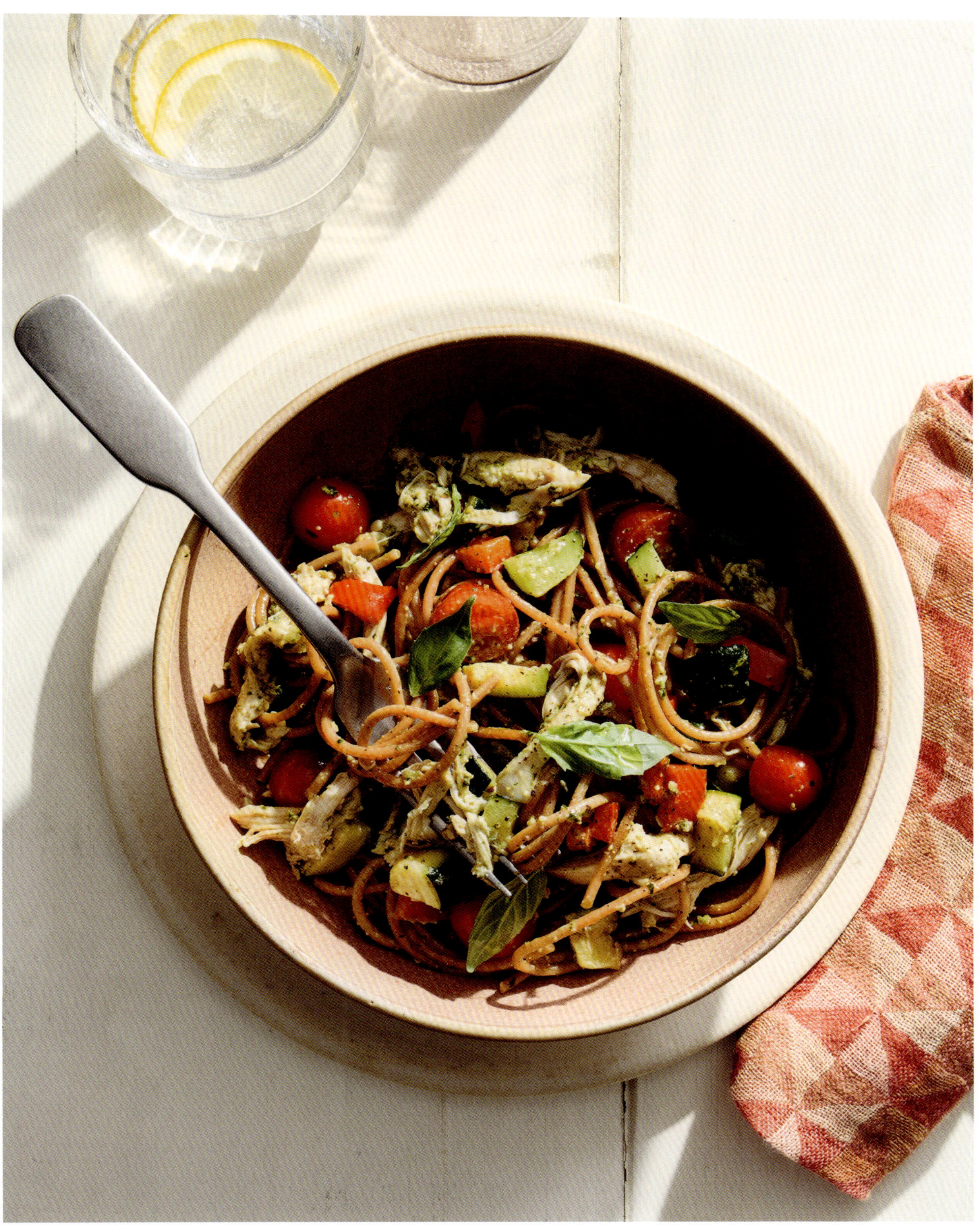

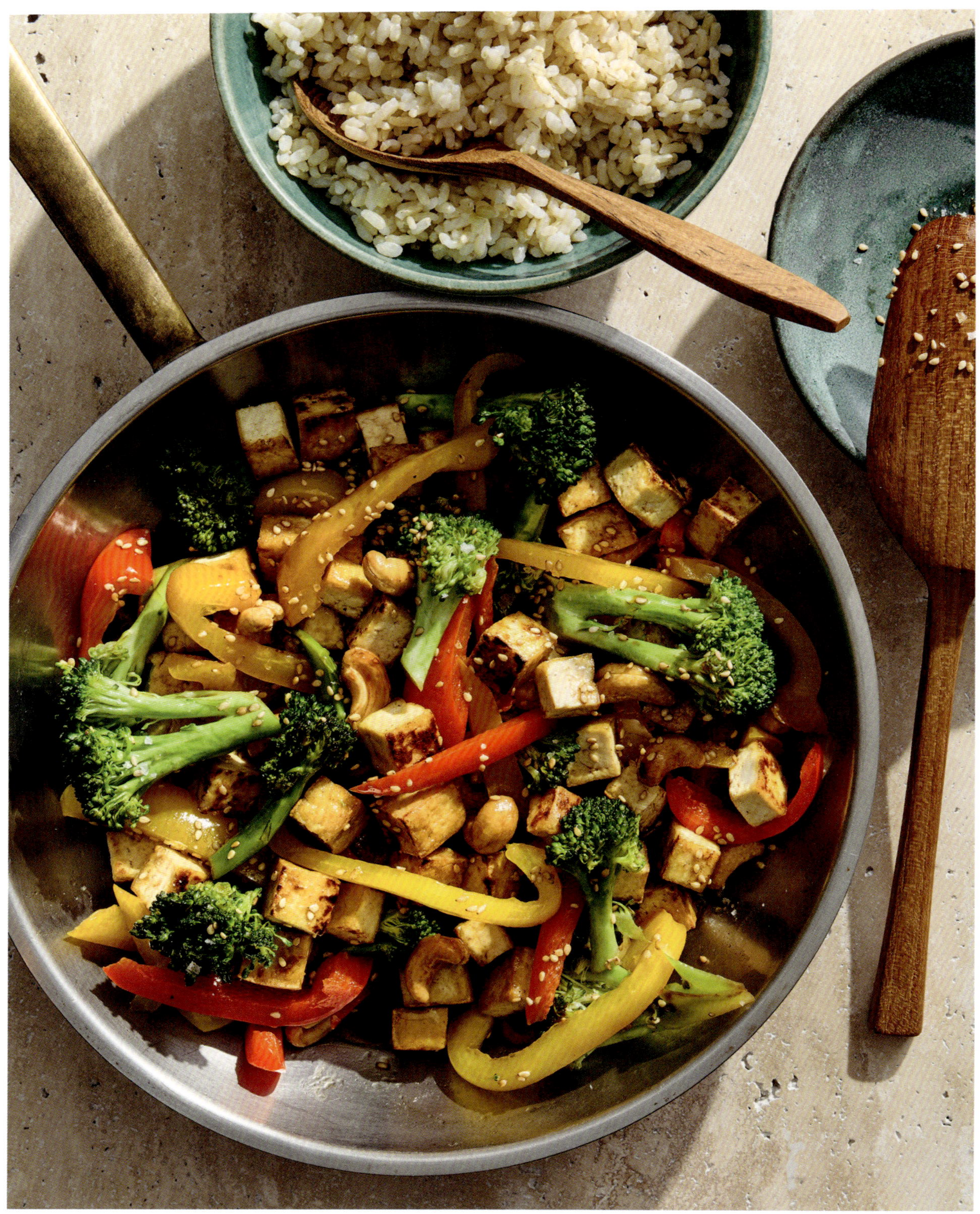

Fresh and Light Tofu and Cashew Stir-Fry

Serves 2

Prep Time: 10 minutes

Cook Time: 15 minutes

I always find myself craving lighter, veggie-forward meals during the follicular phase: something colorful, energizing, and easy to digest. This stir-fry checks all the boxes. The tofu crisps up perfectly; the broccoli and bell peppers bring in that fresh, vibrant crunch; and the coconut aminos tie it all together with that salty-sweet umami flavor. This is also a great way to throw together some of your leftover rice and veggies from an earlier meal-prep or an overstocked veggie drawer.

2 tablespoons olive oil

1 block firm organic tofu, pressed and cut into cubes

2 cups broccoli florets

1 red bell pepper, stemmed, seeded, and thinly sliced

1 yellow bell pepper, stemmed, seeded, and thinly sliced

¼ cup cashews (roasted or raw)

2 tablespoons coconut aminos

1 teaspoon toasted sesame oil (optional)

1 teaspoon sesame seeds (black or white), plus more for garnish

1 cup cooked brown rice, warmed

1 — Heat the olive oil in a large skillet over medium heat. Add the tofu cubes and cook for 5 to 7 minutes, until golden and crispy on all sides. Set aside.

2 — To the same skillet, add the broccoli, bell peppers, and cashews. Stir-fry for 5 minutes, until the vegetables are tender-crisp.

3 — Add the tofu back to the skillet along with the coconut aminos, sesame oil (if using), and teaspoon sesame seeds. Stir to combine and cook for another 2 minutes.

4 — Serve the stir-fry over a bed of brown rice and garnish with the extra sesame seeds!

Ginger Zing Chicken Crunch Salad

Serves 2

Prep Time: 10 minutes

Right after my period ends, I start to feel a little more like myself again—clearer, lighter, and ready to enjoy fresh fruits and veggies. This salad is one I've made repeatedly during that time. It's crunchy, colorful, and tossed in the most addicting sesame-ginger dressing. The rotisserie chicken makes the prep easy, while the cabbage and carrots give your body loads of fiber to keep your digestion moving. I love how it feels so simple yet is so nourishing—exactly the vibe I aim for during the follicular phase when my energy is slowly starting to build.

Chicken Salad

2 cups shredded green or red cabbage

1 cup shredded carrot

1 cup thinly sliced cucumber

½ cup thinly sliced red bell pepper

1 cup shredded rotisserie chicken

¼ cup chopped cilantro

Dressing

3 tablespoons rice vinegar

2 tablespoons coconut aminos

1 tablespoon toasted sesame oil

1 teaspoon pure maple syrup

1 teaspoon grated fresh ginger (or ½ teaspoon ground ginger)

Toppings (optional)

2 tablespoons sesame seeds

¼ cup roasted cashews

1 — Make the salad: In a large bowl, toss together the cabbage, carrot, cucumber, bell pepper, chicken, and cilantro.

2 — Make the dressing: In a small bowl, whisk together the vinegar, coconut aminos, sesame oil, maple syrup, and ginger until well combined.

3 — Finish the salad and top it: Pour the dressing over the salad and toss to combine. Top with the sesame seeds and cashews for added crunch, if desired. Serve immediately and enjoy!

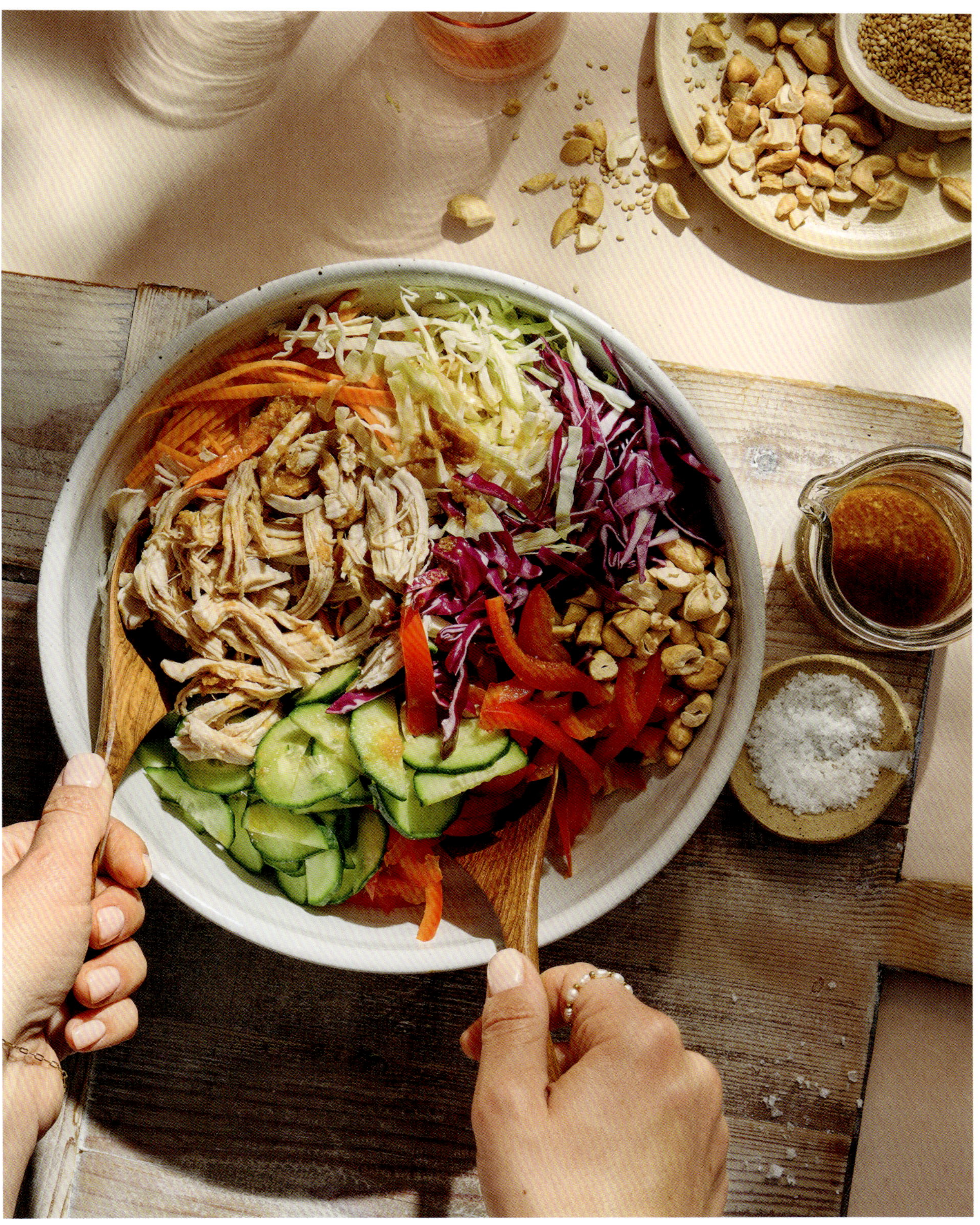

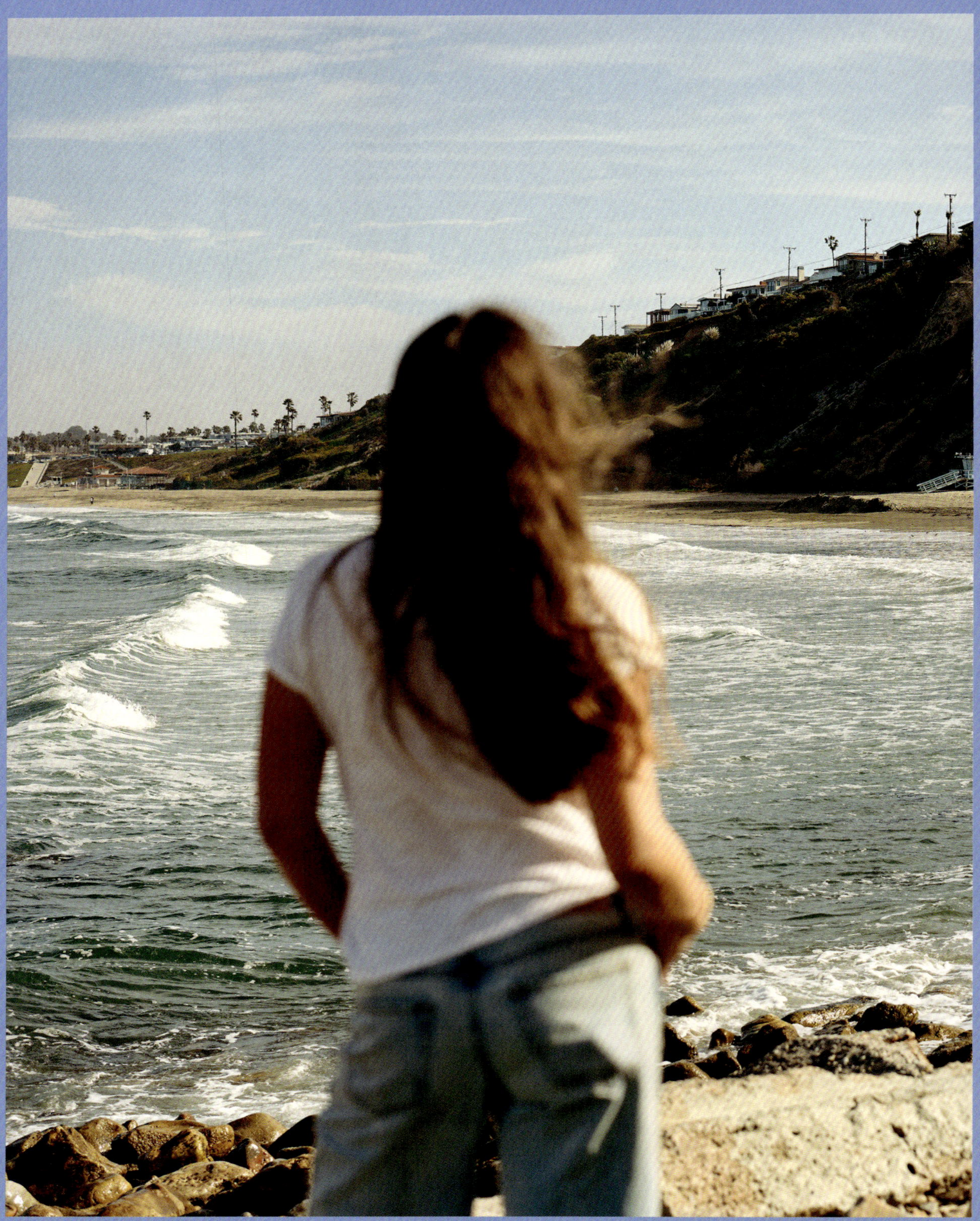

Snacks & Desserts

Chickpea Blondies

Makes 8 blondies
Prep Time: 10 minutes
Cook Time: 25 minutes

I know chickpeas in desserts might seem unconventional, but these blondies are a perfect sweet treat for your follicular phase. Chickpeas are packed with plant-based protein, which helps balance blood sugar and provide steady energy, as well as folate to support cell growth and repair. Almond butter adds those healthy fats we all need to support our hormones, while the maple syrup gives just the right touch of natural sweetness. A little indulgence that celebrates our cyclical bodies!

¼ cup pure maple syrup
1 teaspoon vanilla extract
½ cup almond butter
1 (15-ounce) can chickpeas, drained and rinsed
½ teaspoon baking powder
¼ teaspoon baking soda
¼ teaspoon sea salt
¼ cup dark chocolate chips

1 — Preheat the oven to 350°F. Line an 8 × 8-inch baking dish with parchment paper.

2 — In a food processor, blend the maple syrup, vanilla, almond butter, chickpeas, baking powder, baking soda, and sea salt until the batter is creamy.

3 — Stir in the chocolate chips.

4 — Spread the batter evenly in the prepared dish. Bake for 25 minutes, or until golden brown and set in the center.

5 — Let cool completely before slicing into squares.

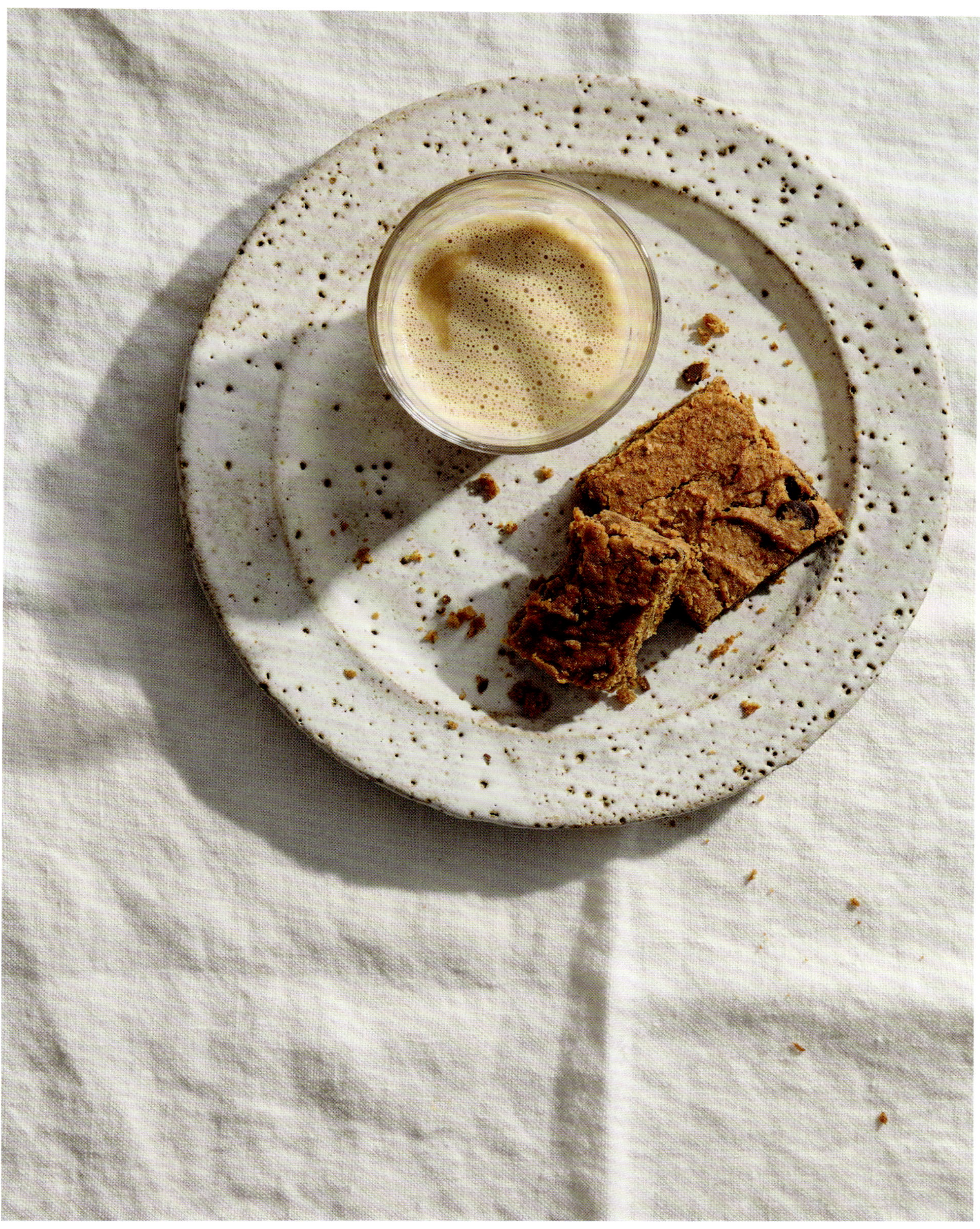

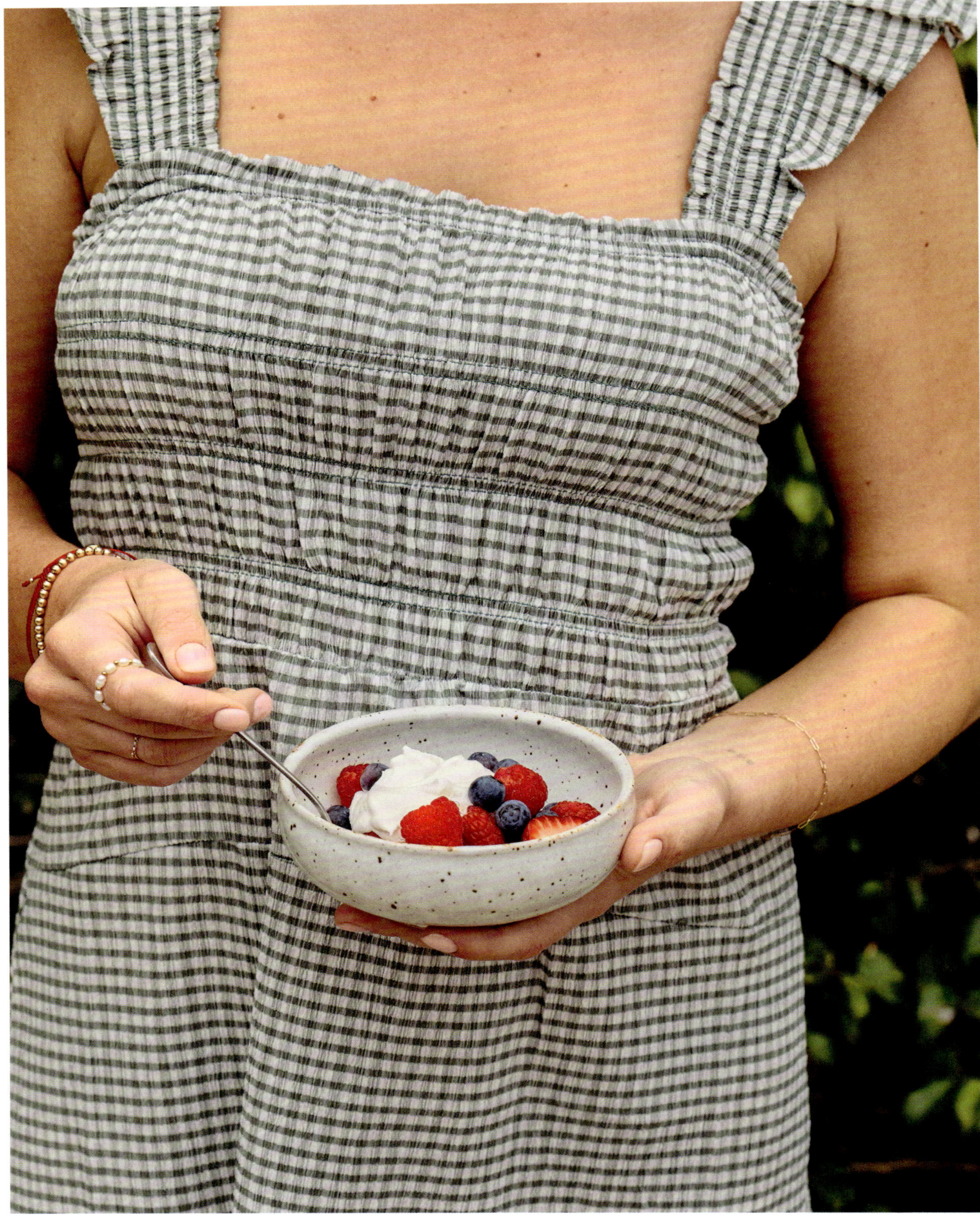

Antioxidants-for-Dessert Berries and Coconut Cream

Serves 2

Prep Time: 5 minutes, plus optional 10 minutes chilling

On those rare nights when I'm not reaching for chocolate, I live for a simple bowl of berries and coconut cream. Berries are packed with antioxidants that support cellular repair and detoxification, while the healthy fats from the coconut cream provide a slow, sustained release of energy—exactly what you need as your body gears up for ovulation.

½ cup coconut cream (chilled overnight)

1 teaspoon pure maple syrup (optional)

½ teaspoon vanilla extract

1 cup mixed fresh berries (blueberries, raspberries, and strawberries)

1 — In a small bowl, whisk together the coconut cream, maple syrup (if using), and vanilla until smooth.

2 — Divide the berries between 2 bowls and top with the whipped coconut cream.

3 — Serve immediately or chill for 10 minutes, if you prefer a firmer texture.

Pro tip

Always keep a can of coconut cream in your fridge so you can throw together coconut whip in minutes. It's a light yet indulgent dessert that feels just as good as it tastes!

Single-Serve Fruit Crisp

Serves 1
Prep Time: 5 minutes
Cook Time: 15 minutes

This single-serve dessert is one I keep coming back to because it's quick, customizable, and so satisfying. After the menstrual phase, cravings for decadent, chocolate-rich desserts often start to subside, and even if you still have a bit of a sweet tooth, you might find yourself more inclined toward lighter sweets. Your body is moving into a phase when it feels more energized and refreshed, making this simple fruit crisp the perfect treat. I love using whatever fruit is in season—apples, pears, and berries are my usual rotation. The natural sugars in the fruit provide a gentle energy boost, while the oats bring fiber to keep the digestion smooth and to support your body's natural detox processes. I like to add a spoonful of coconut yogurt or dairy-free ice cream on top! There's something special about having a dessert that's all yours!

Fruit Blend

½ cup diced fresh fruit (apple, pear, or berries)

½ teaspoon ground cinnamon

½ teaspoon pure maple syrup (optional)

½ teaspoon freshly squeezed lemon juice

Topping

2 tablespoons old-fashioned rolled oats

1 tablespoon almond flour

½ tablespoon coconut oil, melted

½ tablespoon pure maple syrup

Pinch of salt

2 tablespoons coconut yogurt or ice cream (optional)

1 — Preheat the oven to 350°F.

2 — Make the fruit blend: In a small oven-safe ramekin, combine the diced fruit with the cinnamon, maple syrup (if using), and lemon juice.

3 — Make the topping: In another small bowl, use a fork to combine the oats, almond flour, coconut oil, maple syrup, and salt until crumbly.

4 — Bake the dessert: Sprinkle the topping over the fruit mixture in the ramekin. Bake for 12 to 15 minutes, until the fruit is tender and the topping is golden brown. Let cool slightly before enjoying with coconut yogurt or ice cream, if using.

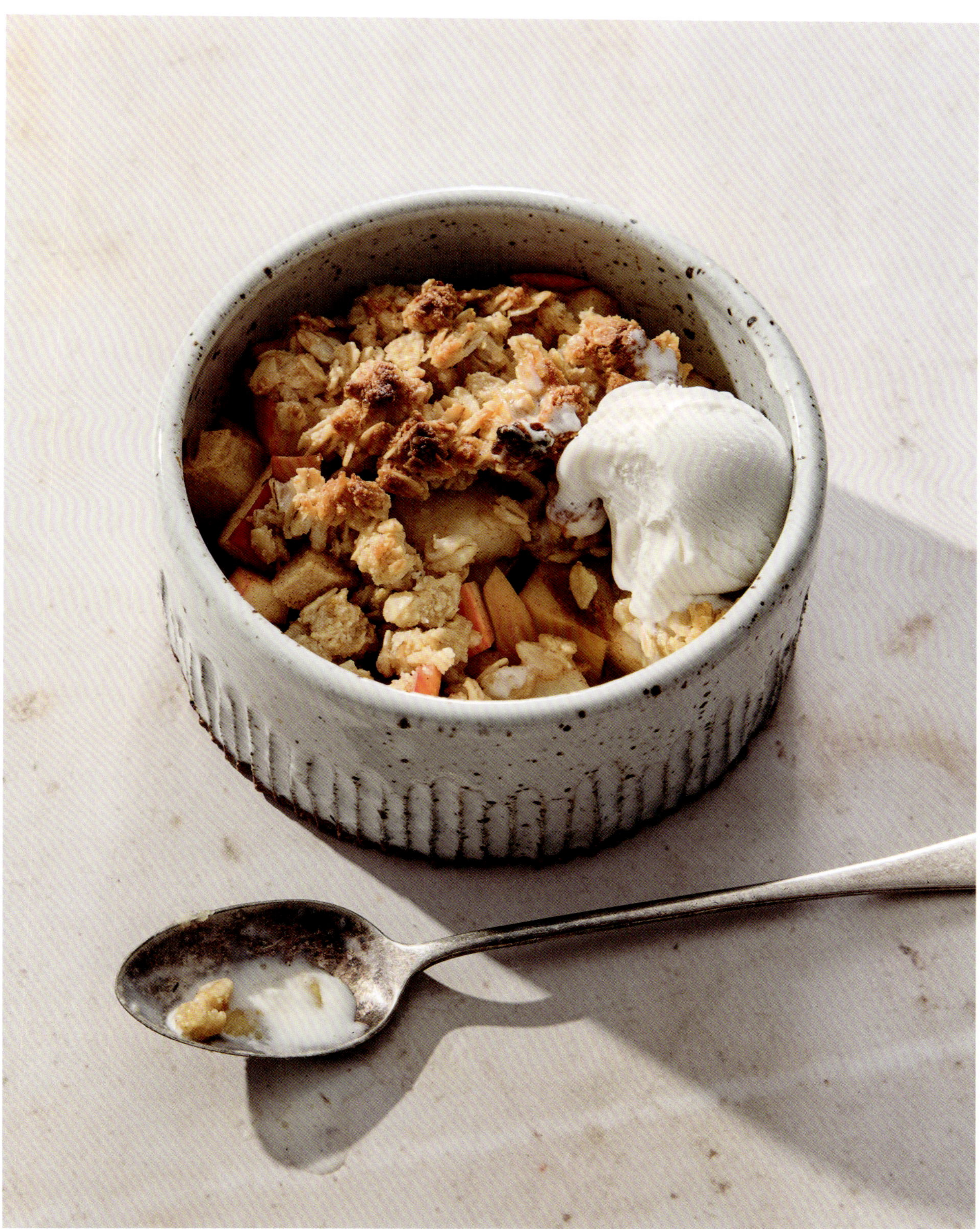

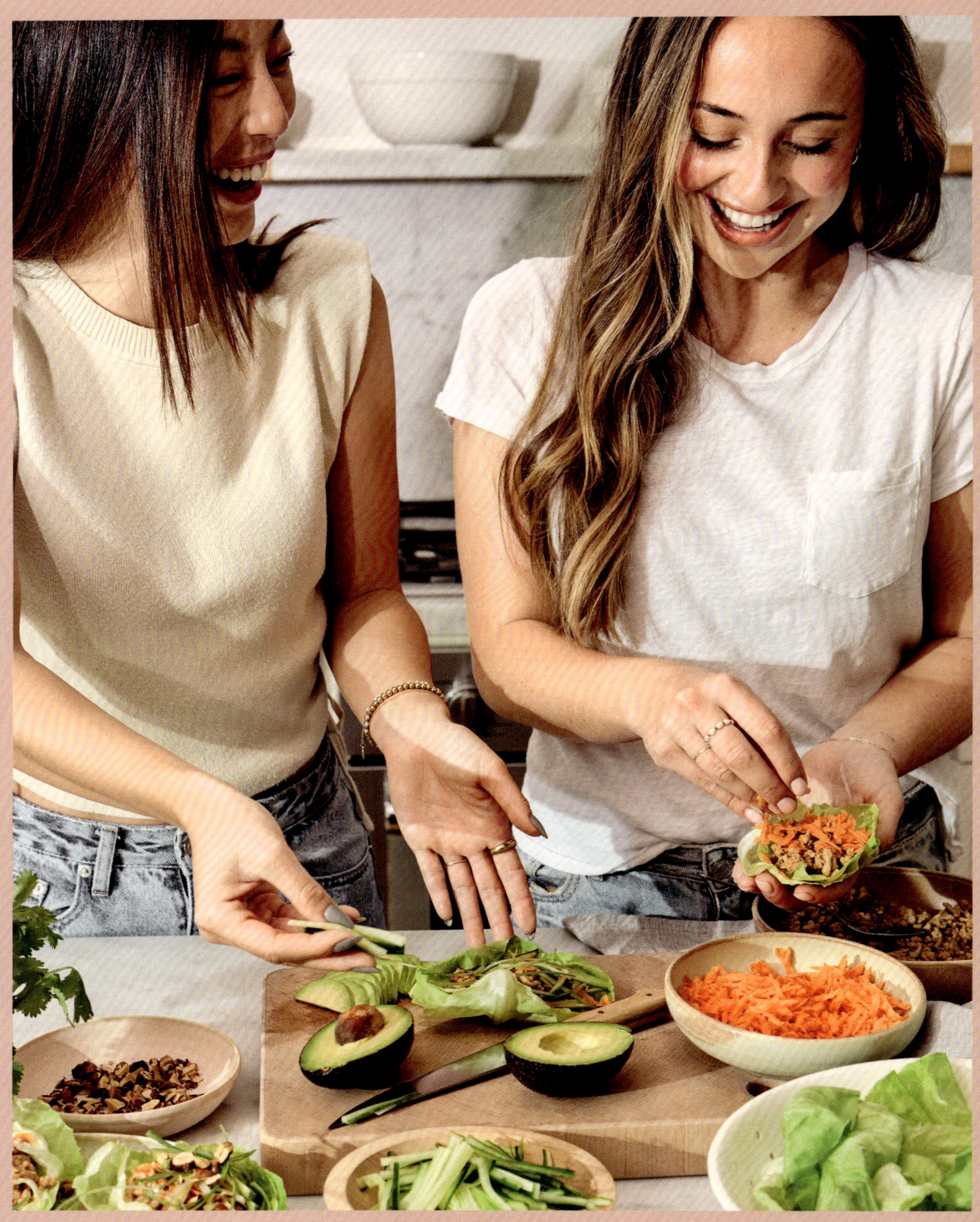

Ovulatory Phase

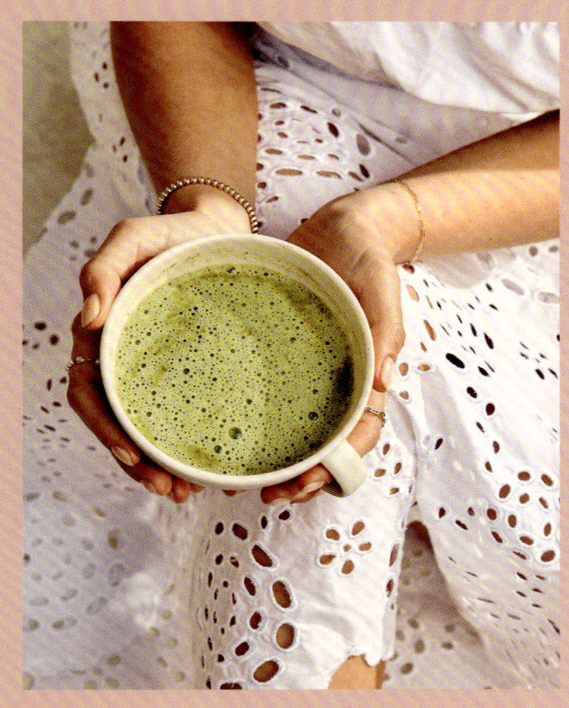

The Peak of Your Cycle

The ovulatory phase is the high point of your cycle, usually happening around days 12 to 16, though it can vary. This is when your body finally releases a mature egg—something it's been gearing up for since the follicular phase. A big surge in luteinizing hormone (LH) triggers this, right as estrogen peaks. While this phase is all about fertility from a biological perspective, it also comes with major perks; think boosted energy, a better mood, and an overall sense of well-being, whether or not you're focused on reproduction!

Hormonal Breakdown: What's Happening

The hormonal landscape during the ovulatory phase is dynamic and powerful. Key players include:

- LUTEINIZING HORMONE (LH) The surge in LH is the trigger for ovulation, signaling the follicle to release the egg. You can use LH test strips to track this surge and pinpoint when you're in your ovulatory phase!

- ESTROGEN Peaking estrogen levels are responsible for many of the vibrant, outward signs of this phase: enhanced skin health, increased energy, and a confident mood.

- TESTOSTERONE Often overlooked as an important female sex hormone, testosterone rises slightly, enhancing libido and physical strength and contributing to a sense of empowerment.

- FERTILE CERVICAL MUCUS You may notice cervical mucus becomes clear, stretchy, and egg-white–like—a key fertility sign.

How Food Can Support You

1 — Support Estrogen Metabolism

Estrogen levels peak during ovulation, which is great for energy and mood, but too much estrogen can lead to bloating, mood swings, and breakouts. Your liver and gut work together to metabolize and clear out excess estrogen, so giving them the right support is key. Fiber binds to excess hormones and helps flush them out through digestion, while cruciferous vegetables like broccoli, kale, and cauliflower contain compounds that enhance liver detoxification. This helps your body process estrogen efficiently and keeps hormone levels balanced.

2 — Reduce Inflammation

Higher estrogen levels can contribute to inflammation, which may show up as puffiness, acne, or general discomfort. Anti-inflammatory foods like berries, turmeric, and omega-3–rich sources (salmon, chia seeds, walnuts) help counteract this by reducing oxidative stress and supporting cellular repair. Omega-3s, in particular, have been shown to lower inflammatory markers and promote healthy skin, mood, and metabolism during this phase.

3 — Balance Blood Sugar

With estrogen at its highest, many people feel a surge in energy, motivation, and even metabolism. However, unstable blood sugar can lead to crashes, irritability, or cravings. To maintain steady energy levels, it's important to pair lean proteins (grilled chicken, salmon, eggs) with fiber-rich foods (quinoa, lentils, leafy greens). Protein and fiber slow down the absorption of sugar into the bloodstream, preventing blood sugar spikes and crashes that can disrupt your mood and energy.

4 — Eat Fresh, Light, and Seasonal Foods

Your body is primed to handle raw, cooling foods during ovulation, unlike the menstrual phase when warmth and slow-cooked meals are more beneficial. This is because digestion is naturally stronger during this phase, meaning your body can efficiently break down raw veggies, fresh fruits, and lighter meals. Plus, cooling foods like salads, smoothies, and spring rolls help balance your body's internal temperature, which can rise slightly during ovulation. Eating hydrating, nutrient-dense foods supports digestion, keeps inflammation low, and helps you feel light and energized.

Top Nutrition Tips for the Ovulatory Phase

With hormones at their peak, your nutritional goals should focus on supporting detoxification, which helps clean out excess hormone levels, combat inflammation, and maintain balanced energy. Proper nutrition during this phase ensures smooth transitions into the next cycle phase—a.k.a. PMS time. Dr. Amersi notes that nutrition can also help optimize fertility and increase your chances of pregnancy in this phase. So if trying for a baby is the goal, increasing consumption of glutathione, folic acid, and omega-3 fatty acids can all help.

Exercise and Lifestyle Tips

Similar to the follicular phase, during the ovulatory phase, your body is naturally primed for high-intensity activity and social connection. Take full advantage of this energy surge by engaging in activities that challenge you physically and mentally.

Self-Care Practices to Support Your Ovulatory Phase

1 — Mindfulness and Breathwork

The sudden burst of energy you get during this time might make you feel positive and social, but it might also lead to some feelings of overstimulation. Grounding yourself with quick breathwork exercises or meditation can help. You can find great free guided breathwork or meditation videos on YouTube!

2 — Skin Care

Stick to gentle, hydrating products. Consider incorporating an antioxidant serum with vitamin C to enhance the natural radiance of your complexion during this phase.

3 — Deepened Connections

Lean into social events or collaborative projects. Your communication skills and charisma are at their peak, making this an ideal time for networking or connecting with loved ones.

Ideal Exercise Split

1 — High-Intensity Interval Training (HIIT)

1 to 2 sessions for maximum energy expenditure and cardiovascular health.

2 — Strength Training:

1 to 2 sessions to capitalize on increased physical resilience and quicker recovery.

3 — Fun Cardio

A dance class or long run to channel your energy into joyful movement.

4 — Restorative Practices

One day of yoga or stretching to balance intense activity.

Sample Ovulatory-Phase Meals

- BREAKFAST A fiber-filled smoothie bowl with spinach, blueberries, flax seeds, and almond butter, topped with chia seeds and cacao nibs.
- LUNCH Quinoa and kale salad with roasted chicken, pumpkin seeds, and a lemon-tahini dressing.
- DINNER Grilled salmon with roasted asparagus, herbed quinoa, and a squeeze of lemon.
- SNACKS Sliced cucumber with hummus or a handful of walnuts and dark chocolate.

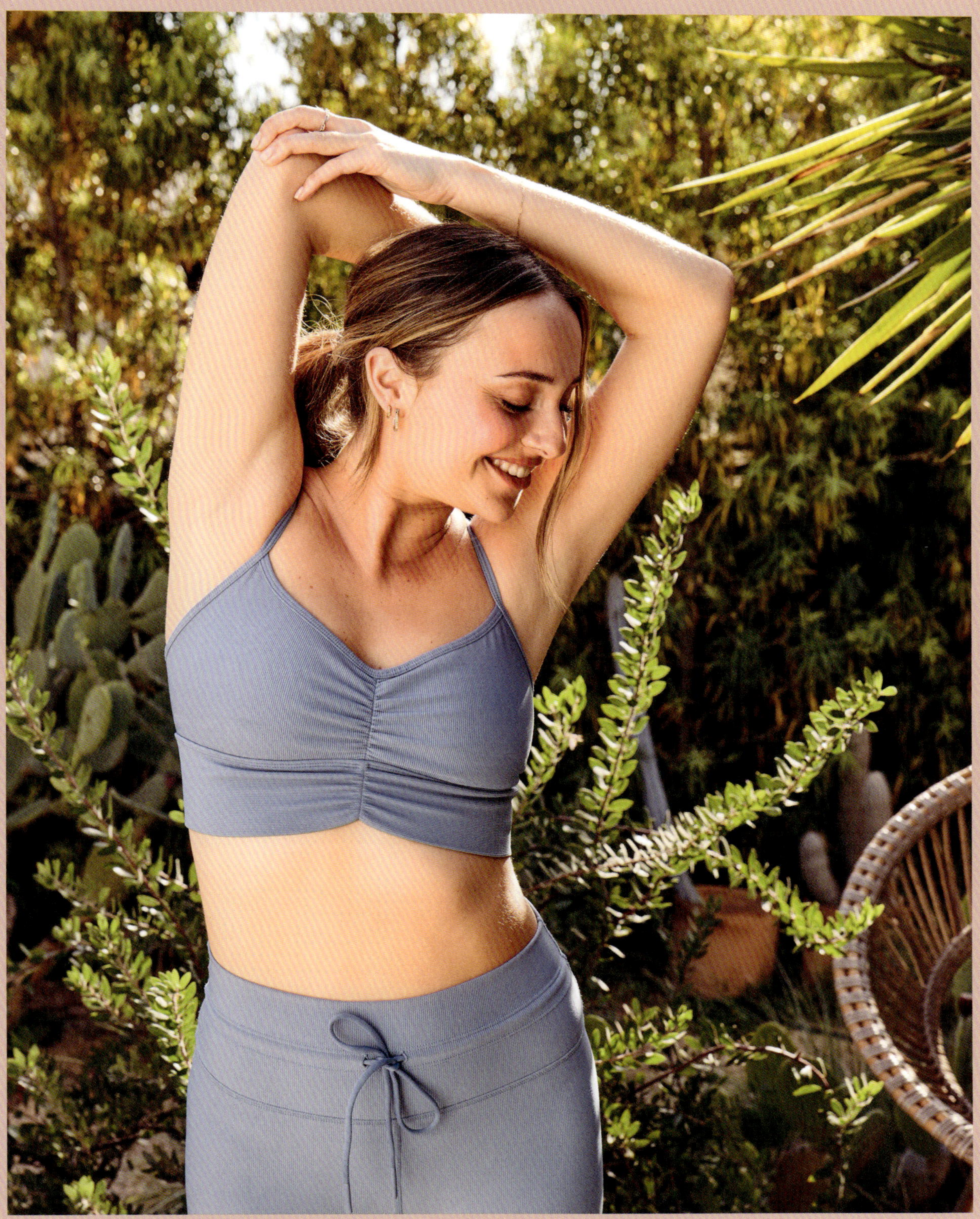

Ovulatory Phase Superfoods

- MACA ROOT POWDER An adaptogen that helps balance hormones and improve energy, libido, and mood.
- CHIA SEEDS High in omega-3 fatty acids and fiber, chia seeds support hormonal health and energy levels.
- EGGS High in protein and essential nutrients like choline, eggs support brain health and energy levels.
- QUINOA A complete protein and rich in fiber, quinoa helps stabilize blood sugar and provide sustained energy.
- KALE Packed with vitamins A, C, and K, as well as calcium, kale supports overall health and hormone balance.
- ALMONDS Rich in magnesium and vitamin E, almonds help reduce PMS symptoms and support skin health.
- CHICKPEAS Great source of plant-based protein and fiber, chickpeas aid in digestion and hormonal balance.
- LENTILS High in protein, iron, and folate, lentils support energy and cellular function.
- KIWI High in vitamin C, antioxidants, and fiber, kiwis support immune health and digestion.
- CRANBERRIES Packed with antioxidants, vitamins C and E, and fiber, cranberries support urinary tract health.
- BROCCOLI Rich in fiber, vitamins C and K, and calcium, broccoli supports bone health and reduces inflammation.
- BERRIES High in antioxidants and fiber, berries aid in digestion and support immune health.
- BRAZIL NUTS High in selenium, Brazil nuts support thyroid function and antioxidant defense.
- TURKEY Excellent source of lean protein, turkey supports muscle repair and satiety.
- BRUSSELS SPROUTS Packed with fiber, vitamins C and K, and folate, Brussels sprouts promote overall health.

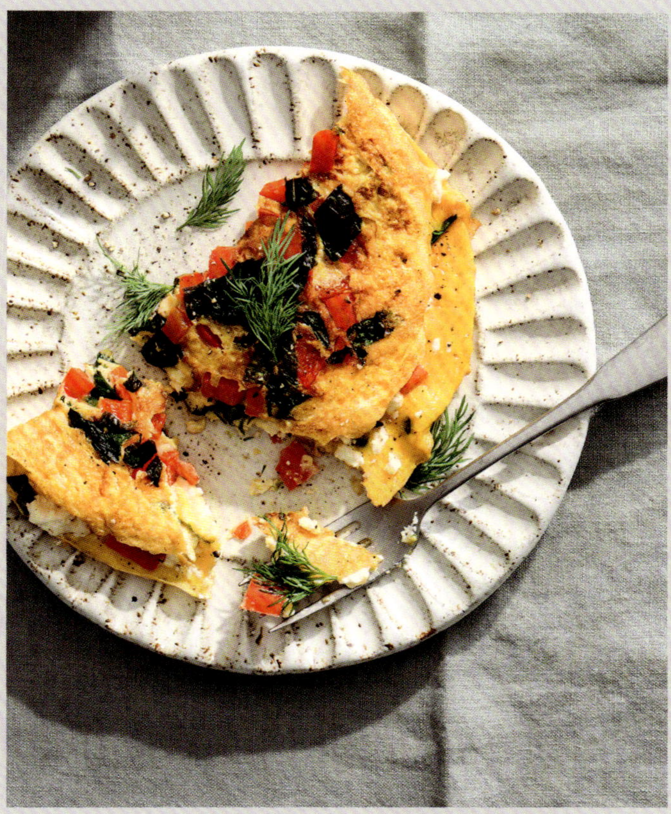

- **SESAME SEEDS** High in calcium, magnesium, and healthy fats, sesame seeds support bone health and reduce cramps.
- **CAULIFLOWER** High in fiber, vitamins C and K, and antioxidants, cauliflower supports overall health.
- **FLAX SEEDS** Rich in lignans and omega-3 fatty acids, flax seeds help to balance hormones.
- **GREEN TEA** Contains antioxidants and catechins, which support metabolism and reduce inflammation.
- **COCONUT OIL** Provides healthy fats that support energy levels and hormone production.
- **CARROTS** High in beta-carotene and fiber, carrots help metabolize excess estrogen.

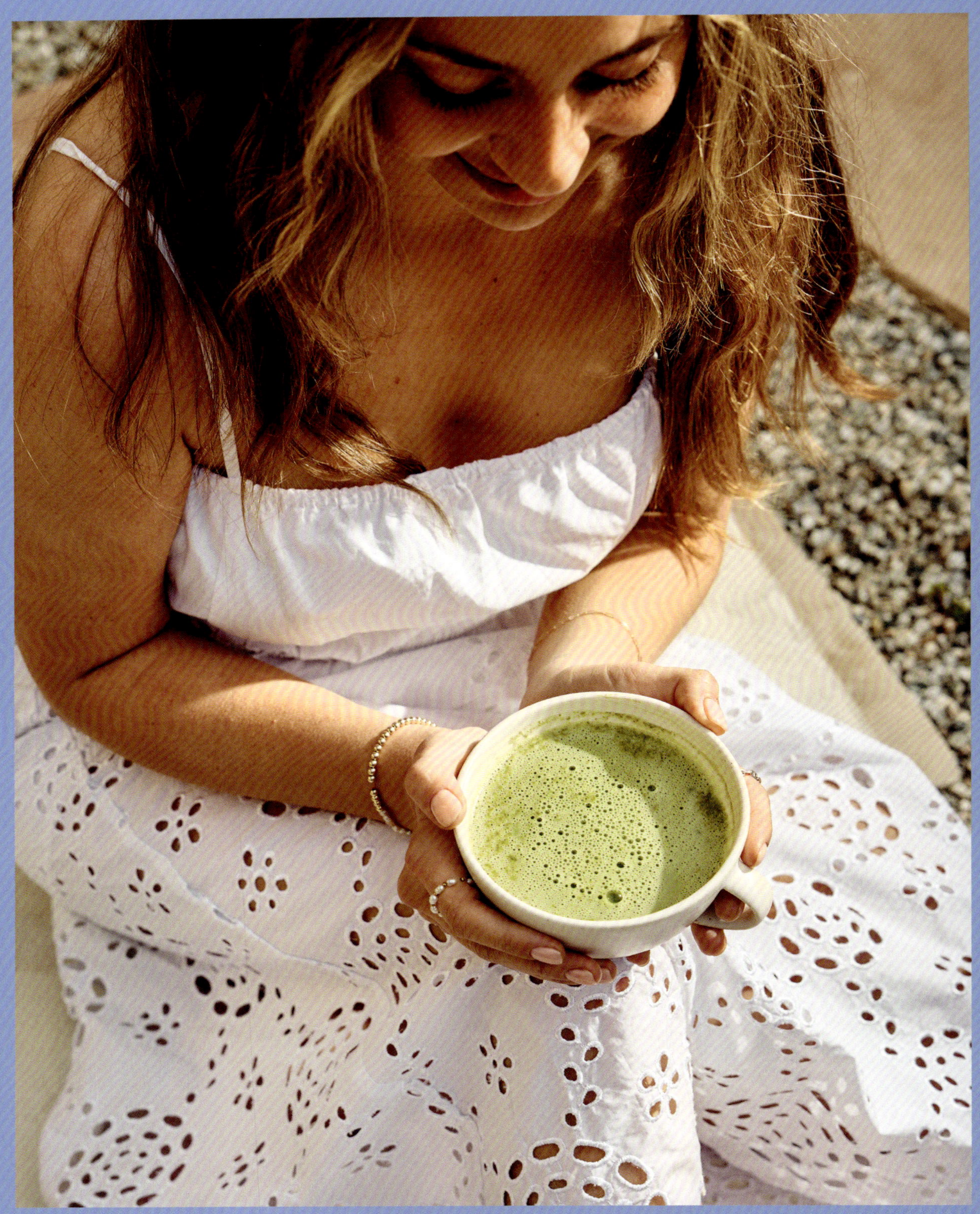

Breakfasts

Glow-and-Go Maca Smoothie

Serves 1
Prep Time: 5 minutes

You're going to hop out of bed feeling energized and ready to tackle the day during this phase, so a smoothie is the perfect grab-and-go breakfast to keep up with your momentum. Maca is a powerful adaptogen, meaning it helps your body adapt to stress by supporting the hypothalamic-pituitary-adrenal (HPA) axis—the communication network between your brain and adrenal glands that regulates stress and hormone balance. (I grab my maca from Amazon or Whole Foods.) The combination of banana and almond butter provides quick-digesting carbs and healthy fats to fuel your morning, while cinnamon and protein powder help stabilize blood sugar. It doesn't hurt that this smoothie tastes like a decadent shake while every ingredient is working hard for your body!

1 frozen peeled banana
1 teaspoon maca powder
1 cup unsweetened almond milk
1 scoop vanilla protein powder
1 tablespoon almond butter
½ teaspoon ground cinnamon
Handful of small ice cubes

Place the banana, maca powder, almond milk, protein powder, almond butter, ground cinnamon, and ice cubes in a high-speed blender. Blend on high speed until smooth and creamy. Pour into a glass and enjoy immediately.

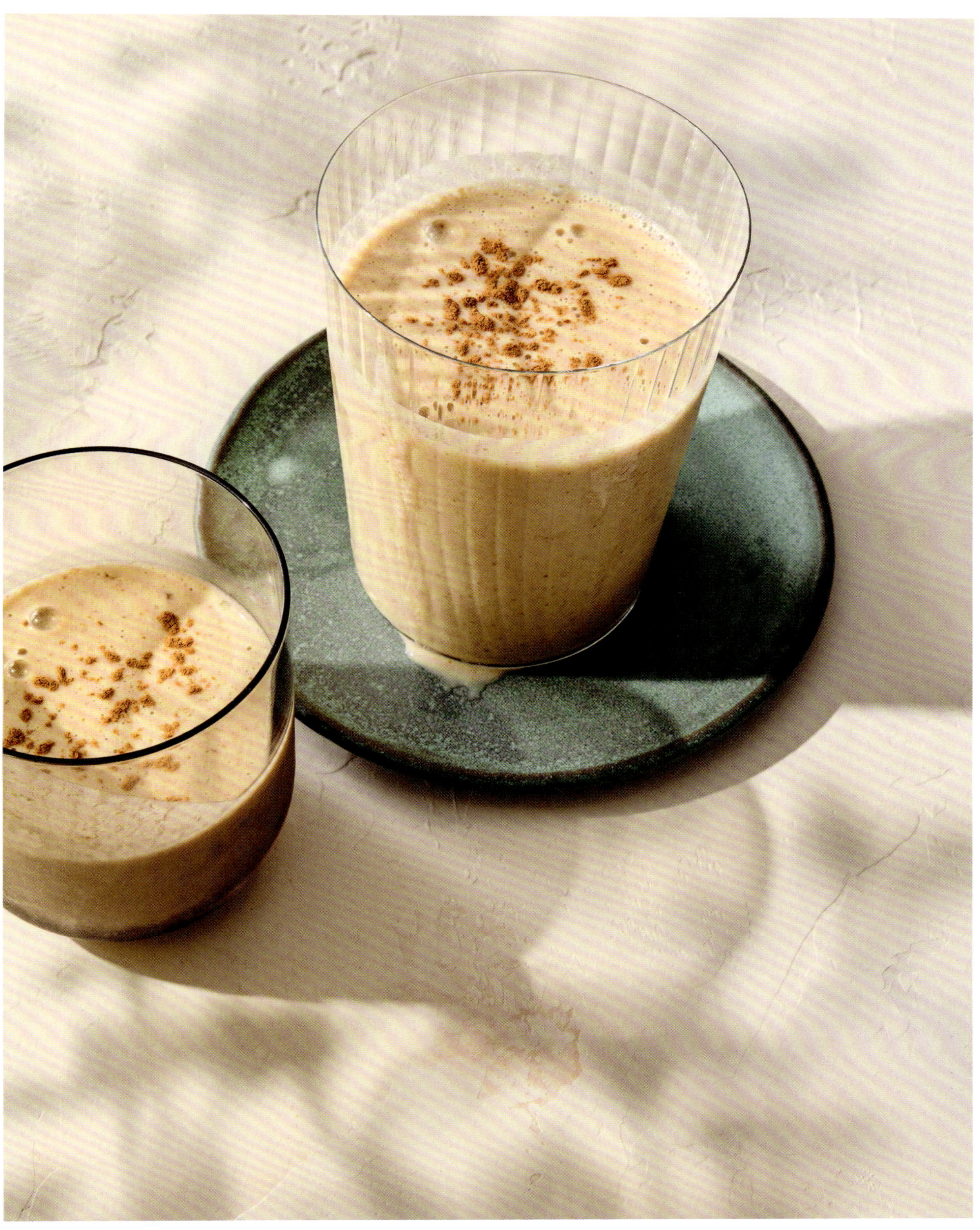

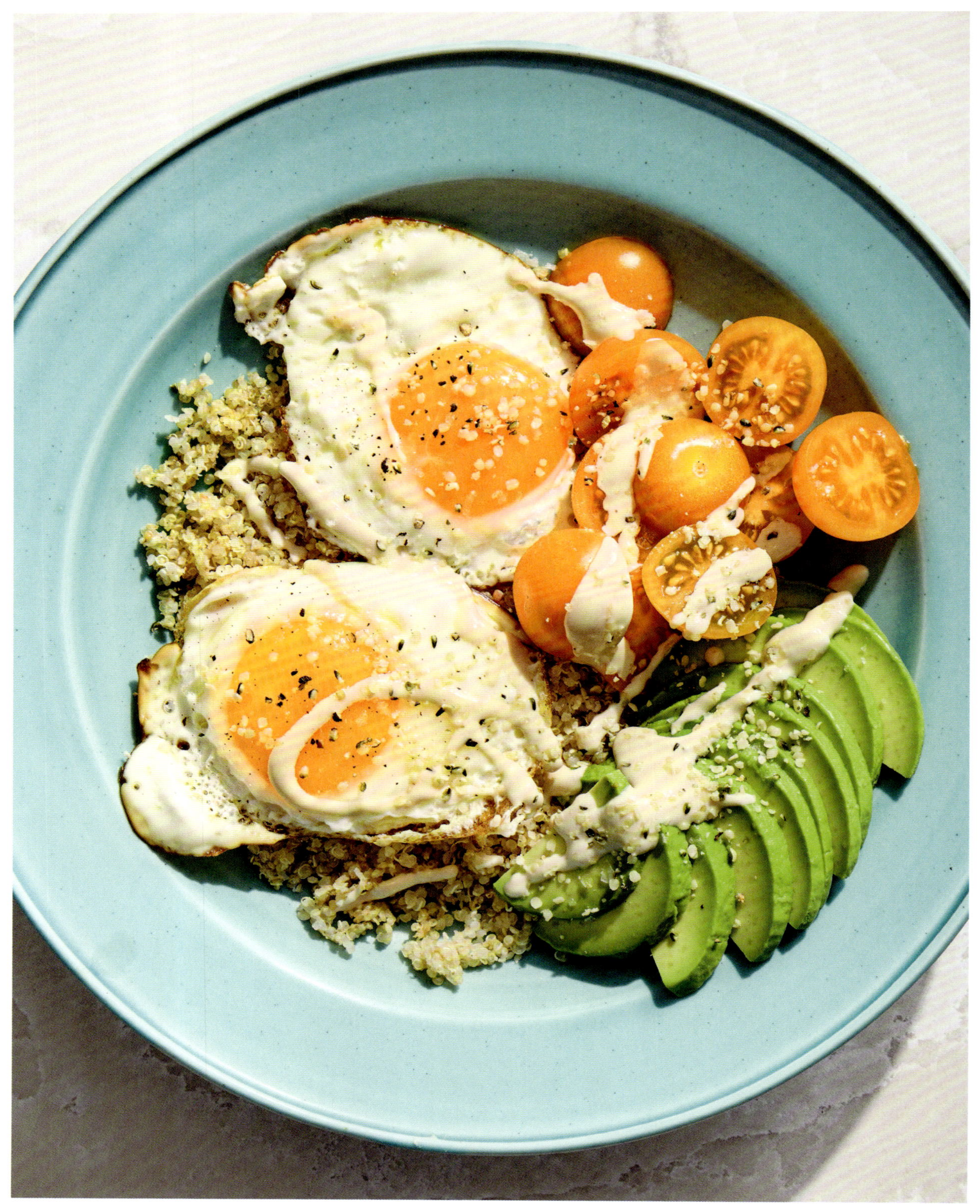

Quinoa Breakfast Bowl with Lemon-Tahini Drizzle

Serves 1

Prep Time: 10 minutes

This bowl is the perfect balance of protein, healthy fats, and fiber—a.k.a. the basis for blood sugar balance. You made a similar breakfast bowl in your follicular phase, but this one gets a glow-up with a creamy, tangy lemon-tahini drizzle that ties everything together beautifully. Tahini is a key ingredient here, not just for its flavor but also for its seed-cycling benefits during the ovulatory phase (see page 20 for more on seed cycling). Made from sesame seeds, tahini is rich in zinc, which supports progesterone production and balances estrogen levels. You'll see tahini popping up in a few of the recipes in this chapter because of its prime role in nourishing your body during this phase. Quinoa serves as the perfect grain base, with all nine essential amino acids and a solid dose of fiber for steady energy. The eggs deliver choline to aid in estrogen synthesis, the avocado provides healthy fats to keep you satisfied, and the hemp seeds and cherry tomatoes add a burst of nutrients and omega-3s to reduce inflammation!

Lemon-Tahini Drizzle

2 tablespoons tahini

Juice of ½ lemon

½ teaspoon honey or pure maple syrup

Pinch of salt

Breakfast Bowl

½ cup cooked quinoa, warmed

2 large eggs, poached or fried, kept warm

½ avocado, pitted and sliced

¼ cup halved cherry tomatoes

1 tablespoon hemp seeds

Salt and freshly ground black pepper

1 — Make the drizzle: In a small bowl, whisk together the tahini, lemon juice, honey, and a pinch of salt. Add a little warm water, 1 to 2 tablespoons at a time, until the sauce reaches your desired consistency.

2 — Assemble the breakfast bowl: Place the cooked quinoa into a serving bowl. Add the eggs, avocado slices, cherry tomatoes, and hemp seeds.

3 — Drizzle the lemon-tahini sauce over the bowl, season with salt and pepper to taste, and serve immediately.

Future-Is-Bright Veggie Omelet with Lemon Zest

Serves 1
Prep Time: 5 minutes
Cook Time: 10 minutes

Your ovulatory phase is like your inner summer—a time when you're naturally energized and glowing. This light and vibrant omelet is the perfect match for how you're feeling right now. The bell peppers and spinach bring fiber and antioxidants to support digestion, while a pop of lemon zest adds brightness to wake up your taste buds. I feel most satisfied when I serve this with a carb, so I usually opt for a slice of gluten-free sourdough or some roasted sweet potato on the side!

2 large eggs
Salt and freshly ground black pepper
½ teaspoon grated lemon zest
1 teaspoon olive oil
¼ cup diced bell pepper
¼ cup chopped baby spinach
1 tablespoon crumbled feta cheese (optional)
Fresh herbs, like parsley or dill, for garnish

1 — Crack the eggs into a small bowl and lightly whisk with a pinch of salt and pepper, then add the lemon zest for added brightness.

2 — Heat the olive oil in a large nonstick skillet over medium heat. Add the bell pepper and sauté for 2 to 3 minutes, until softened. Add the spinach and cook for 1 minute, until just wilted.

3 — Pour the whisked eggs over the veggies in the skillet. Gently swirl the pan to distribute the eggs evenly and cook for 2 to 3 minutes, until edges of the omelet begin to set.

4 — Sprinkle the feta on one side of the omelet (if using), then fold the omelet in half and cook for another minute, until the cheese is slightly melted.

5 — Slide the omelet onto a plate, garnish with the fresh herbs, and enjoy warm for a bright, energizing start to your day.

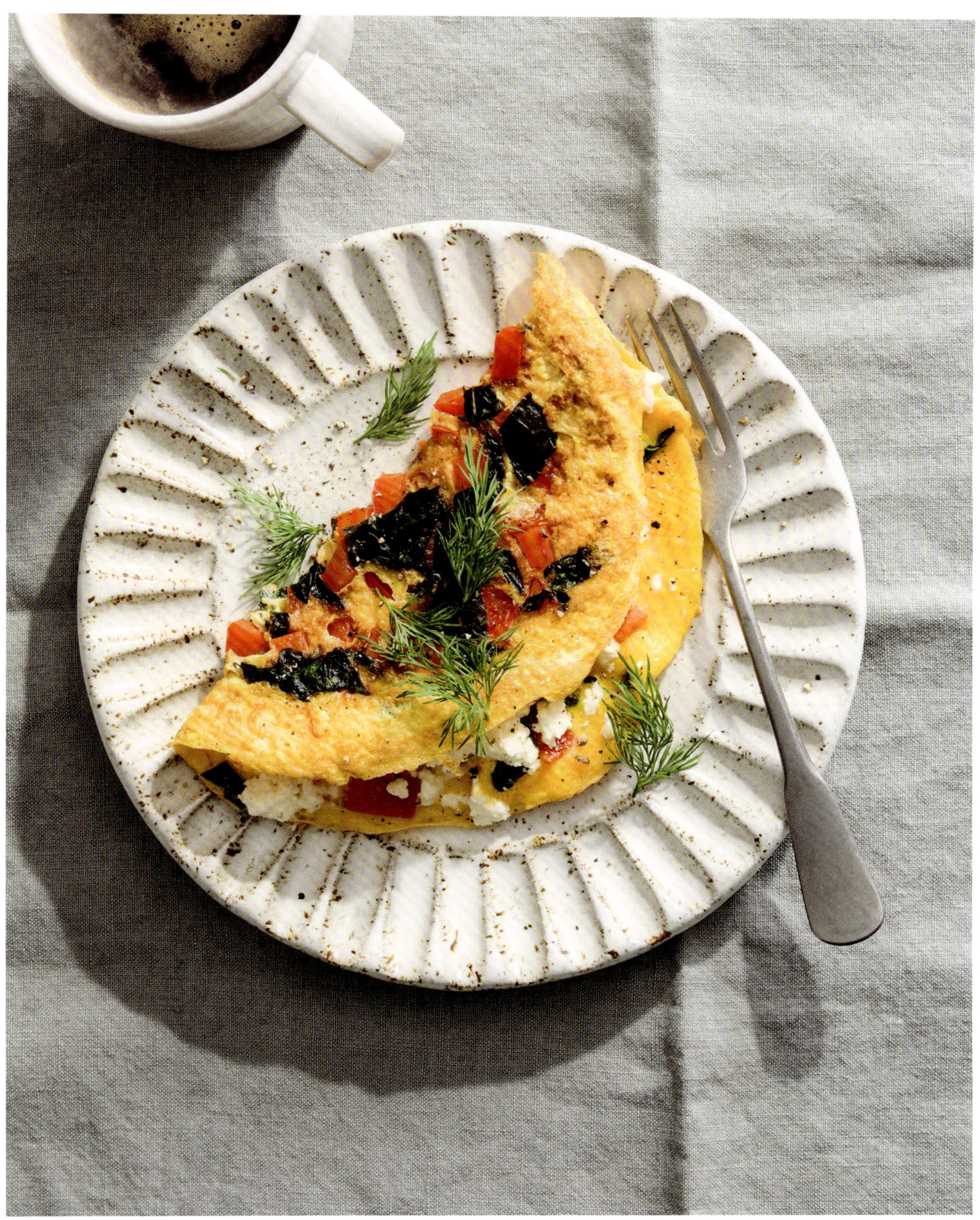

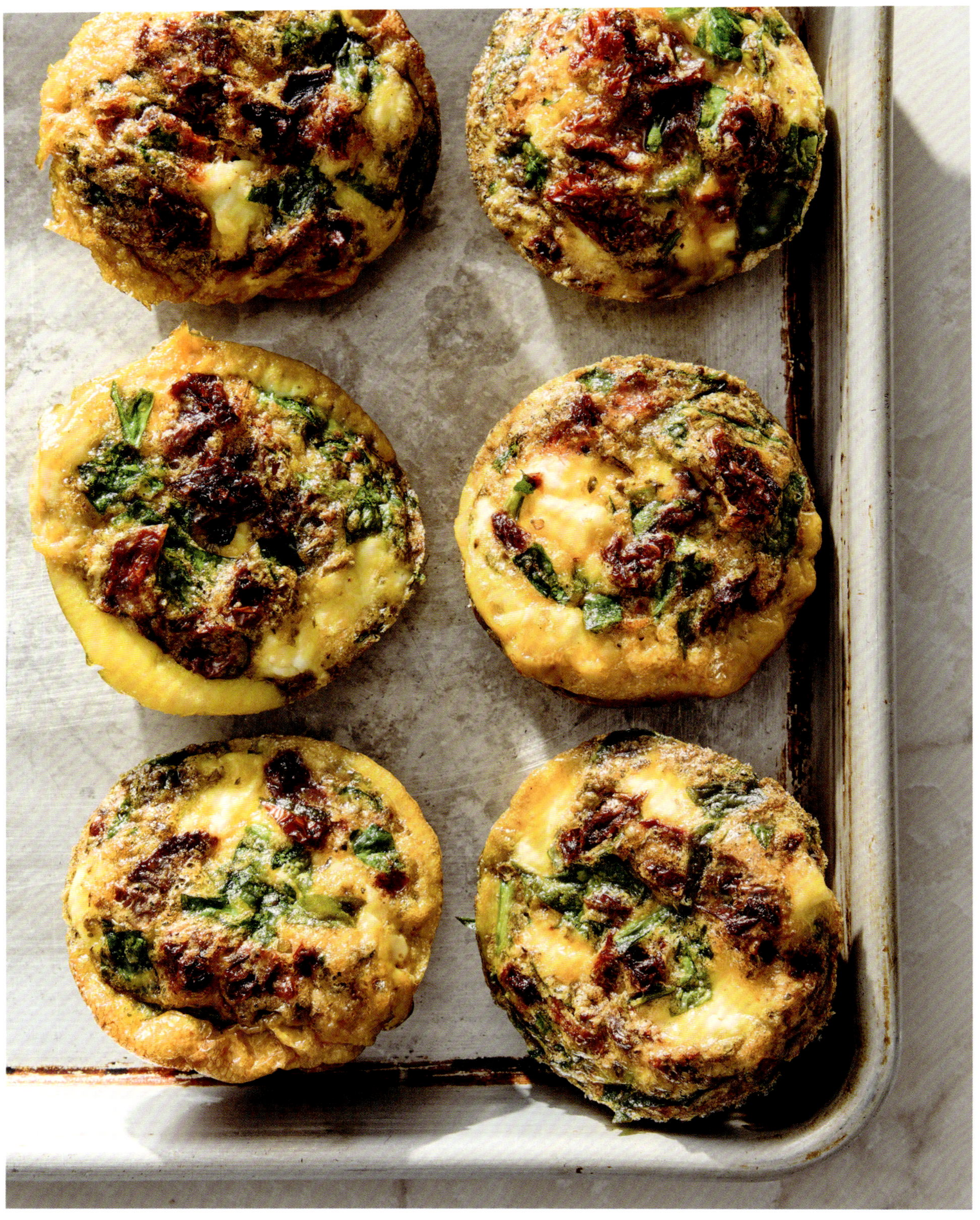

Mediterranean Egg Muffins

Makes 12 muffins
Prep Time: 10 minutes
Cook Time: 20 minutes

I'm all about breakfasts that feel a little fancy but take basically no effort, and these egg muffins are exactly that. Packed with sun-dried tomatoes, spinach, and goat cheese, they're a Mediterranean-inspired bite that's perfect for your ovulatory phase. During this time, your body is operating at its best; your energy is at its highest, and your digestion is working efficiently, meaning you can easily absorb and utilize the protein and nutrients in these muffins. The muffins are also meal-prep friendly, freeing up your mornings for sunlight, a walk with friends, a workout class, or journaling instead of cooking. Pair these with avocado for hormone-supporting healthy fats or roasted sweet potatoes for extra fiber to keep blood sugar balanced. Note: A serving is 2 muffins.

---

12 large eggs
2 teaspoons dried oregano
Salt and freshly ground black pepper
½ cup sun-dried tomatoes, diced
½ cup chopped baby spinach
½ cup crumbled goat cheese

1 — Preheat the oven to 375°F. Grease a 12-cup muffin tin.

2 — In a large bowl, lightly whisk the eggs and season them with the oregano and salt and pepper to taste. Fold in the tomatoes, spinach, and goat cheese.

3 — Pour the mixture into the muffin cups, filling each cup about three-fourths full.

4 — Bake the muffins for 20 minutes, until set; test to see that a toothpick inserted in the center comes out clean.

5 — Allow the muffins to cool briefly and then pop them out of the tin. Place 2 muffins on your plate and enjoy. (Store the extra muffins in an airtight container for up to 4 days. Reheat them in the microwave for 20 to 30 seconds or in a toaster oven at 350°F for 5 minutes, until warmed through.)

Vanilla Berry Bliss Protein Smoothie Bowl

Serves 1

Prep Time: 5 minutes

During the ovulatory phase, your body is naturally in a higher-energy state and your metabolism is running at its peak. This makes it easier to handle cooler foods like smoothies, unlike the luteal and menstrual phases, when warming, grounding meals feel best to support energy and digestion. Mixed berries here provide antioxidants, which help combat oxidative stress and support cellular health, especially important during ovulation, when your body is releasing an egg and estrogen levels are at their highest. Chia seeds offer fiber and omega-3s to help metabolize estrogen. I like my smoothie bowl topped with cacao nibs for more of a fiber boost, shredded coconut for healthy fats, and a low-sugar granola for a crunch!

1 cup frozen mixed berries

½ cup almond milk

½ cup plain Greek yogurt or coconut yogurt

1 scoop vanilla protein powder

1 tablespoon chia seeds

1 cup crushed ice

Granola, cacao nibs, bee pollen, or shredded coconut, for garnish

Place the berries, almond milk, yogurt, protein powder, chia seeds, and ice in a high-speed blender. Blend on high speed until smooth. Pour the mixture into a bowl and add your desired toppings.

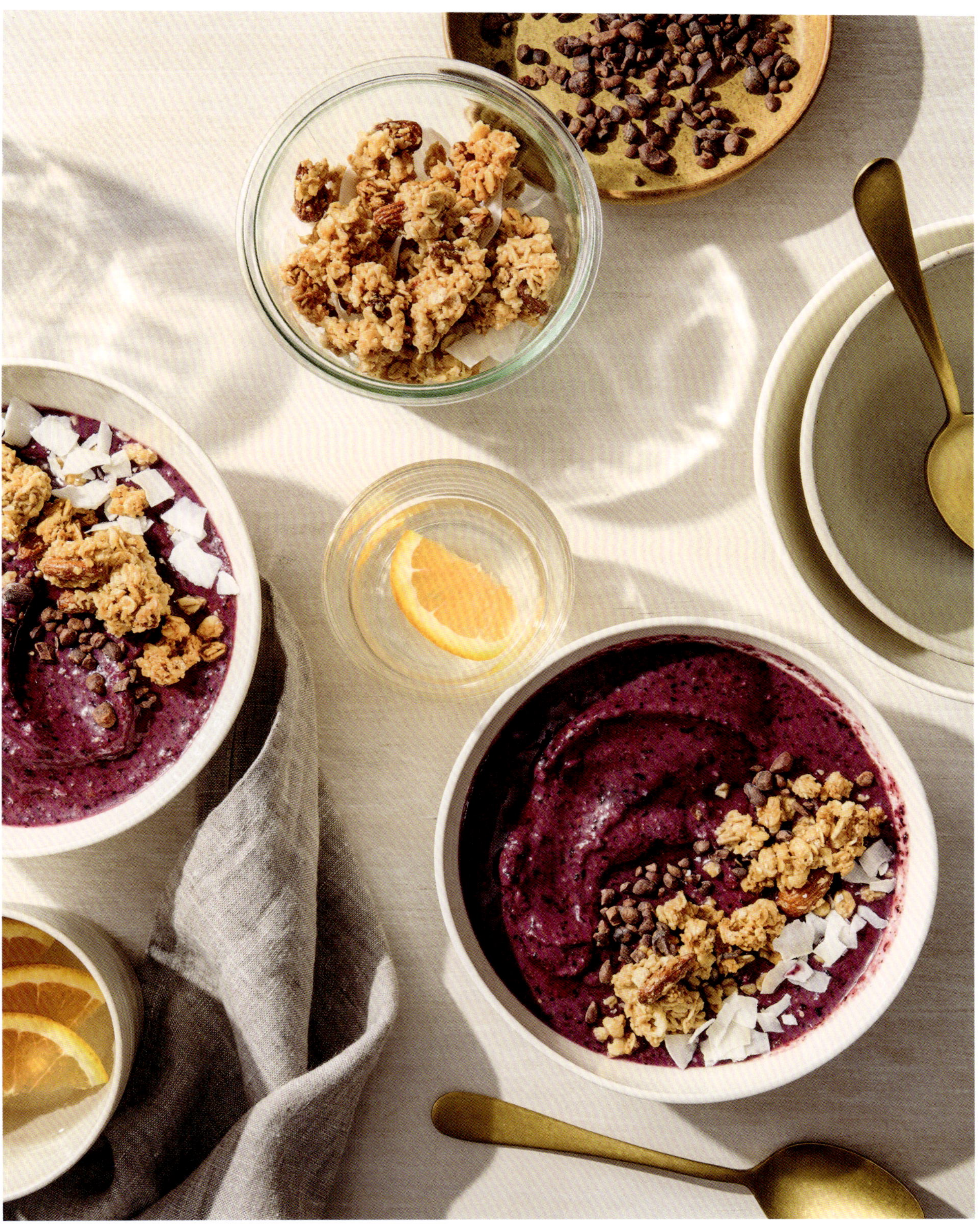

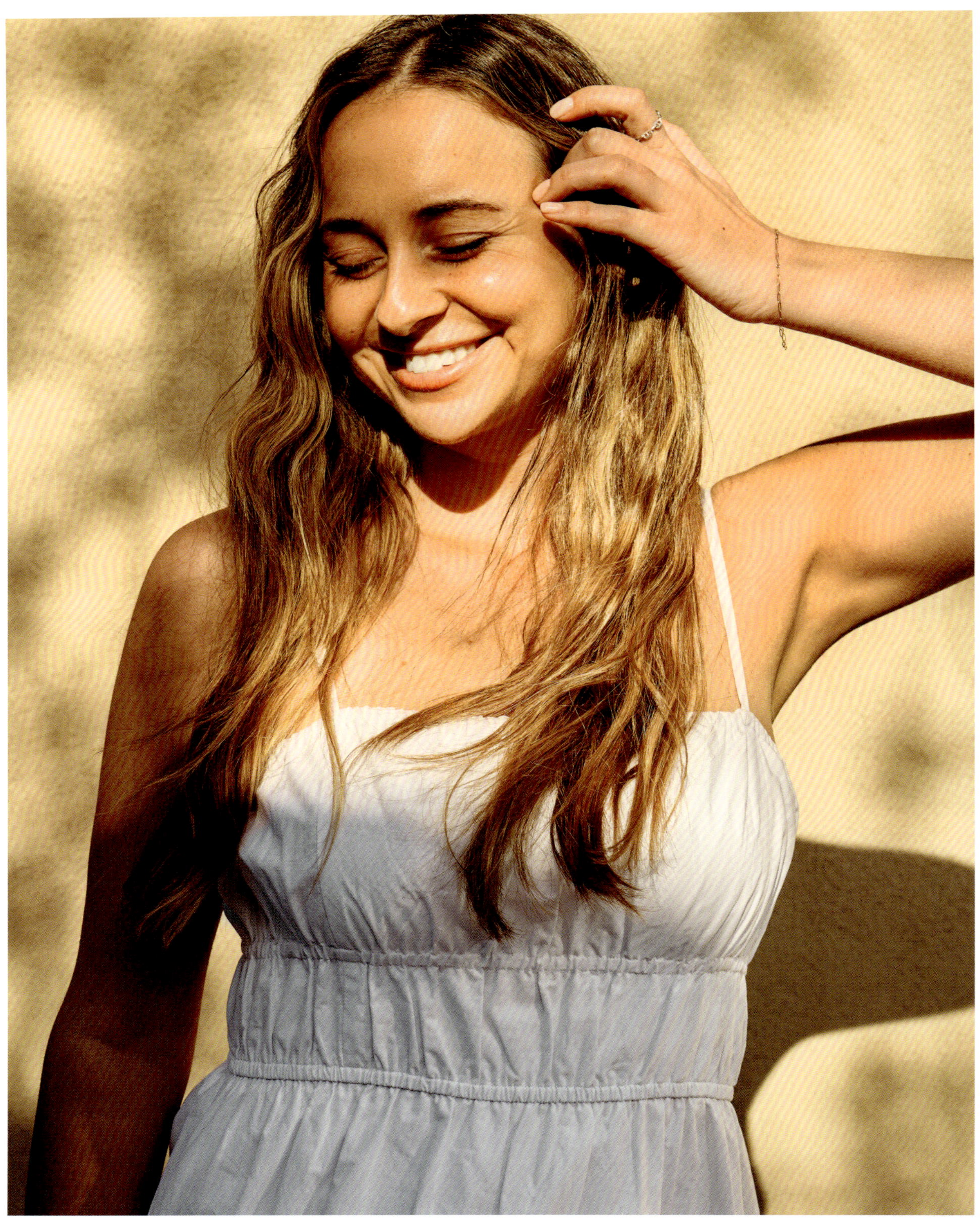

Dressed-Up Avocado Toast

Serves 1
Prep Time: 5 minutes
Cook Time: 1 minute

As much as I love romanticizing unique breakfasts, avocado toast will always have a place in my rotation, no matter the phase. It's the perfect balance of carbs from the toast and healthy fats from the avocado, but it's often missing a solid protein source. To keep my blood sugar steady and stay full longer, I usually top mine with eggs. If I'm not feeling like having eggs, though, I'll switch to turkey bacon, mash in some cottage cheese, or sprinkle on some hemp seeds for an extra boost. My motto is to never restrict foods; just find creative ways to make them work better for your body!

½ avocado, pitted and sliced
1 teaspoon freshly squeezed lemon juice
Salt and freshly ground black pepper
1 slice whole-grain or sourdough bread
2 large eggs, hardboiled and sliced, over easy, poached, or scrambled
1 tablespoon hemp seeds
Red pepper flakes

1 — In a small bowl, place the avocado, lemon juice, and salt and pepper to taste and mash with a spoon or potato masher.

2 — Toast the bread and spread it with the mashed avocado.

3 — Top with the eggs, hemp seeds, and a sprinkle of red pepper flakes.

Sunny Days Sunflower Seed Parfait

Serves 2
Prep Time: 5 minutes

If you follow me on social media, you know I'm all about Greek yogurt bowls. Greek yogurt is one of my go-to protein sources, and I love that it's packed with probiotics, which is why I think I digest it so much better than many other dairy products. I make a Greek yogurt bowl every week, just varying the toppings based on the phase. During the ovulatory phase, I often add sunflower seeds or sunflower seed butter. Sunflower seeds are a key part of seed cycling, as they're rich in zinc, which supports estrogen regulation and healthy ovulation. Zinc also helps maintain hormonal balance by supporting progesterone production during this phase. This is another perfect example of how you can keep enjoying your favorite foods with subtle tweaks to make them more supportive of whatever phase you're in!

1 cup plain Greek yogurt (or dairy-free alternative)

½ cup Maple-Walnut Superseed Granola (page 45), or your favorite store-bought low-sugar granola

2 tablespoons sunflower seeds or sunflower seed butter

¼ cup pomegranate seeds or mixed fresh berries

1 tablespoon honey (optional)

In two glasses, layer the yogurt, granola, sunflower seeds or butter, and pomegranate seeds or mixed berries. Drizzle each glass with a bit of honey (if desired) and serve immediately. (Alternatively, prepare the parfaits in glass jars, then cover and refrigerate for up to 5 days.)

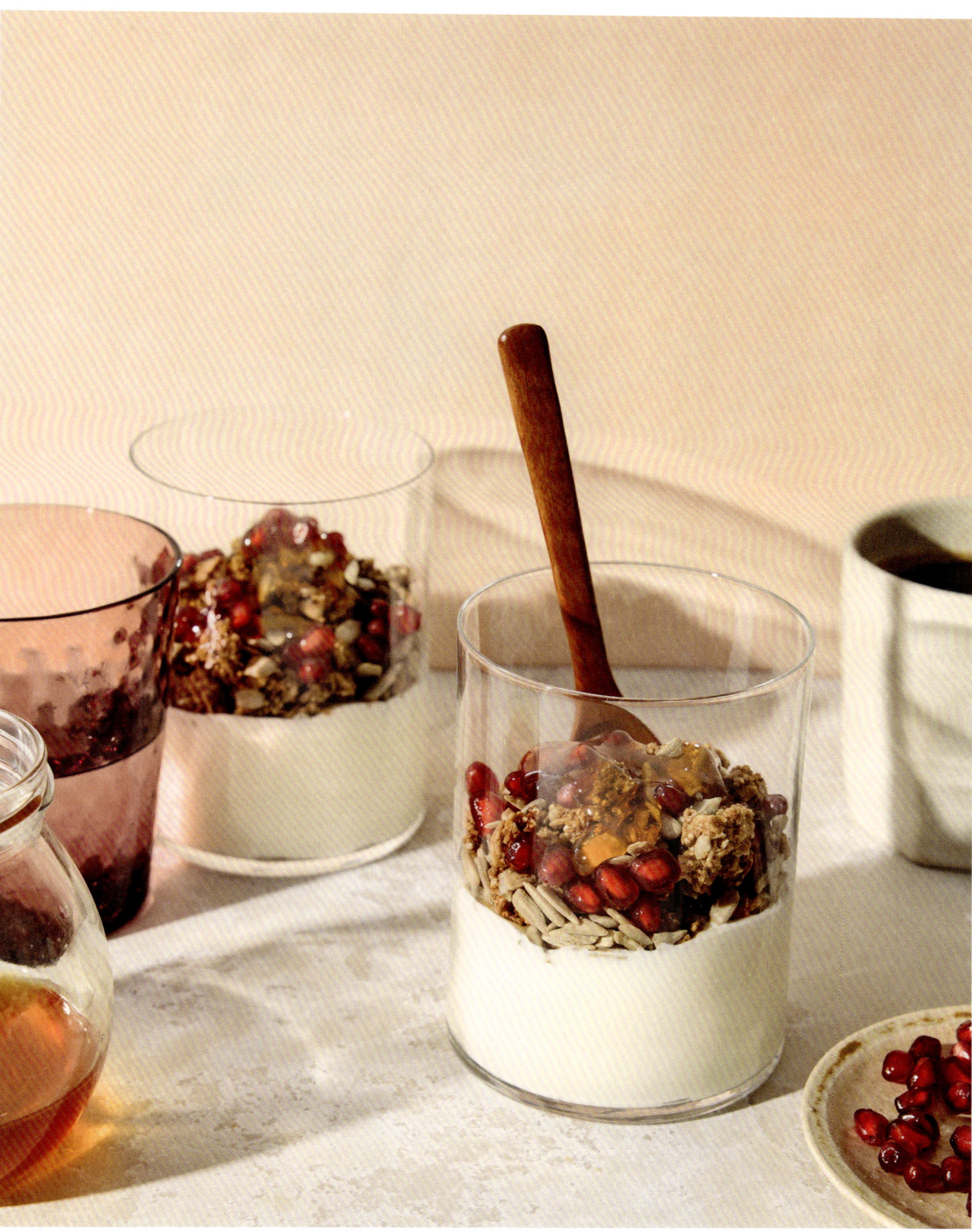

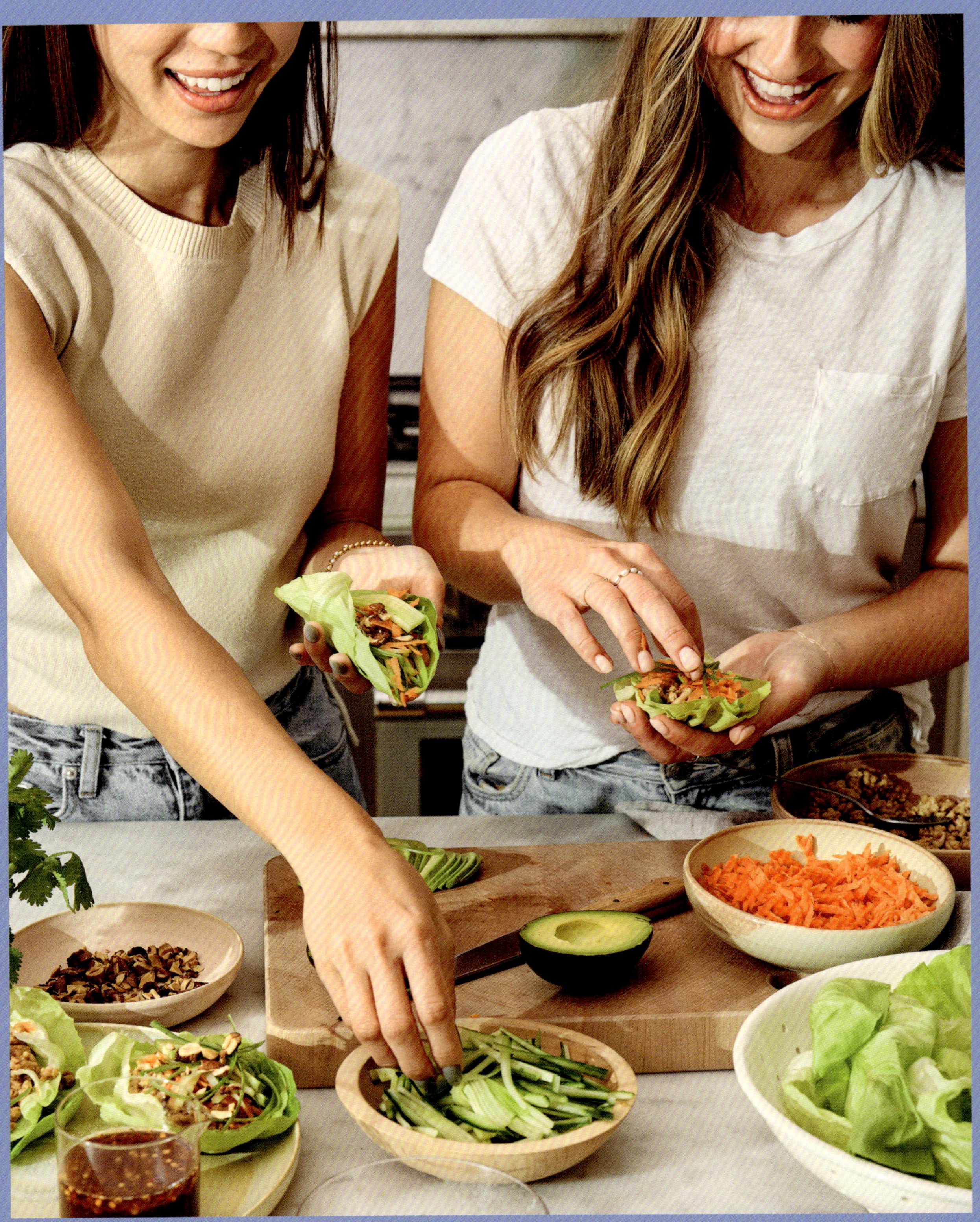

Lunches & Dinners

Peak Energy Chickpea Pasta Salad

Serves 4
Prep Time: 10 minutes
Cook Time: 10 minutes

Chickpea pasta is a total game-changer, turning a traditionally carb-heavy dish into one that's loaded with protein and fiber to keep you full, support digestion, and balance blood sugar. This pasta salad is light yet satisfying, with a mix of crisp veggies, a tangy dressing, and the perfect bite from the chickpea pasta, which is slightly nutty, hearty, and so good at soaking up flavors. Make a big batch of this at the beginning of the week, and you've got yourself a quick, protein-packed lunch that'll keep you fueled!

1 (8-ounce) package chickpea pasta
1 cup cherry tomatoes, halved
½ cup diced cucumber
¼ cup pitted Kalamata olives, sliced
¼ cup crumbled feta cheese
2 tablespoons olive oil
1 tablespoon freshly squeezed lemon juice
1 teaspoon dried oregano
Salt and freshly ground black pepper

1 — Cook the pasta according to the package instructions, until al dente. Drain and let cool.

2 — Place the pasta in a large bowl and toss in the tomatoes, cucumber, olives, and feta.

3 — Drizzle on the olive oil and lemon juice, and season with the oregano and salt and pepper to taste.

4 — Give another toss, and serve.

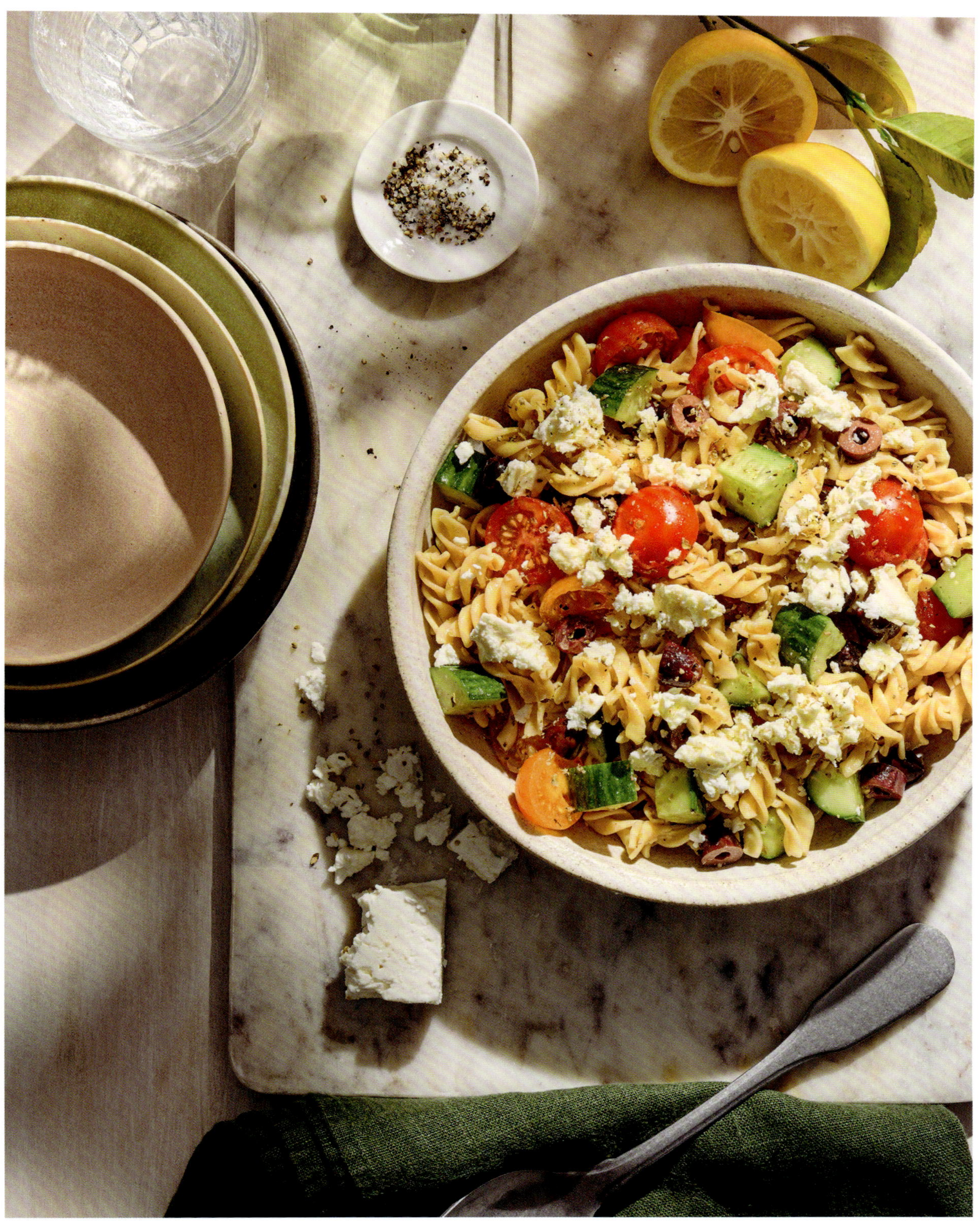

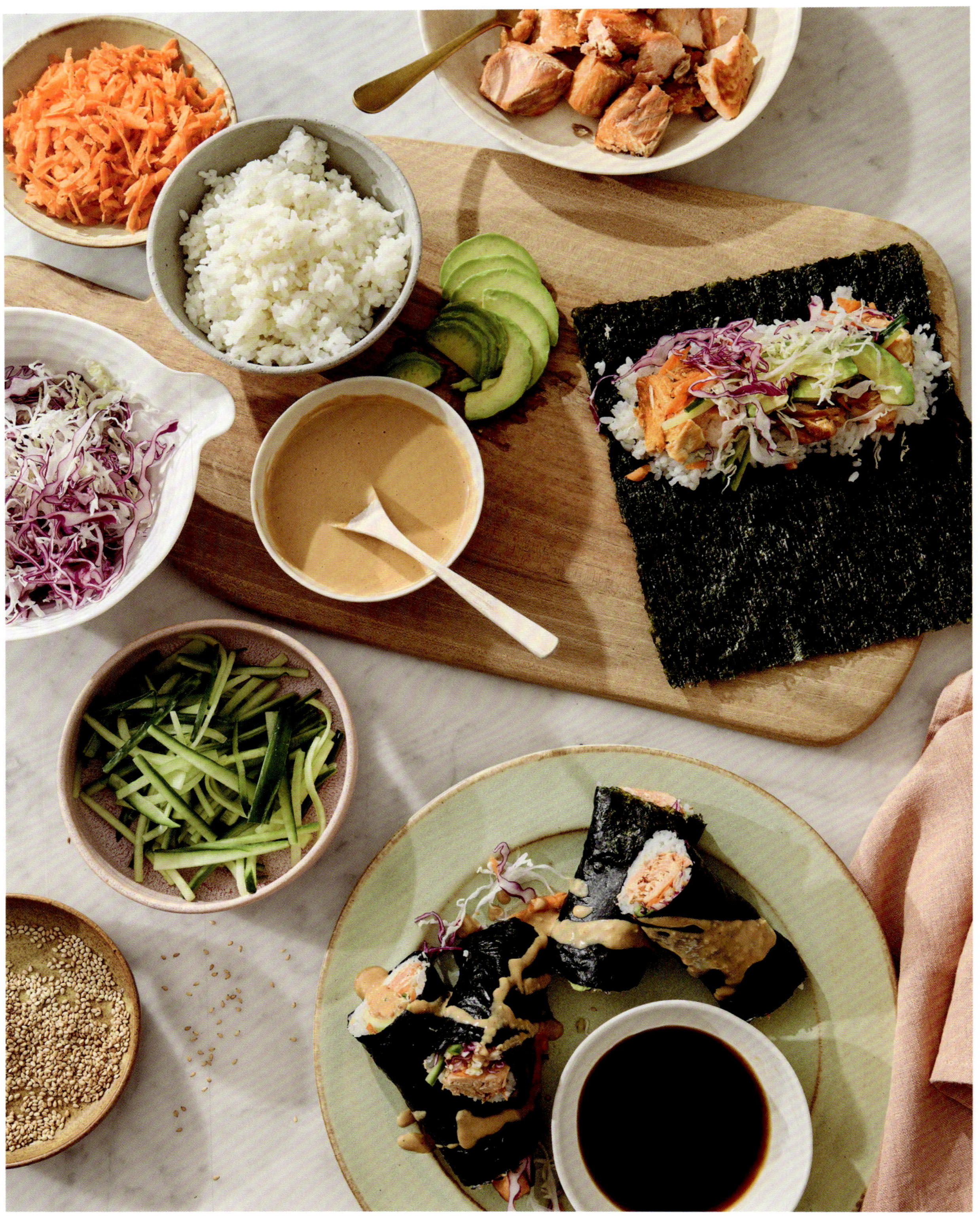

Salmon and Avocado Nori Wraps with a Spicy Ginger-Miso Drizzle

Serves 2
Prep Time: 20 minutes
Cook Time: 10 minutes

This recipe is one of my favorite ways to enjoy salmon! During the ovulatory phase, the body is preparing for potential pregnancy, and the increased need for energy and hormonal support (whether your intention is to get pregnant or not) makes healthy fats and protein essential. Healthy fats, like those found in avocado and salmon, help support progesterone production, which is necessary for ovulation. Wrapping everything up in a nori sheet makes this easy to eat, but nori is also a great source of iodine, which supports thyroid health—essential for keeping your metabolism and hormones balanced. So many good things in one wrap! Note: A serving is 2 wraps.

Salmon

1 (4-ounce) wild-caught salmon fillet (or piece of smoked salmon for a no-cook option)

Salt and freshly ground black pepper

1 tablespoon olive or avocado oil

Spicy Ginger-Miso Drizzle

1 tablespoon tahini

1 teaspoon white miso paste

½ teaspoon grated fresh ginger

½ teaspoon sriracha hot sauce, or more as desired

1 teaspoon rice vinegar

1 teaspoon coconut aminos

Assembly

4 sheets of nori

1 cup cooked sushi rice (or cauliflower rice, for a veggie boost)

1 avocado, halved, pitted, and sliced

¼ cup julienned cucumber

¼ cup shredded carrot

2 tablespoons microgreens or shredded cabbage, for extra crunch (optional)

1 tablespoon sesame seeds (black or white)

Tamari or coconut aminos, for dipping

1 — Make the salmon for the filling: Place a medium nonstick skillet or cast-iron skillet over medium-high heat and allow the skillet to heat for a couple of minutes.

2 — Pat the salmon fillet dry with a paper towel, and season with a pinch of salt and pepper on both sides.

3 — Add the oil to the hot skillet, then place the salmon fillet skin side down in the pan. Let it cook for 4 to 5 minutes without moving it to allow the skin to crisp up. Flip the fillet over and allow to cook for another 2 to 3 minutes, depending on thickness, until it reaches your desired doneness. The salmon should be golden brown and crisp on the outside, but still tender and moist inside.

4 — Remove the salmon from the pan and let it rest for a couple of minutes on a plate. When cooled slightly, flake the salmon with a knife into bite-size pieces. (Alternatively, if you are using the smoked salmon, break it up into small pieces.) If you cooked the salmon with skin on, you can discard the skin now.

5 — Make the drizzle: In a small bowl, whisk together the tahini, miso, fresh ginger, sriracha, rice vinegar, and coconut aminos until the dressing is smooth. Adjust the consistency with 1 to 2 teaspoons of warm water, if needed.

continued

Salmon and Avocado Nori Wraps with a Spicy Ginger-Miso Drizzle, *continued*

6 — Assemble the wraps: Lay a sheet of nori on a flat surface. Spread one-fourth of the rice in a thin layer across the bottom third.

7 — Add about one-fourth of the salmon bits, the avocado slices, cucumber julienne, shredded carrot, and a pinch of the microgreens or cabbage (if using). Sprinkle with some of the sesame seeds. Roll up the nori sheet tightly and slice it in half.

8 — Continue to make the remaining 3 nori wraps, using the remaining ingredients.

9 — Arrange the wraps on a serving plate and drizzle with the spicy ginger-miso sauce. Serve with the tamari or coconut aminos for dipping.

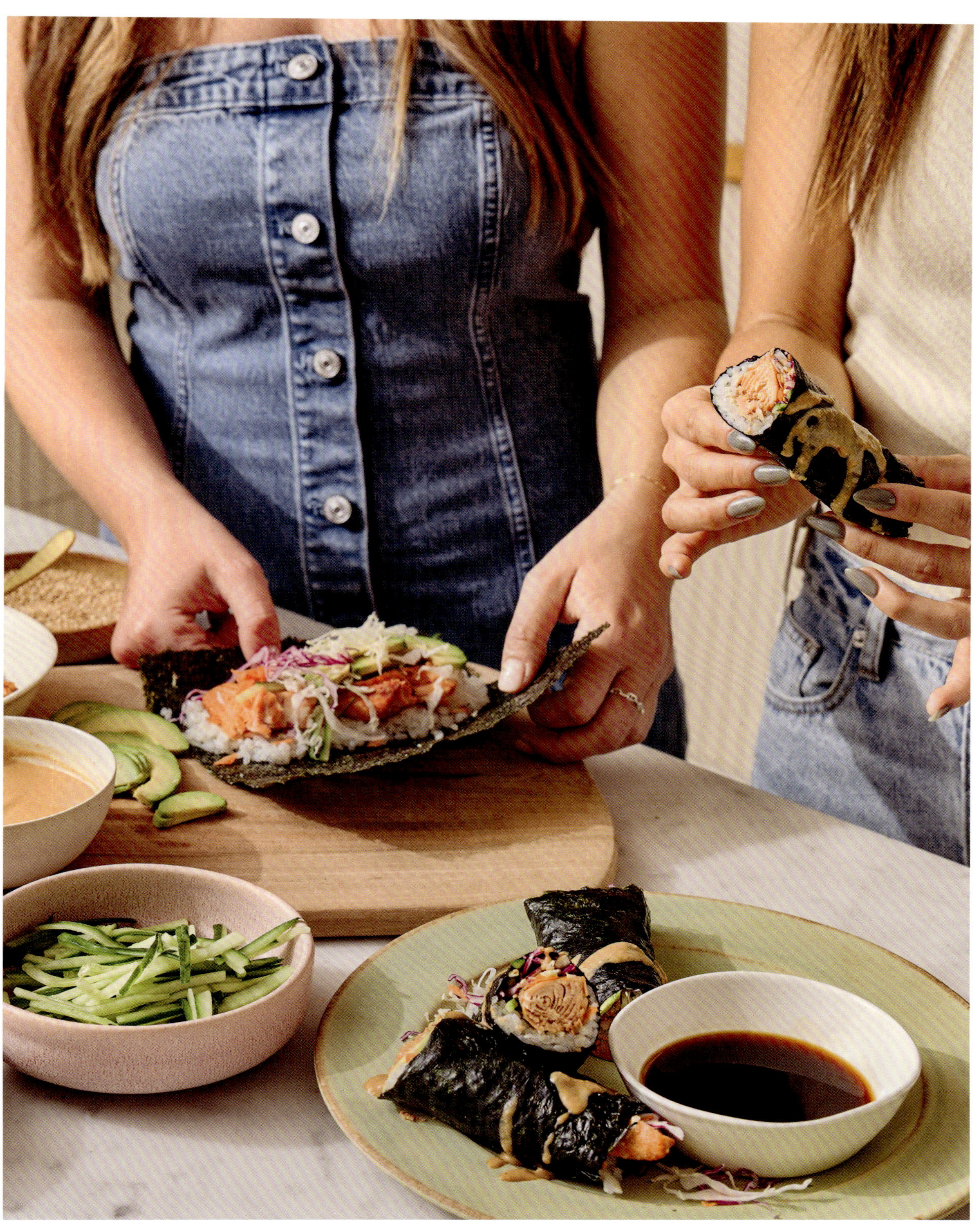

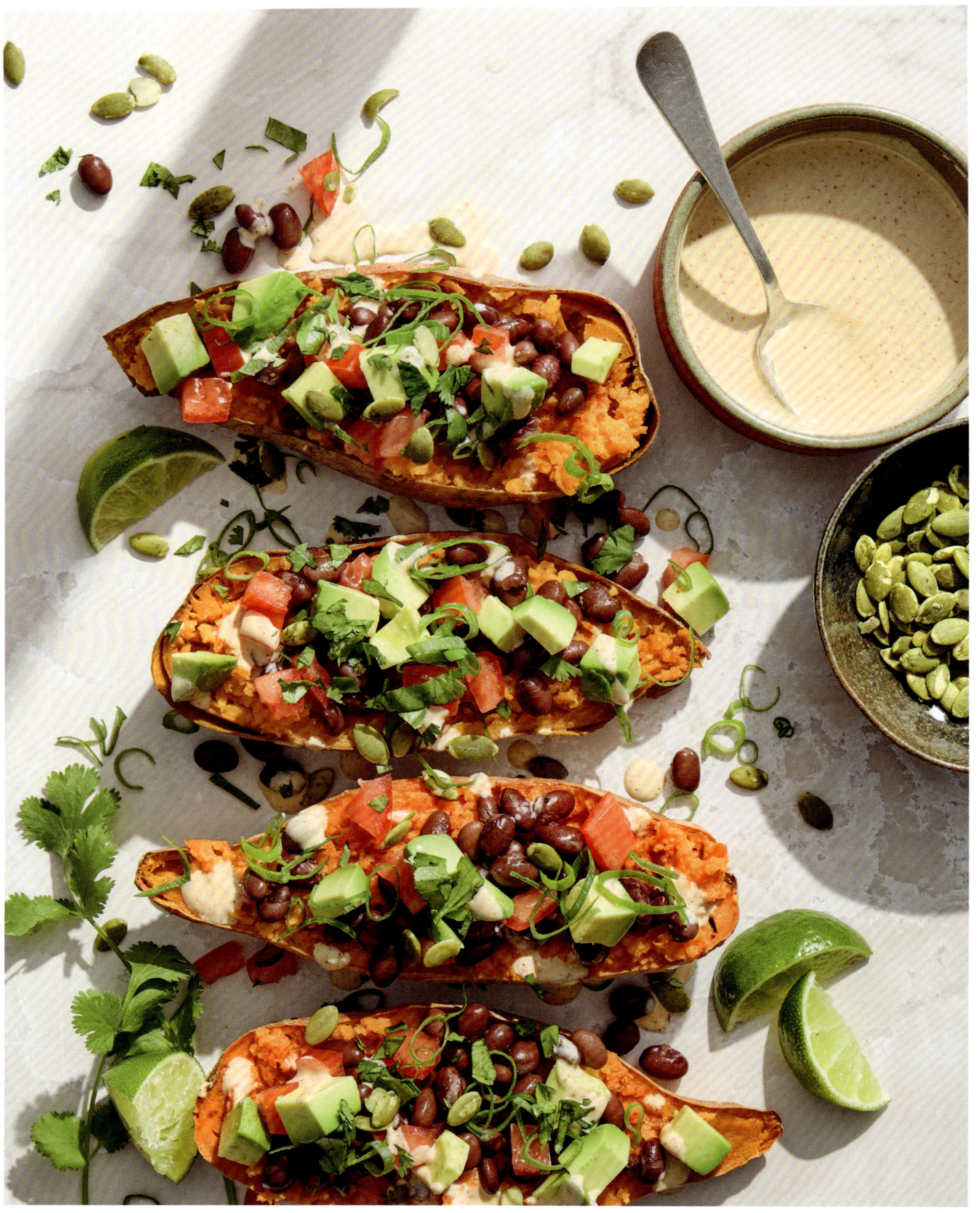

Loaded Sweet Potato with Smoky Chipotle-Lime Crema

Serves 4

Prep Time: 20 minutes

Cook Time: 45 minutes

This is one of those simple, go-to meals you can whip up with ingredients you probably already have in your kitchen. Sweet potatoes are a total staple for me in every phase—they're a powerhouse of long-lasting energy, perfect for this time when your body naturally feels more active and energized. Black beans bring in even more fiber and plant-based protein to help keep your blood sugar steady. Cumin doesn't just add a warm, cozy flavor; it's also amazing for digestion. In fact, cumin is known to help break down food in the stomach, which can reduce bloating and make it easier for your body to absorb all the good stuff, especially when beans are involved. Also, using a sweet potato as a bowl is just so much fun!

Sweet Potatoes

4 medium sweet potatoes

2 teaspoons ground cumin

1 teaspoon smoked paprika

Salt and freshly ground black pepper

Smoky Chipotle-Lime Crema

½ cup plain Greek yogurt (or coconut yogurt for dairy-free)

1 teaspoon chipotle powder (or smoked paprika for milder spice)

1 tablespoon freshly squeezed lime juice

2 teaspoons coconut aminos

1 teaspoon honey or maple syrup

Toppings

2 cups canned black beans, rinsed

½ cup diced ripe tomato

1 avocado, halved, pitted, and diced

¼ cup chopped cilantro

2 tablespoons sliced green onion tops

¼ cup toasted pepitas (pumpkin seeds, for crunch)

1 — Preheat the oven to 400°F.

2 — Bake the sweet potatoes: Scrub the sweet potatoes, pat them dry, and prick them a few times with a fork. Place them on a baking sheet and bake for about 45 minutes, until they are fork-tender and caramelized on the edges. Remove from the oven and let cool enough to handle.

3 — Slice open the potatoes lengthwise. Fluff the insides with a fork and sprinkle with the cumin, smoked paprika, and salt and pepper to taste.

4 — Make the crema: In a small bowl, whisk together the yogurt, chipotle powder, lime juice, coconut aminos, and honey until smooth. Adjust seasoning to taste.

5 — Top the potatoes: Top each sweet potato with some of the beans, tomato, avocado, and cilantro. Sprinkle with some of the green onion tops.

6 — Drizzle the stuffed sweet potatoes generously with the crema and finish with a sprinkling of the toasted pepitas for crunch. Enjoy!

Kale and Quinoa–Stuffed Bell Peppers with Garlic-Lemon-Yogurt Sauce

Serves 4
Prep Time: 15 minutes
Cook Time: 30 minutes

I absolutely love this spin on classic stuffed peppers. Growing up in California, I think of them as a Mexican dish, but I swapped in some Italian flavors here for a fun twist that works wonders for your body during the ovulatory phase. Quinoa and kale bring the fiber and antioxidants to fuel your energy and support hormone metabolism, while the bell peppers, full of vitamin C, help your body absorb the iron from the ground beef. You can also substitute ground chicken or turkey for the beef, or skip the meat and add cooked lentils to keep it veggie-based!

Bell Peppers

4 large bell peppers
1 tablespoon olive oil
1 pound ground beef (preferably grass-fed)
1 cup cooked quinoa
1 cup chopped fresh kale
½ cup cherry tomatoes, diced
1 teaspoon Italian seasoning
Salt and freshly ground black pepper
½ cup shredded mozzarella (or dairy-free cheese)

Garlic-Lemon-Yogurt Sauce

1 cup plain Greek yogurt (or dairy-free alternative)
1 garlic clove, finely grated or minced
1 tablespoon freshly squeezed lemon juice
1 teaspoon grated lemon zest
1 tablespoon olive oil
½ teaspoon ground cumin, for warm flavor (optional)
½ teaspoon salt, or more as desired
¼ teaspoon freshly ground black pepper
1 tablespoon finely chopped fresh dill or parsley (optional)

1 — Preheat the oven to 375°F.

2 — Stuff the peppers: Slice off the top third of each bell pepper and remove the stem, seeds, and ribs. Lightly brush the outside of the peppers with olive oil and place the peppers upright in an 8 × 8-inch baking dish.

3 — Heat a large skillet over medium heat. Add the ground beef to the pan and cook for about 5 minutes, until browned and fully cooked, breaking up any clumps as it cooks. If necessary, drain off any grease, and set the meat aside.

4 — In a large bowl, combine the quinoa, kale, cherry tomatoes, Italian seasoning, and salt and pepper to taste. Stir in the meat and blend well.

5 — Spoon the filling evenly into the bell peppers, gently pressing it down to compact it. Sprinkle the shredded cheese over the tops to create a golden layer.

6 — Cover the pan loosely with foil and bake the peppers at 375°F for 25 minutes. Remove the foil and bake for another 5 minutes, until the peppers are tender and the cheese is melted and slightly golden.

7 — Meanwhile, make the yogurt sauce: In a medium bowl, whisk together the yogurt, garlic, lemon juice, lemon zest, olive oil, cumin, salt, and pepper. Stir in the dill or parsley, if using. If the sauce is too thick, add a little water, a tablespoon at a time, until you reach your desired consistency. Let the sauce sit for at least 10 minutes (or chill for up to 1 hour) to allow the flavors to meld.

8 — Carefully transfer the stuffed peppers to serving plates and pour the sauce over the baked peppers and enjoy.

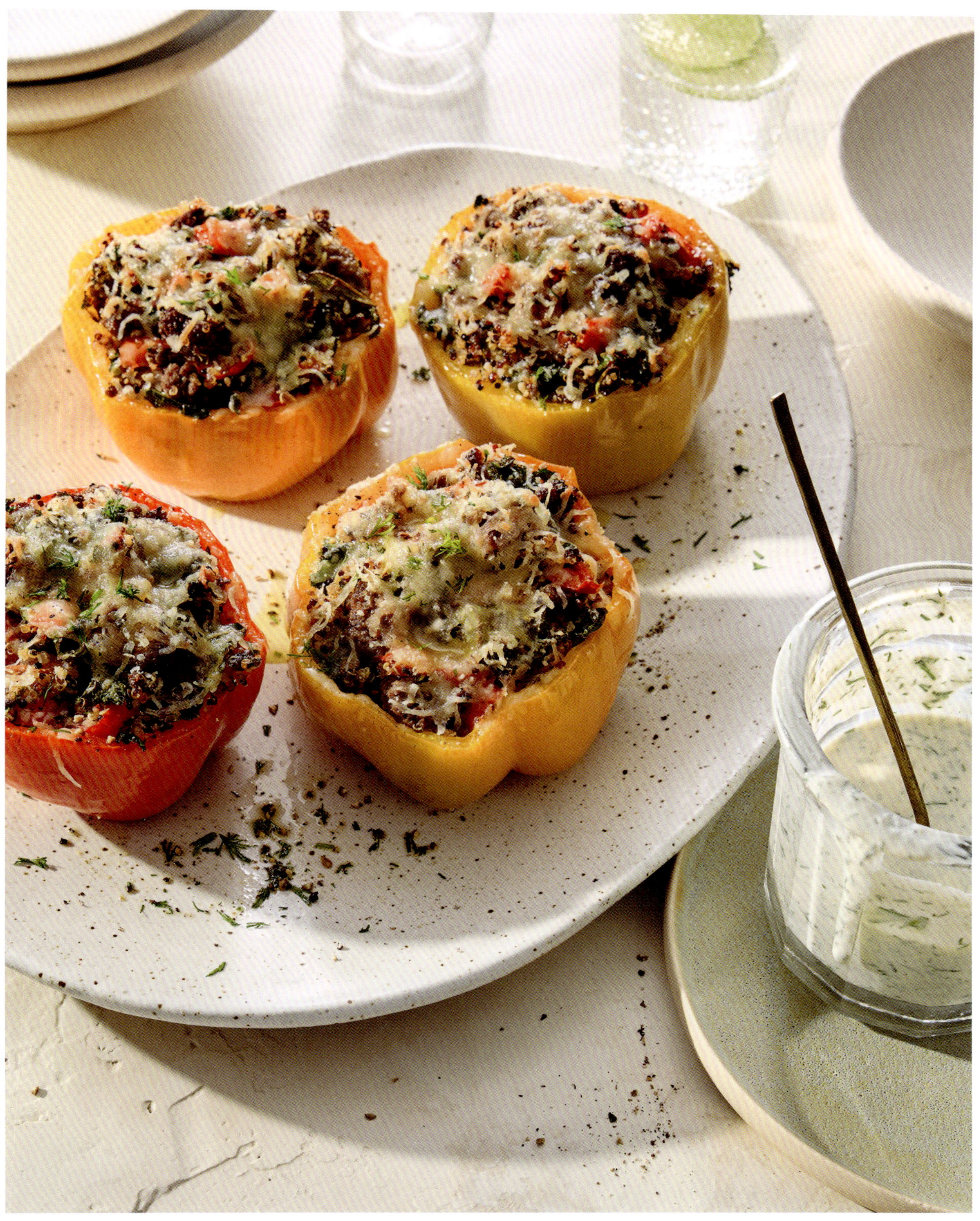

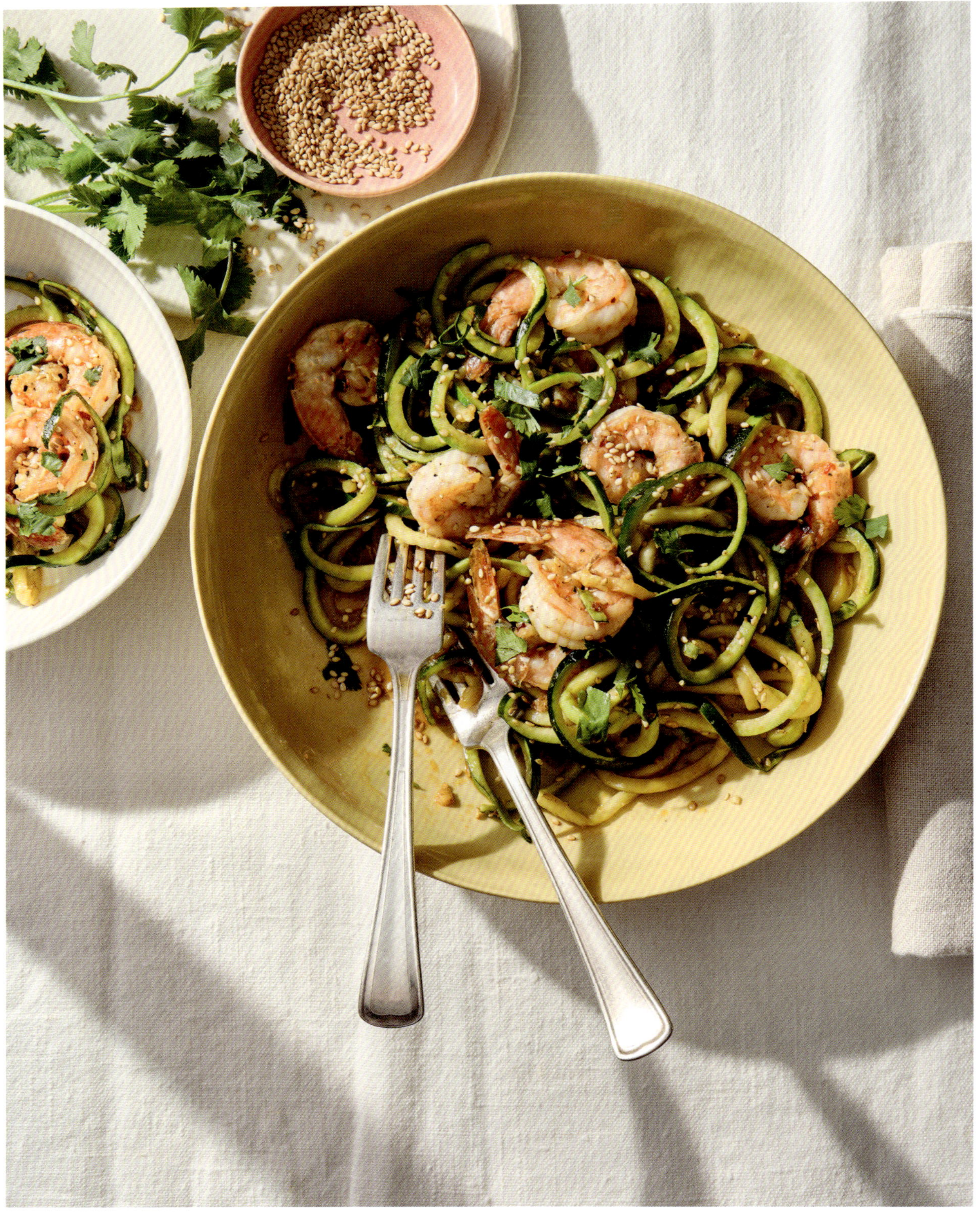

Spicy Shrimp and Zucchini Noodles with Chile-Lime Butter

Serves 4

Prep Time: 10 minutes

Cook Time: 12 minutes

Shrimp is such an underrated powerhouse! It's packed with lean protein and iodine, which is crucial for thyroid health. The thyroid is like the body's hormone control center—when it's happy, everything else stays in balance. I love pairing shrimp with zucchini noodles to sneak in extra veggies and fiber to support digestion. This version takes it up a notch with a chile-lime butter sauce that coats every bite with bold, zesty flavor. A handful of toasted sesame seeds and chopped cilantro add the perfect finishing touch. And I never shy away from the red pepper flakes, which add a little metabolism-boosting heat!

2 tablespoons olive oil

2 pounds raw large shrimp, peeled and deveined

2 teaspoons red pepper flakes, or as desired

4 garlic cloves, minced

2 tablespoons butter or ghee

Juice of 2 limes

2 teaspoons coconut aminos or tamari

1 teaspoon smoked paprika

4 medium zucchini, spiralized into noodles

Salt and freshly ground black pepper

2 tablespoons toasted sesame seeds

¼ cup chopped cilantro

1 — Add the olive oil to a large skillet and heat over medium heat. Add the shrimp, red pepper flakes, and garlic, and cook 2 to 3 minutes per side, until the shrimp turn pink and opaque. Remove from the skillet and set aside.

2 — In the same skillet, reduce the heat to low and add the butter, lime juice, coconut aminos, and smoked paprika. Stir until melted and combined.

3 — Toss the zucchini noodles into the skillet, cooking them for 2 to 3 minutes, until slightly softened but still firm. Add the shrimp and toss to coat everything in the sauce.

4 — Taste and season with the salt and pepper, then sprinkle with the toasted sesame seeds and cilantro. Serve immediately!

Garlic-Ginger-Tofu Stir-Fry with Bok Choy and Sesame Rice

Serves 4
Prep Time: 15 minutes
Cook Time: 30 minutes

I wanted to include a tofu dish in this book, but since I don't cook with it often, I took my time perfecting the recipe. With bok choy and ginger in mind, it took me four test runs to get it just right—and now it's a staple! Earlier in this chapter I explained how, during ovulation, your liver works overtime to process excess estrogen and prepare for the next phase of your cycle. Supporting that detox process with fiber and calcium-rich foods, like tofu and bok choy, can really help your body do its thing. Fiber helps eliminate waste and toxins, while calcium supports healthy liver function and overall detoxification. Paired with healthy fats and carbs from the sesame rice, this dish is totally blood sugar balanced. It also makes great leftovers for lunch the next day!

Sesame Rice

1 cup jasmine rice, rinsed until water runs clear

1 (15-ounce) can low-fat coconut milk

¼ cup water

2 teaspoons toasted sesame oil

2 teaspoons sesame seeds

Stir-Fry

2 tablespoons toasted sesame oil

2 (14-ounce) blocks extra-firm organic tofu, pressed and cubed

4 garlic cloves, minced

2 tablespoons grated fresh ginger

6 baby bok choy, halved

2 cups sugar snap peas

2 tablespoons coconut aminos

2 teaspoons rice vinegar

2 teaspoons honey or pure maple syrup

Chopped green onions (white and green parts), for garnish (optional)

1 — Prepare the rice: In a medium saucepan, combine the rice with the coconut milk and water. Bring to a boil over medium-high heat, then reduce the heat to low, cover, and simmer for 12 to 15 minutes, until the water is all absorbed by the rice. Remove from the heat and let sit, covered, for 5 minutes. Fluff with a fork, then toss with the sesame oil and sesame seeds. Cover to keep warm.

2 — Make the stir-fry: Heat 1 tablespoon of the sesame oil in a large skillet or wok over medium heat. Add the tofu cubes in a single layer and cook for 6 to 8 minutes, flipping occasionally, until golden brown on all sides. Remove from the pan and set aside.

3 — In the same skillet, add the remaining tablespoon sesame oil, followed by the garlic and ginger. Sauté for about 1 minute, stirring frequently, until fragrant. Add the bok choy and peas, and stir-fry for 3 to 4 minutes, until the vegetables are tender-crisp but still vibrant in color.

4 — Stir in the coconut aminos, rice vinegar, and honey. Cook for another 2 minutes, allowing the sauce to coat the vegetables. Add the tofu to the skillet, tossing everything together until well coated and warmed through.

5 — Divide the warm sesame rice among 4 servings bowls, then top with the tofu and vegetable stir-fry. Garnish with the green onions, if desired. (Alternatively, meal-prep by dividing the rice mixture into containers, covering, and saving for another time.)

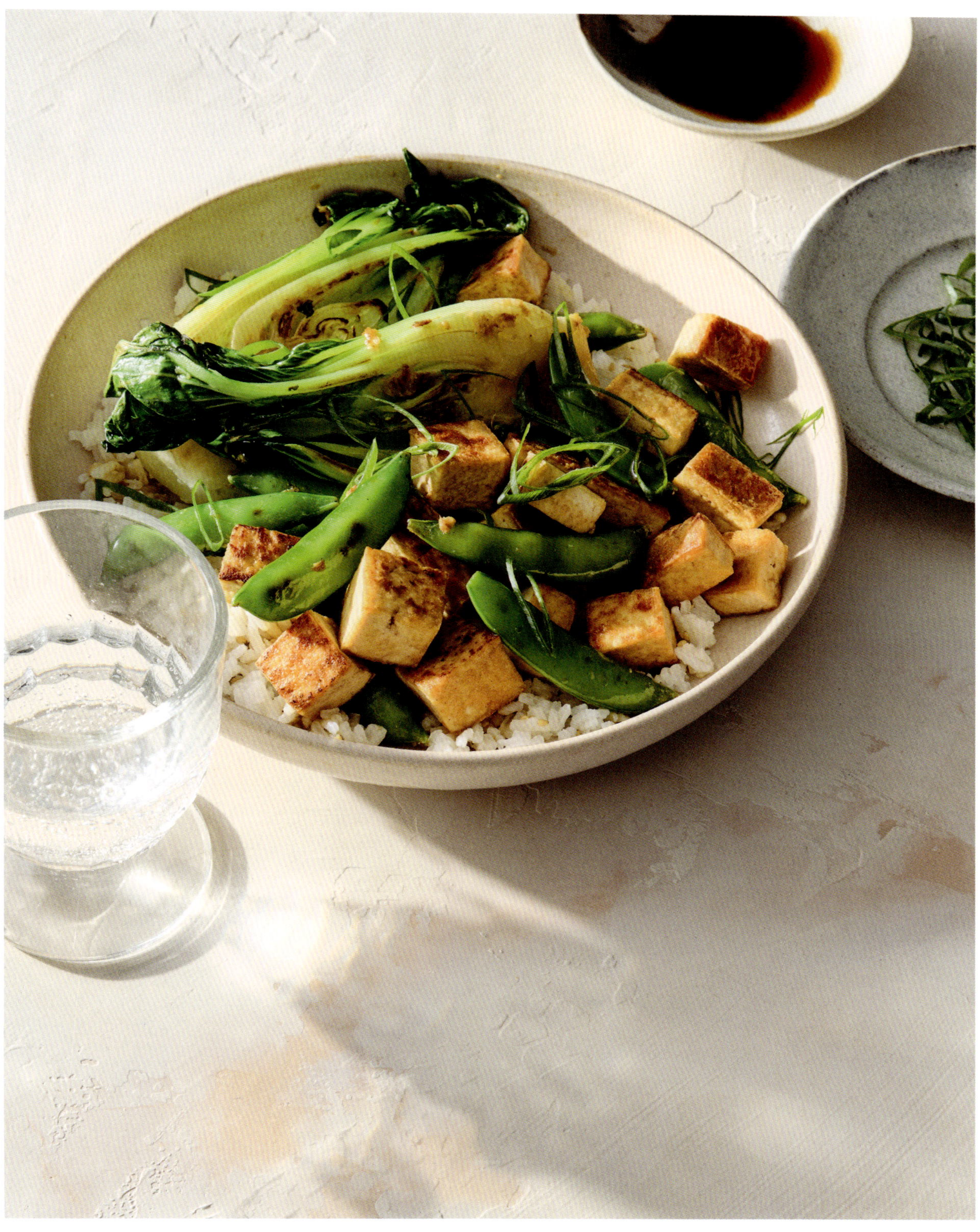

Mediterranean Quinoa Salad with Grilled Chicken

If it's not already a habit, it's time to start prepping a big batch of quinoa for each ovulatory phase—trust me, you'll thank me later! If quinoa isn't your thing, you can use rice or cauliflower rice instead. This Mediterranean-inspired salad is loaded with flavor, and the creamy lemon-tahini dressing adds a rich, nutty taste while providing healthy fats that help keep your blood sugar steady and your energy levels high during your ovulatory phase. Tahini's sesame seeds are packed with calcium and magnesium—two essential minerals for hormone health. Calcium helps regulate hormone release, which is key during ovulation when your body is releasing the egg. Magnesium balances the blood sugar, supports your nervous system, and reduces stress to keep your hormones in check. Together, these minerals help ensure your body is primed for ovulation and your hormones stay balanced.

Serves 4
Prep Time: 15 minutes
Cook Time: 15 minutes

Salad

2 cups cooked quinoa
2 cups mixed baby greens
1 cup cherry tomatoes, halved
¼ cup crumbled feta cheese
¼ cup sliced, pitted Kalamata olives
2 boneless, skinless chicken breasts (about 8 ounces total)
1 tablespoon olive oil
Salt and freshly ground black pepper

Lemon-Tahini Dressing

3 tablespoons tahini
2 tablespoons olive oil
1 tablespoon freshly squeezed lemon juice
1 teaspoon honey or pure maple syrup
1 small garlic clove, minced
Salt and freshly ground black pepper

1 — Prepare the salad: In a large bowl, toss together the quinoa, greens, cherry tomatoes, feta, and olives.

2 — Heat a grill pan or large skillet over medium-high heat. Lightly brush the chicken breasts with olive oil and season to taste with salt and pepper.

3 — Place the chicken on the grill pan or in the skillet and cook for 6 to 7 minutes per side, until the internal temperature reaches 165°F. Remove from the pan and let rest for a few minutes, then thinly slice. Add the chicken slices to the salad.

4 — Make the dressing: In a small bowl, whisk together the tahini, olive oil, lemon juice, honey, garlic, and salt and pepper to taste. Add a tablespoon or so of warm water to adjust to your desired consistency (dressing should be smooth and pourable).

5 — Drizzle the dressing over the salad and toss to combine. Serve immediately. (Alternatively, store in an airtight container for up to 2 days and dress when consuming.)

Thai Peanut Chicken Lettuce Wraps with a Chile-Lime Drizzle

Serves 4
Prep Time: 10 minutes
Cook Time: 12 minutes

This recipe has quickly become one of my all-time favorite lunches or dinners! It's loaded with protein from the ground chicken, healthy fats from the creamy peanut butter, fiber from the shredded carrots, and gut support from the ginger. As an alternative, I use coconut aminos instead of soy sauce here because it's gluten-free, lower in sodium, and still packs that savory umami flavor. Shredded carrots are an ovulatory-phase superstar, packed with beta-carotene to help support hormone health by promoting healthy estrogen metabolism. I'm extra excited for you to try this recipe—these wraps are absolutely perfect! Note: A serving is 2 wraps.

Chicken Wraps

1 tablespoon coconut oil

1 pound ground chicken

¼ cup creamy peanut butter (or almond butter)

2 tablespoons coconut aminos

1 tablespoon freshly squeezed lime juice

1 teaspoon grated fresh ginger

1 teaspoon Thai fish sauce (optional)

1 teaspoon honey

8 large lettuce leaves

Chile-Lime Drizzle

1 tablespoon freshly squeezed lime juice

½ teaspoon red pepper flakes or sriracha hot sauce

1 teaspoon coconut aminos

1 teaspoon sesame oil

½ teaspoon honey

Toppings

½ cup shredded carrot

¼ cup chopped peanuts (or cashews)

½ small cucumber, julienned

½ avocado, pitted and sliced

2 tablespoons chopped cilantro

2 tablespoons thinly sliced green onions (green and white parts)

1 — Make the wraps: Heat the coconut oil in a large skillet over medium heat. Add the chicken and cook for 5 to 7 minutes, until lightly browned, breaking up any clumps with a spatula.

2 — Stir the peanut butter, coconut aminos, lime juice, ginger, fish sauce (if using), and honey into the chicken. Simmer for 3 to 4 minutes, until thick and creamy.

3 — Turn off the burner and let mixture cool for 5 minutes, then spoon the skillet mixture into the lettuce leaves.

4 — Make the drizzle: In a small bowl, whisk together the lime juice, pepper flakes, coconut aminos, sesame oil, and honey.

5 — Finish the wraps: Top the filled wraps with your choice of toppings: the shredded carrot, peanuts, cucumber, avocado, cilantro, and green onions. Spoon the drizzle over the tops for an extra flavor punch.

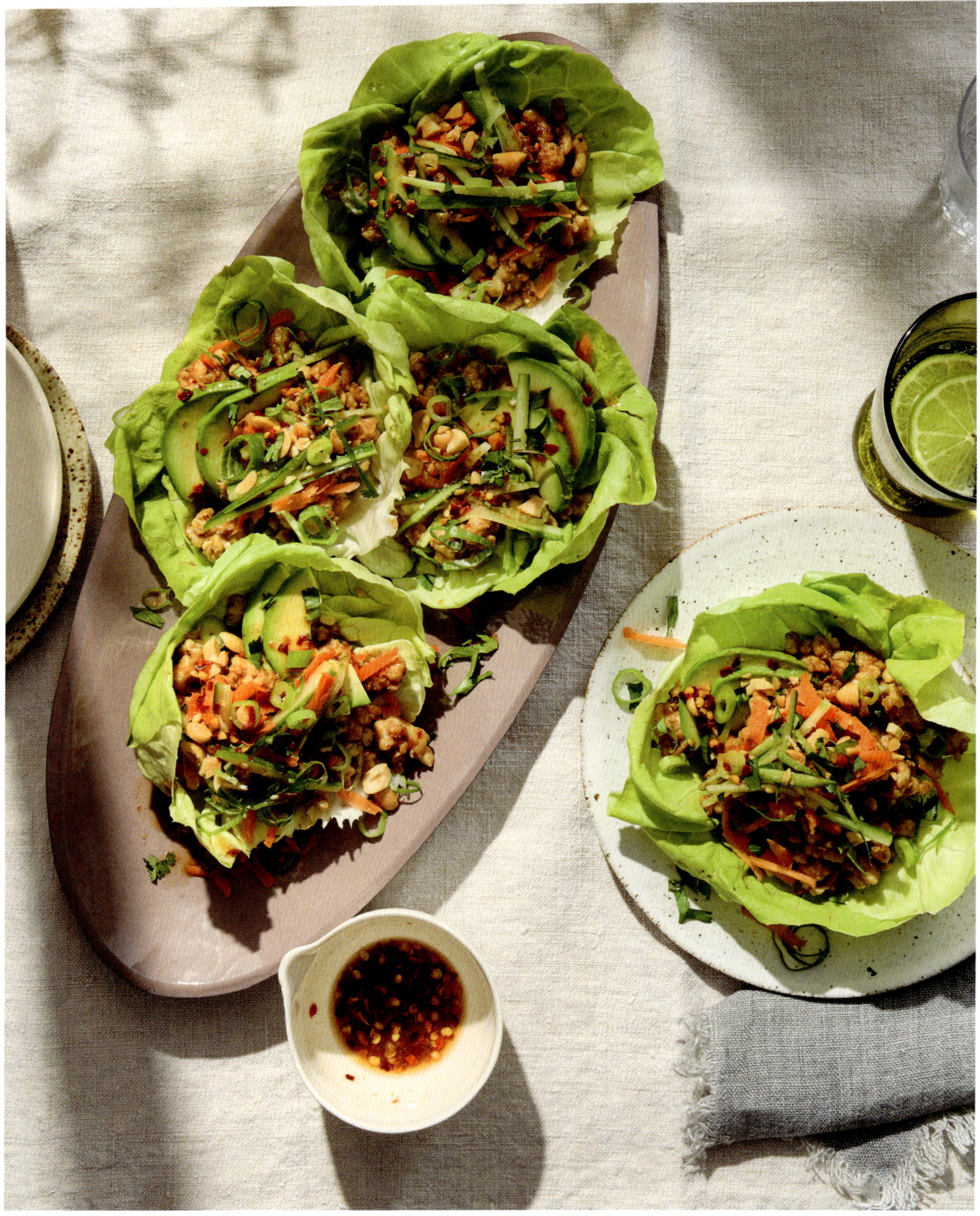

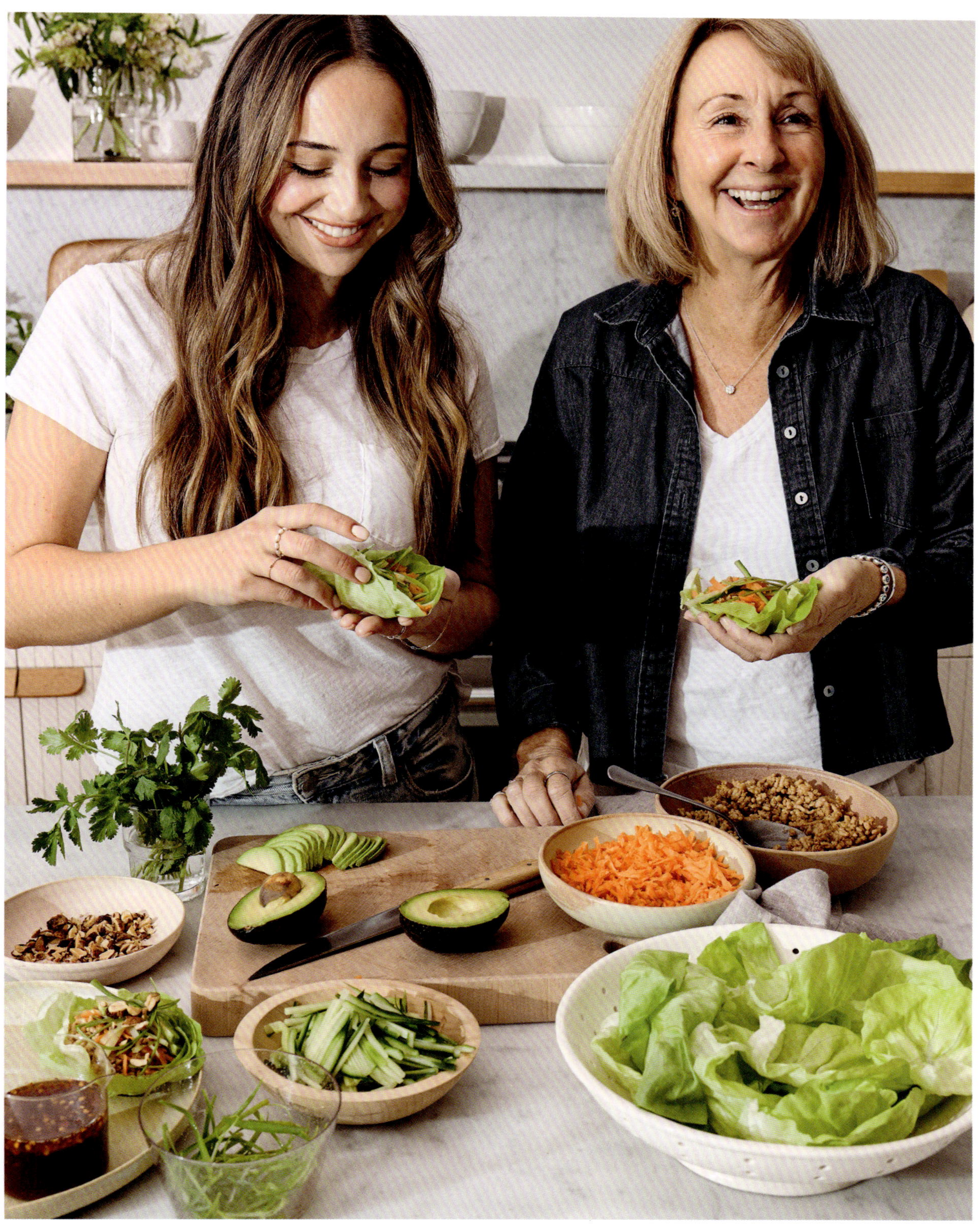

Sweet Potato and Black Bean Tacos with Avocado Crema

During your ovulatory phase, you're likely feeling your most outgoing, confident, and energized—this is the time to say yes to dinner with friends, plan a fun night out, or host a little gathering! I recently hosted a taco night, and I wanted to make a version that some of my vegetarian friends would love. That's when these sweet potato and black bean tacos were born! They are packed with fiber to support digestion and hormone metabolism, and the avocado crema adds the perfect creamy balance while providing healthy fats to keep your blood sugar stable. If you want to bulk them up a bit, add some rotisserie chicken or leftover ground beef to make them even heartier. Whether you're enjoying them solo or sharing with friends, these tacos are fresh, flavorful, and perfect for this vibrant phase of your cycle! Note: A serving is 2 tacos.

Serves 4
Prep Time: 15 minutes
Cook Time: 25 minutes

Sweet Potato Cubes

2 medium sweet potatoes, peeled and diced

1 tablespoon olive oil

1 teaspoon ground cumin

Avocado Crema

1 ripe avocado, halved, pitted, and sliced

2 tablespoons freshly squeezed lime juice

¼ cup plain Greek yogurt (or dairy-free alternative)

Salt and freshly ground black pepper

Tacos

8 (6-inch) corn tortillas

1 cup canned or cooked black beans, drained and rinsed

Chopped cilantro

1 lime, cut into wedges (optional)

1 — Preheat the oven to 400°F.

2 — Bake the sweet potatoes: In a medium bowl, toss the diced sweet potatoes with the olive oil and cumin. Spread them out in an even layer on a baking sheet and roast for about 20 minutes, tossing halfway through, or until tender and slightly crispy on the edges.

3 — Make the crema: Add the avocado slices, lime juice, and yogurt to a food processor or blender and process until smooth. Season to taste with salt and pepper, adding a bit of water if needed to reach a creamy, smooth consistency.

4 — Assemble the tacos: Warm the tortillas in a dry skillet over medium heat for about 30 seconds on each side, or wrap them in a damp paper towel and microwave for 30 seconds until soft and pliable.

5 — Layer the tacos with the roasted sweet potatoes, the black beans, and a generous drizzle of the avocado crema. Garnish with the cilantro and serve with lime wedges, if desired. Serve immediately. (Alternatively, pack them up for lunch the next day!)

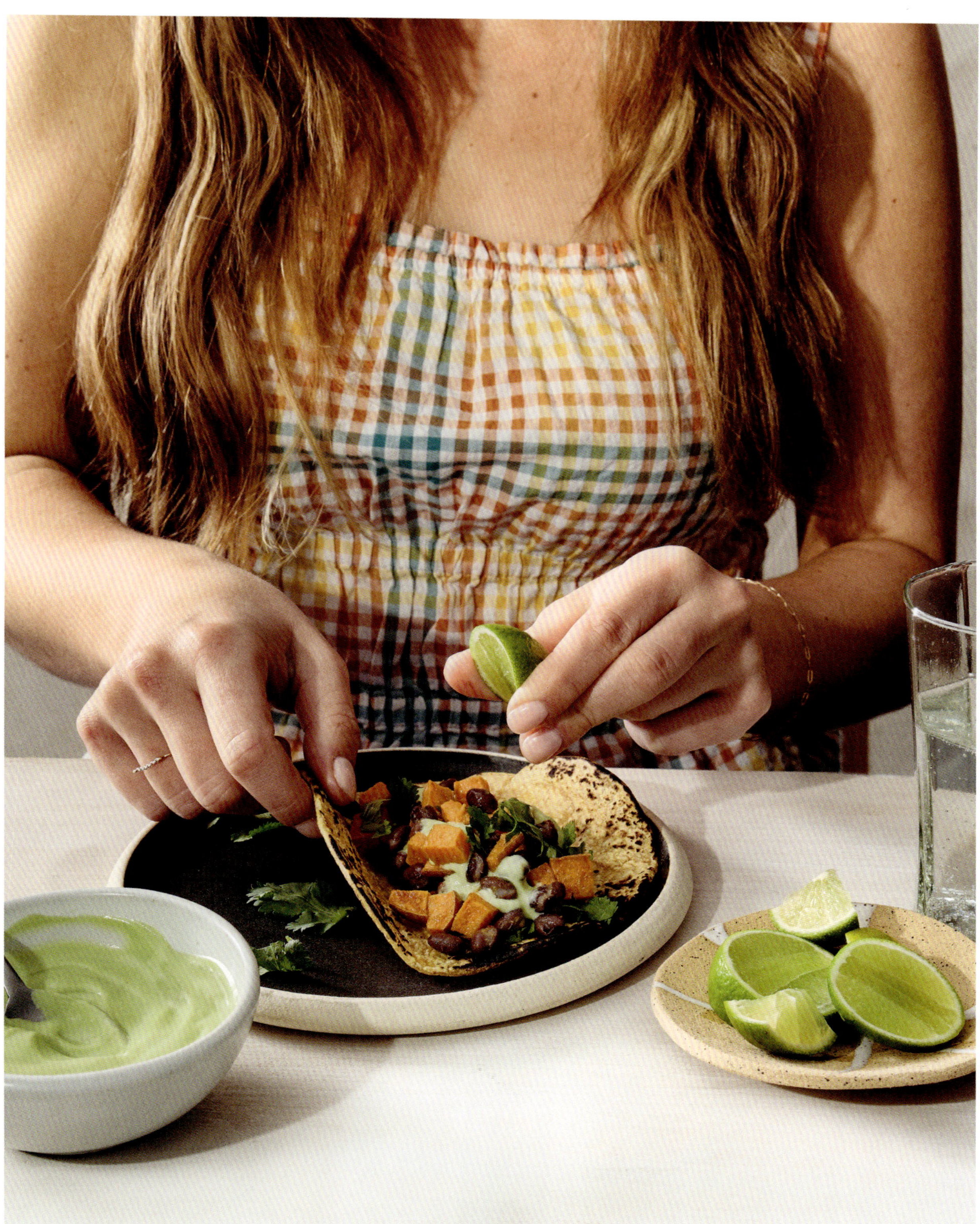

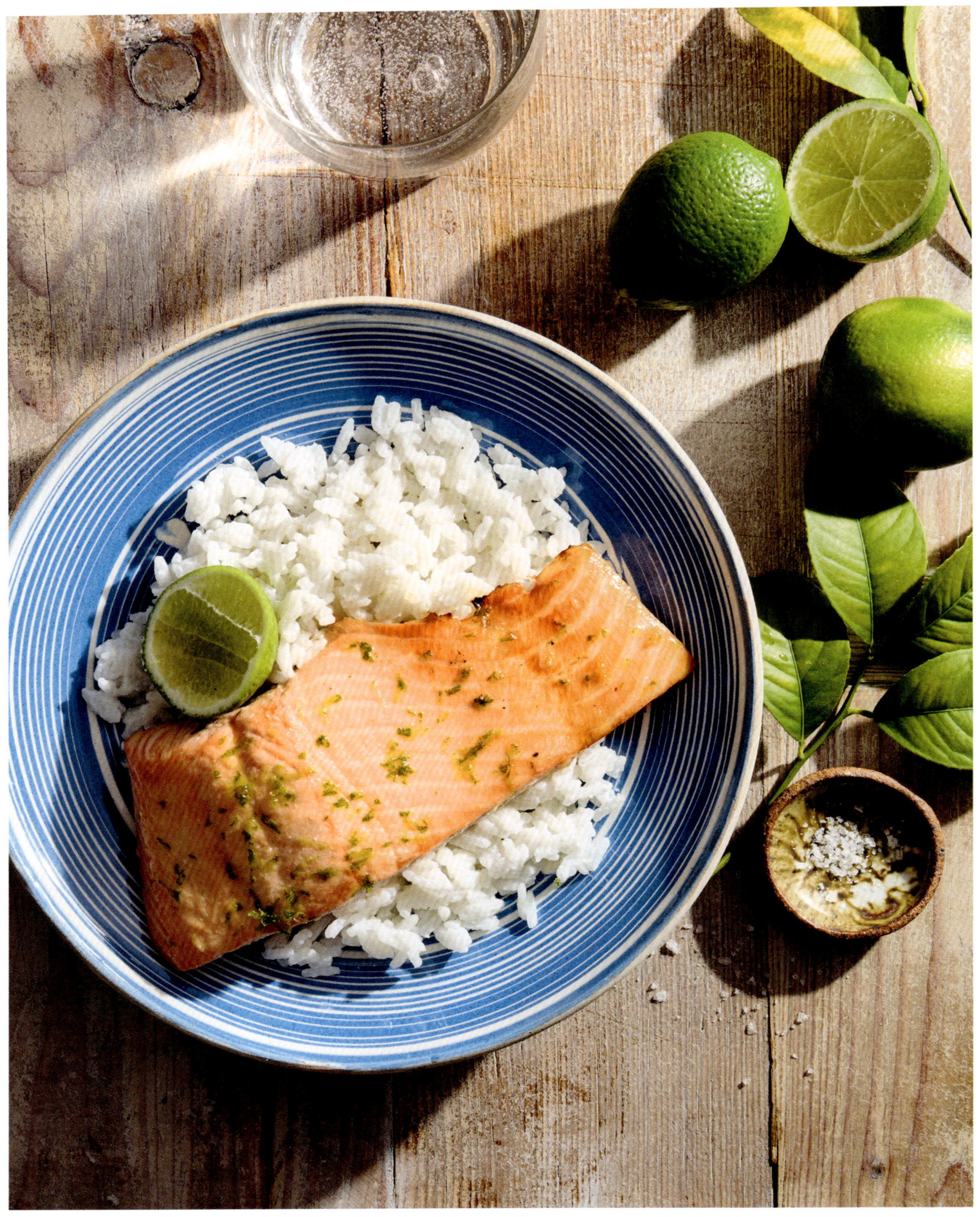

Honey-Lime Salmon and Coconut Rice

This meal just feels like summer to me. Picture a warm evening, the sun setting late, and you're having a cozy dinner outside with friends or family—that's the vibe. Since the ovulatory phase is our "inner summer," I knew this one had to be featured in this chapter. The honey-lime glaze is the perfect mix of sweet and tangy, balancing the richness of the salmon and making every bite feel light and fresh. And once you try the coconut rice, you'll never want to eat rice another way! It's creamy, a little sweet, and the perfect base to keep blood sugar steady and energy high. I love serving this with garlic-sautéed broccolini for a little extra green. I'm really excited for you guys to add this one to your meal rotation!

Serves 4
Prep Time: 10 minutes
Cook Time: 20 minutes

2 tablespoons honey
2 tablespoons freshly squeezed lime juice
1 teaspoon garlic powder
4 salmon fillets (about 1 pound total)
1 cup jasmine rice
1 cup full-fat coconut milk
1 cup water
1 lime, cut into wedges

1 — Preheat the oven to 400°F. Lightly grease a sheet pan.

2 — In a small bowl, mix the honey, lime juice, and garlic powder. Brush the honey-lime mixture over the salmon fillets, coating them evenly.

3 — Place the salmon, skin side down, on the sheet pan and bake for 15 to 20 minutes, until the salmon is cooked through and flakes easily with a fork.

4 — Meanwhile, in a medium saucepan, combine the jasmine rice, coconut milk, and water. Bring to a boil, then reduce to a simmer. Cover and cook for about 15 minutes, until the rice is tender and the liquid is absorbed. Fluff with a fork.

5 — Spread the coconut rice on 4 plates and top each with a salmon fillet. Garnish with the lime wedges for an extra burst of citrus, and serve.

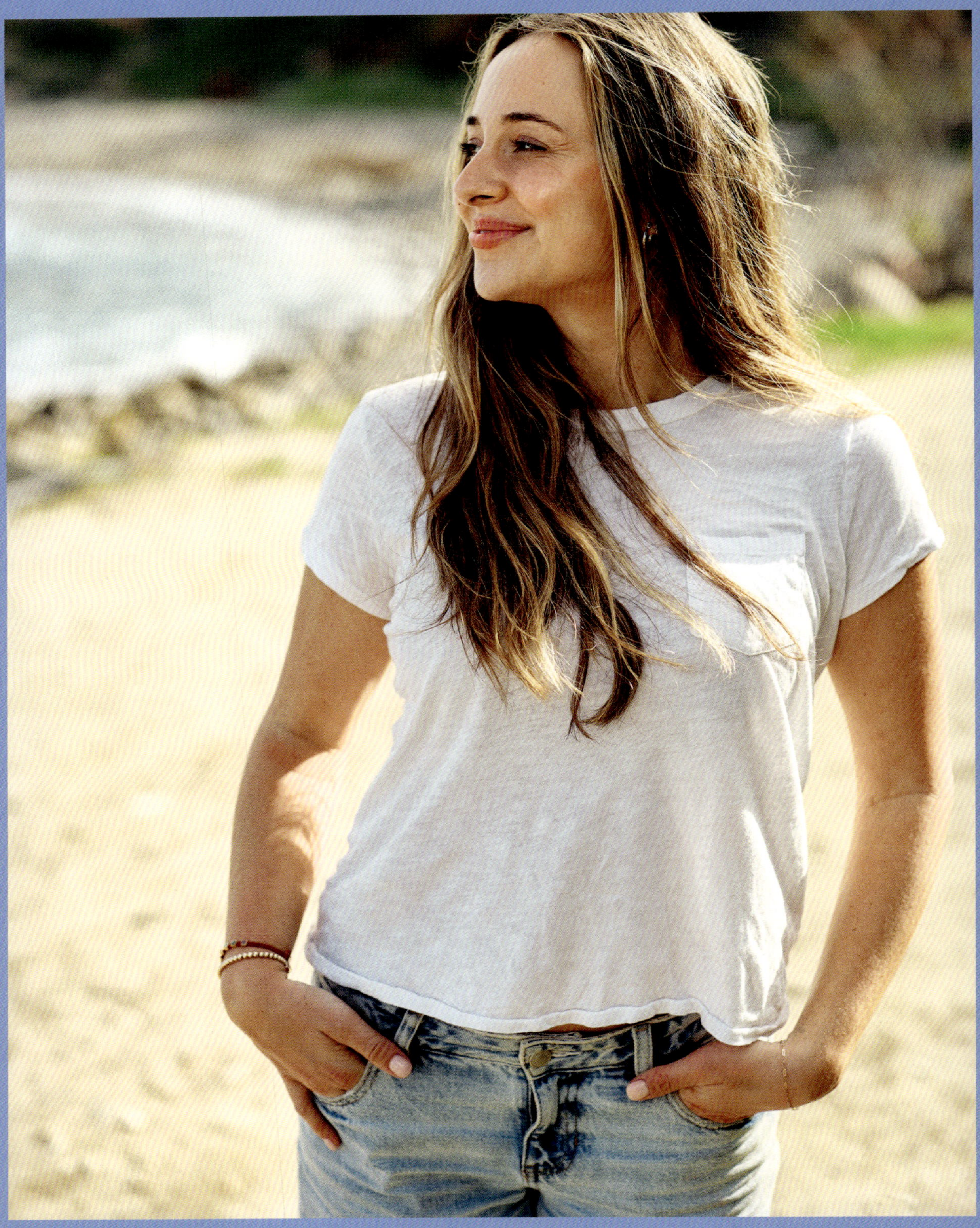

Snacks & Desserts

Collagen Blender Muffins

Makes 12 muffins
Prep Time: 10 minutes
Cook Time: 22 minutes

As you've been making the dishes from this book, I'm sure you can tell I'm all about simple recipes that deliver big benefits. These muffins are the epitome of that. They're made in a blender, so cleanup is a breeze, and they sneak in collagen, which is full of amino acids that support skin elasticity, reduce joint inflammation, and promote overall connective tissue health. I reach for these as a snack to stabilize my energy between meals or as a post-workout treat to help my body recover. They also make a great breakfast—just warm one up and top it with a little nut butter or toss it into a yogurt bowl! If you want to save some for later, simply wrap and freeze them. Note: A serving is 1 muffin.

3 ripe bananas
3 large eggs
⅓ cup almond butter
⅓ cup honey or pure maple syrup
⅔ cup oat flour
4 scoops collagen powder
1¼ teaspoons baking powder
1 teaspoon ground cinnamon
⅓ cup dark chocolate chips (optional)

1 — Preheat the oven to 350°F. Line a 12-cup muffin tin with paper liners.

2 — Place all the ingredients except the chocolate chips into a blender and blend until smooth.

3 — Fold in the chocolate chips, if using, and pour the batter into the muffin cups, filling them about three-fourths full.

4 — Bake for 18 to 22 minutes, until a toothpick inserted into the center of a muffin comes out clean. Let cool slightly before popping out of the tin, then cool completely before enjoying!

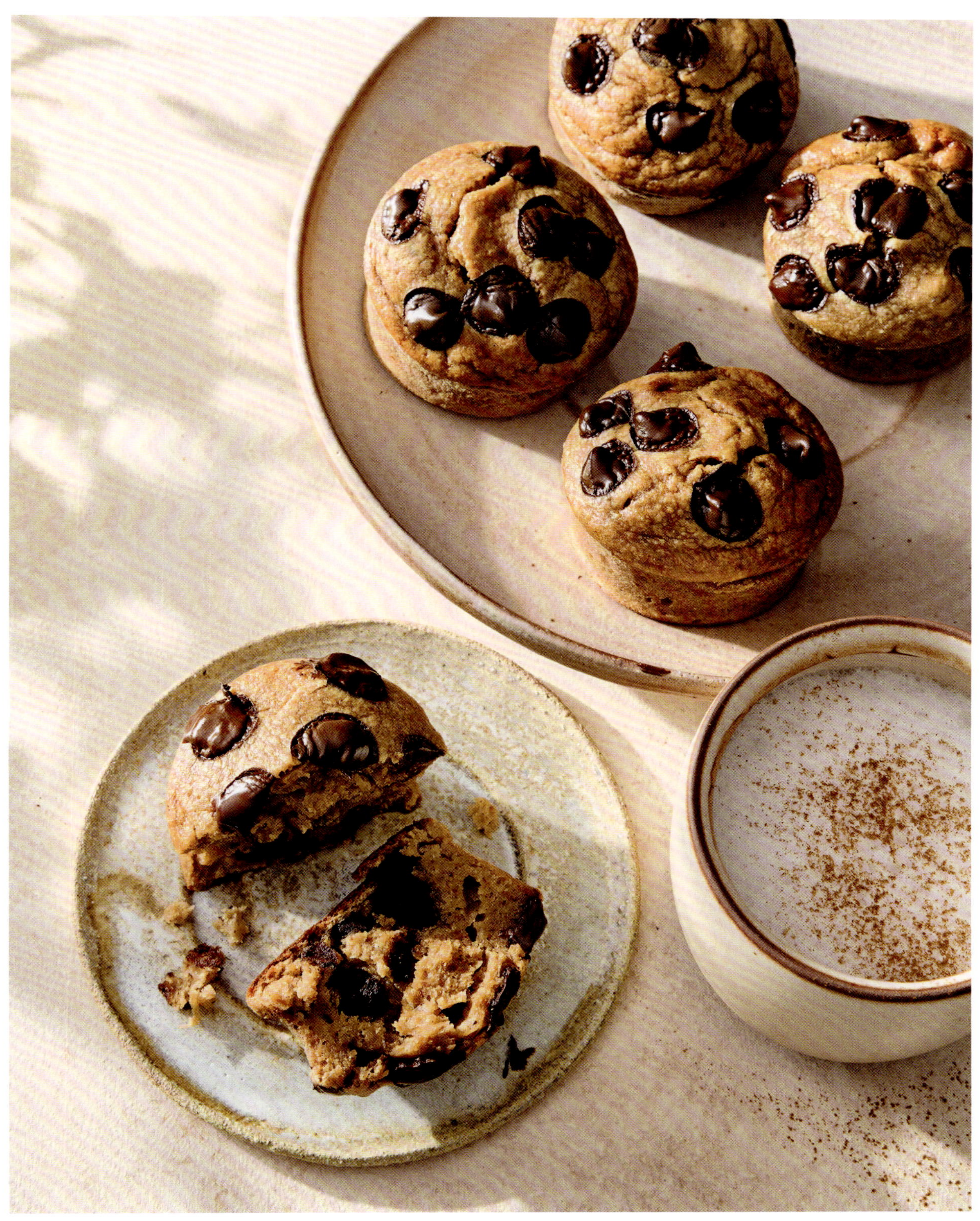

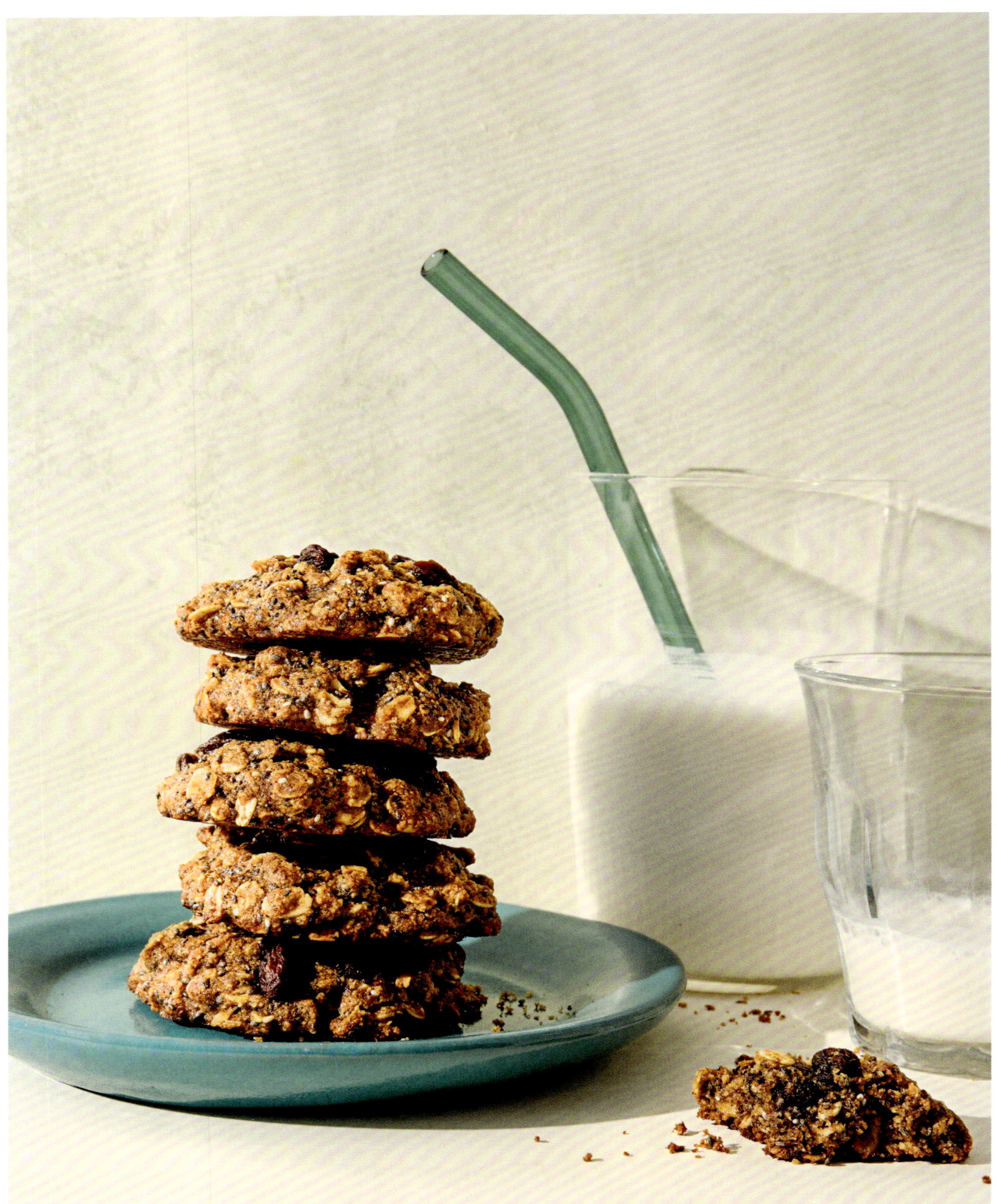

Gut-Loving Oatmeal Cookies

Makes 10 to 12 cookies
Prep Time: 10 minutes
Cook Time: 12 minutes

Baking is my therapy, and I find so much comfort in making sweet treats that support my body's fluctuations each week. Fiber is obviously the name of the game in this phase, and these oatmeal cookies get their fiber from oats, flaxseed, and chia seeds. Naturally sweetened with honey and full of healthy fats from coconut oil, the cookies taste as good as they make you feel. I love turning baking into a relaxing ritual; put on some music or your favorite podcast and really enjoy the process. This phase is all about energy, but I love finding ways to slow down and savor the little moments.

1 cup old-fashioned rolled oats
½ cup almond flour
3 tablespoons ground flaxseed
3 tablespoons chia seeds
½ teaspoon baking soda
1 teaspoon ground cinnamon
¼ cup coconut oil, melted
¼ cup honey
1 large egg
¼ cup raisins or dark chocolate chips

1 — Preheat the oven to 350°F. Line a baking sheet with parchment paper.

2 — In a medium bowl, combine the oats, almond flour, flaxseed, chia seeds, baking soda, and cinnamon.

3 — In a small bowl, whisk together the coconut oil, honey, and egg.

4 — Pour the wet ingredients into the dry ingredients and stir to combine, then fold in the raisins or chocolate chips.

5 — Scoop tablespoon-size amounts of dough onto the baking sheet, leaving 1 inch between them, then gently press to flatten.

6 — Bake for 10 to 12 minutes, or until golden brown. Let cool slightly on a rack before enjoying.

Chocolate-Almond Energy Bites

Makes 12 bites

Prep Time: 10 minutes, plus 20 minutes chilling

Energy bites are one of my go-to snacks when I need quick pre-workout fuel, something to pair with my coffee, or just a little treat to cleanse my palate after a meal. Dates are my secret weapon for natural sweetness and that quick energy boost, while the healthy fats from almonds and chia seeds help stabilize blood sugar. I experience chocolate cravings all month long, and the cacao powder here satisfies that craving while packing in antioxidants and a little bit of natural caffeine. These are one of those things you'll always find prepped in my fridge!

1 cup raw almonds
½ cup chopped pitted dates
2 tablespoons cacao powder
1 tablespoon chia seeds
½ teaspoon vanilla extract

1 — In a food processor, combine the almonds and dates and process until crumbly.

2 — Add the cacao powder, chia seeds, and vanilla and blend again, until smooth. If the mixture feels too dry, add a little water, 1 teaspoon at a time, until it holds together.

3 — Roll the mixture into bite-size balls and place the balls on a parchment-lined tray. Chill in the fridge or freezer for at least 20 minutes before enjoying.

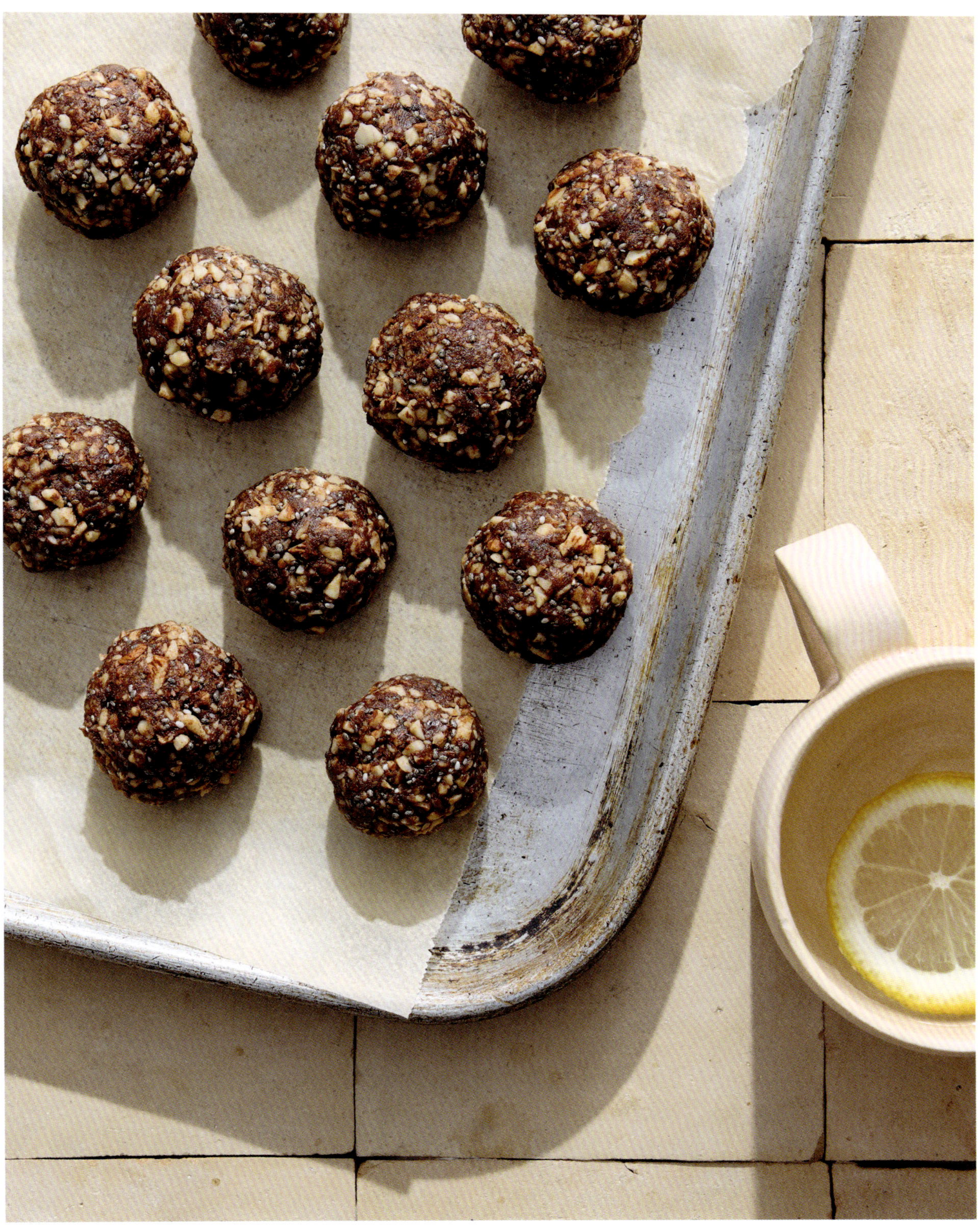

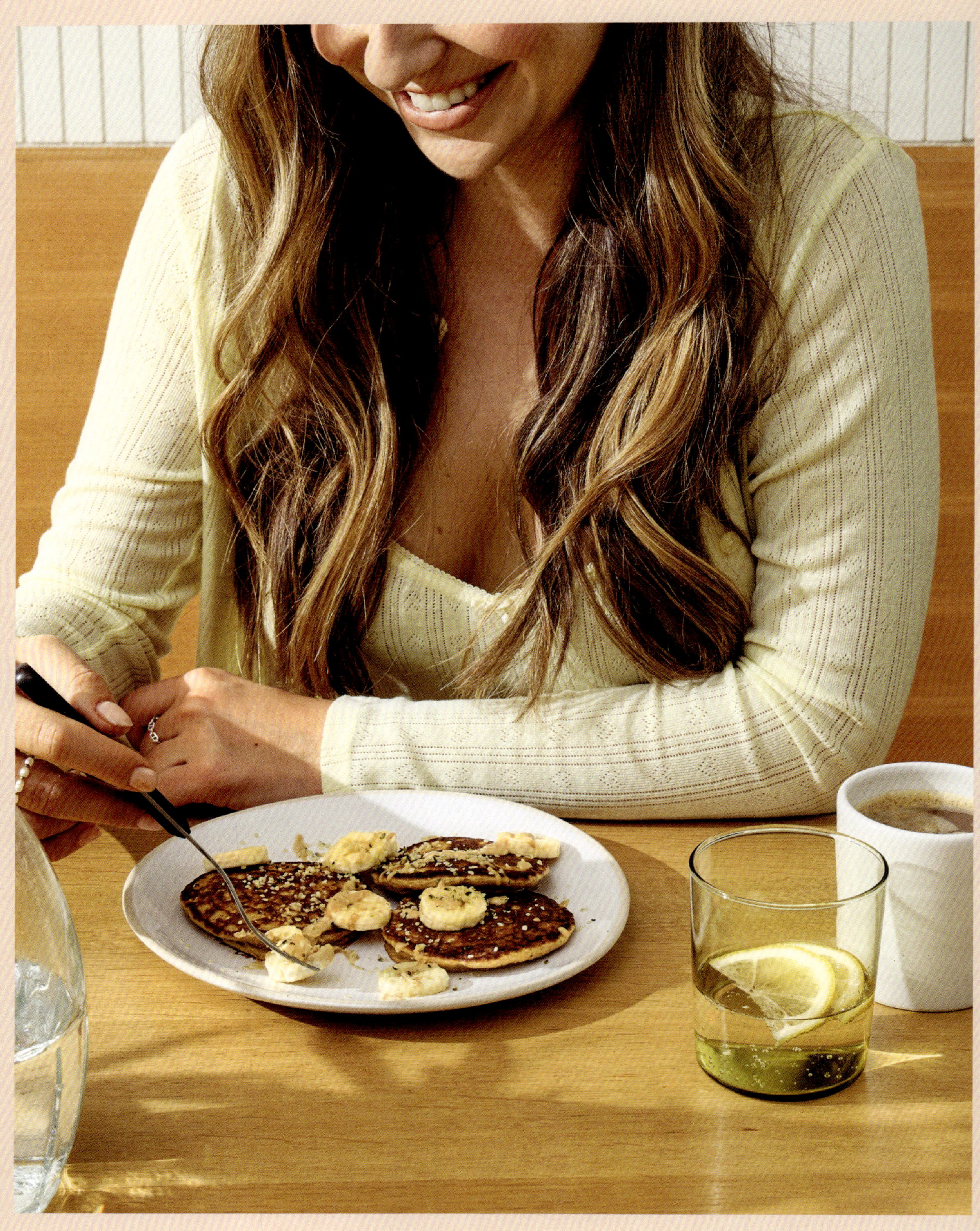

Luteal Phase

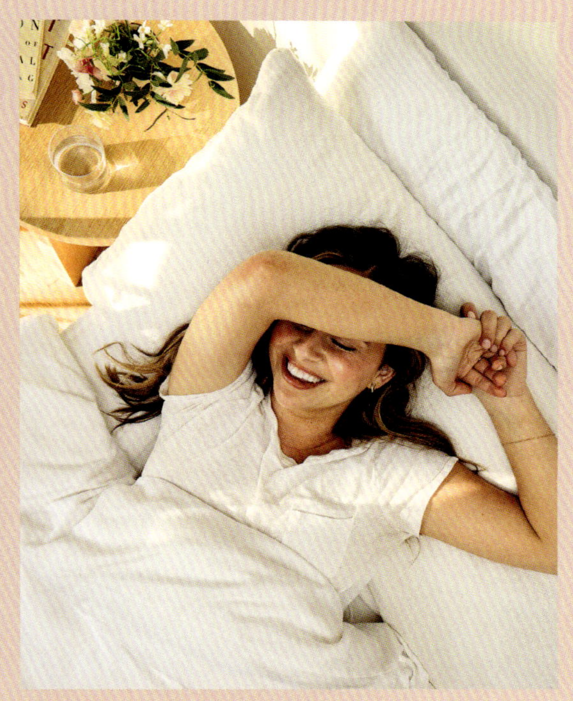

Preparing for Your Body's Reset

The luteal phase is the second half of the menstrual cycle, spanning from ovulation to the onset of your period, typically lasting 10 to 14 days. It's a time of transition, when your body prepares for a potential pregnancy or the natural reset for your next cycle. Progesterone takes center stage in this phase, bringing with it a host of physical and emotional shifts. This is also when PMS symptoms—such as bloating, fatigue, mood swings, and cravings—often show up as hormone levels fluctuate. While this phase may feel challenging, understanding its hormonal landscape and tailoring your nutrition and lifestyle can help you thrive during this time.

Hormonal Breakdown: What's Happening

The luteal phase is marked by intricate hormonal changes that influence your energy levels, mood, and physical state:

- PROGESTERONE After ovulation, the follicle that released the egg morphs into the corpus luteum, a temporary structure that produces progesterone. Progesterone has a calming effect on the nervous system, which we love, however these rising progesterone levels can also contribute to bloating, fatigue, and increased appetite.

- ESTROGEN Estrogen dips immediately after ovulation but rises slightly in the middle of the luteal phase, before tapering off again. This secondary rise supports mood and energy levels before its final decline signals the body to prepare for menstruation.

- PMS SYMPTOMS As progesterone and estrogen decline in the latter half of this phase, symptoms such as irritability, cravings, bloating, breast tenderness, and fatigue may emerge, signaling the body's shift toward menstruation. These symptoms are a sign of your body's changing needs and an invitation to focus on nourishment and rest.

These hormonal fluctuations may feel overwhelming, but by responding to your body with the right foods, movement, and self-care practices, you can minimize discomfort and make the most of this phase. Nutrition plays a huge role here: Focusing on anti-inflammatory foods, plenty of fiber, and healthy fats can help balance hormones and stabilize blood sugar, reducing symptoms like bloating, fatigue, and mood swings. Incorporating stress-reducing activities, like gentle movement, deep breathing, or even taking time for rest, can also have a profound impact. Listening to your body and nourishing it with the right fuel can not only alleviate symptoms but also empower you to feel more in tune with your natural rhythm. By making small changes to support your body during this phase, you can ease those uncomfortable symptoms and feel more balanced, energized, and focused.

How Food Can Support You

Supporting your body during the luteal phase involves balancing blood sugar, reducing inflammation, and managing common PMS symptoms. Choosing nutrient-dense, warming foods can help stabilize your mood, reduce bloating, and support hormonal detoxification. Dr. Amersi shares that eating foods high in magnesium at this time can help mitigate cramps, while magnesium is also thought to boost low energy and libido during this phase.

1 — Focus on Healthy Fats

During the luteal phase, your body's metabolic rate increases, and it requires more energy. Healthy fats are crucial for maintaining energy levels, balancing blood sugar, and supporting hormone production. Incorporating omega-3-rich foods like wild-caught salmon, flax seeds, chia seeds, walnuts, and avocado can help keep your hormones balanced and reduce inflammation, which is common during this phase. These fats also support healthy progesterone levels, helping to alleviate mood swings and cramps.

2 — Crave Complex Carbs

In the luteal phase, your body's increased need for energy often leads to cravings for carbohydrates. Opt for complex carbs such as sweet potatoes, quinoa, brown rice, and legumes to provide steady energy without spiking your blood sugar. These carbs are rich in fiber, which helps stabilize blood sugar levels and can prevent the irritability and fatigue that many experience during this phase. Pairing these with healthy fats and proteins will also help keep you feeling full and satisfied.

3 — Magnesium for Muscle Relaxation

Magnesium is especially helpful during the luteal phase, as it plays a key role in reducing muscle cramps and supporting restful sleep. Incorporate magnesium-rich foods like spinach, pumpkin seeds, dark chocolate, and almonds to ease tension in your muscles and support overall mood. Magnesium also helps manage the bloating and discomfort that may occur during this phase, promoting relaxation and balance.

4 — B Vitamin Boost

B vitamins, especially B6, are vital during the luteal phase to support your body's stress response and maintain balanced mood levels. Foods like eggs, poultry, avocados, and leafy greens are rich in B vitamins and can help alleviate symptoms like irritability, fatigue, and low energy. In particular, B6 can help manage PMS symptoms and support your body in producing serotonin, which helps stabilize mood.

5 — Hydrate with Herbal Teas

Hormonal fluctuations during the luteal phase can lead to increased water retention, causing feelings of bloating and discomfort. Drinking plenty of water and incorporating herbal teas such as peppermint, ginger, and chamomile can help reduce bloating, improve digestion, and provide soothing relief. These teas also have calming properties, which can help you unwind and combat stress.

Top Nutrition Tips for the Luteal Phase

1 — Balance Blood Sugar

The luteal phase often brings cravings for quick energy from sugary or processed foods. Combat these fluctuations by prioritizing meals rich in protein, fiber, and healthy fats to keep blood sugar steady and avoid energy crashes.

2 — Reduce Inflammation

Increased inflammation during this phase can contribute to bloating, cramps, and fatigue. Omega-3-rich foods like salmon, chia seeds, and walnuts, along with anti-inflammatory spices like turmeric and ginger, help soothe the body and promote hormonal balance.

3 — Support Progesterone Production

During the luteal phase, your progesterone levels rise, and while this is a natural and necessary part of your cycle, it can also contribute to symptoms like bloating and fatigue. To support healthy progesterone production without overstimulating it, focus on key nutrients like magnesium, vitamin B6, and zinc. These nutrients help ensure that progesterone functions optimally without exacerbating symptoms. Foods like spinach, bananas, sesame seeds, and pumpkin seeds provide these essential building blocks, supporting your body's natural balance and helping you feel your best during this phase.

4 — Warming, Easy-to-Digest Foods

During the luteal phase, your digestion naturally slows down a bit as your body prepares for potential pregnancy. This means your gastrointestinal system isn't as efficient at breaking down food, and it may take a bit longer for food to pass through. Incorporating warming, long-cooked foods like soups, stews, roasted vegetables, and cooked greens can be especially soothing during this time. These foods are easier on the digestive system because the cooking process breaks down fiber and complex compounds, making them simpler to digest and absorb. Additionally, the warmth of these foods helps promote circulation and support a calm, grounded energy, reducing bloating and keeping you feeling nourished and balanced.

Exercise and Lifestyle Tips

During the luteal phase, your body often craves a slower, more restorative pace. While moderate exercise is still beneficial, it's important to listen to your body and scale back intensity as needed. I often find myself scheduling in two to three non-negotiable full rest days at the end of my luteal phase, right before my period arrives, to make sure I give my body the rest it needs. You might find you need the rest more on days 1 and 2 of your cycle (the first two days of your period), or you might need more than three days of rest. What's important is that you honor what *your* body needs.

Self-Care Practices to Support Your Luteal Phase

Your body is working hard to prepare for the next cycle, making self-care an essential part of feeling balanced and supported.

- PRIORITIZE SLEEP Progesterone's rise can make you feel more fatigued, so honor your body by going to bed earlier and creating a relaxing nighttime routine.
- MANAGE STRESS This phase can amplify stress sensitivity. Engage in breathwork, meditation, or journaling to stay grounded and centered.
- EMBRACE WARMTH AND COMFORT A heating pad or warm Epsom salt bath can soothe cramps and help you unwind during the premenstrual days.
- STAY HYDRATED Combat bloating by drinking plenty of water and incorporating herbal teas like ginger, peppermint, or dandelion root.

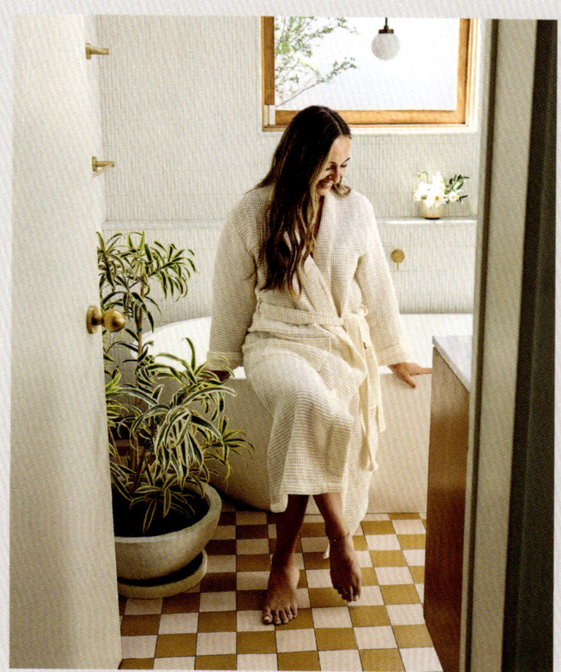

Understanding your luteal phase is about more than just managing symptoms; it's also about working with your body instead of against it. By prioritizing nourishing foods, gentle movement, and intentional self-care, you can enter each new cycle feeling more balanced, energized, and in tune with your body's natural rhythms.

Ideal Exercise Split

- STRENGTH TRAINING Focus on moderate-intensity sessions at the beginning of the luteal phase to maintain muscle health and support hormonal stability. Prioritize exercises with a steady, intentional pace, fully engaging your muscles through each movement rather than rushing through reps. Avoid excessive strain or high-impact training during this phase.
- YOGA OR PILATES As the phase progresses, transition into gentle, restorative activities like yoga or Pilates. These movements improve circulation, ease bloating, and help release physical and mental tension.
- LOW-IMPACT CARDIO Brisk walks or light jogging can help reduce cramps, boost mood, lower stress, and support overall well-being without overwhelming your system.

Sample Luteal Phase Meals

- BREAKFAST Sweet potato and kale hash with a fried egg or pumpkin spice overnight oats.
- LUNCH Moroccan chickpea tagine with quinoa or mushroom risotto with roasted asparagus.
- DINNER Salmon tacos or creamy butternut squash pasta with sautéed spinach.
- SNACKS Pumpkin seed date bark or chocolate-covered banana bites.

Luteal Phase Superfoods

- SESAME SEEDS Rich in zinc and healthy fats, which support progesterone production and help balance hormones.
- EGGS High in protein and essential nutrients, supporting energy levels and hormone production.
- AVOCADO Rich in healthy fats, fiber, and potassium, supporting hormone balance and reducing bloating.
- PUMPKIN SEEDS High in magnesium and zinc, which help reduce PMS symptoms and support hormone health.
- SALMON Packed with omega-3 fatty acids, which reduce inflammation and support mood regulation.
- SWEET POTATOES High in complex carbohydrates and fiber, providing sustained energy and supporting digestion.
- DARK CHOCOLATE Contains magnesium and antioxidants, helping to reduce cravings and improve mood.
- BANANAS Excellent source of potassium, which helps reduce bloating and muscle cramps.
- SPINACH Rich in iron, magnesium, and vitamins A and C, promoting energy and reducing inflammation.

- WALNUTS High in omega-3 fatty acids and antioxidants, supporting brain health and reducing inflammation.
- CHIA SEEDS Packed with omega-3 fatty acids, fiber, and protein, supporting hormonal health and satiety.
- GINGER Anti-inflammatory and can help alleviate menstrual cramps and nausea.
- SUNFLOWER SEEDS Rich in vitamin E, magnesium, and selenium, aiding in hormonal balance and reducing inflammation.
- TURMERIC Contains curcumin, which has powerful anti-inflammatory properties.
- MUSHROOMS Rich in B vitamins and antioxidants, supporting immune health and reducing inflammation.
- BUTTERNUT SQUASH High in fiber and in vitamins A and C, supporting immune health and digestion.
- BLACK BEANS Great source of plant-based protein, fiber, and iron, supporting energy levels and digestion.
- APPLE Rich in fiber and antioxidants, aiding in digestion and reducing inflammation.
- CINNAMON Contains antioxidants and has anti-inflammatory properties, supporting blood sugar regulation.
- PUMPKIN High in fiber and in vitamins A and C, supporting immune health and digestion.
- COLLAGEN Supports skin, hair, nails, and joint health.
- BLUEBERRIES Packed with antioxidants and vitamin C, supporting immune health and reducing inflammation.
- DATES High in fiber, potassium, and antioxidants, supporting energy levels and digestion.
- CHICKPEAS Great source of plant-based protein and fiber, aiding in digestion and hormonal balance.

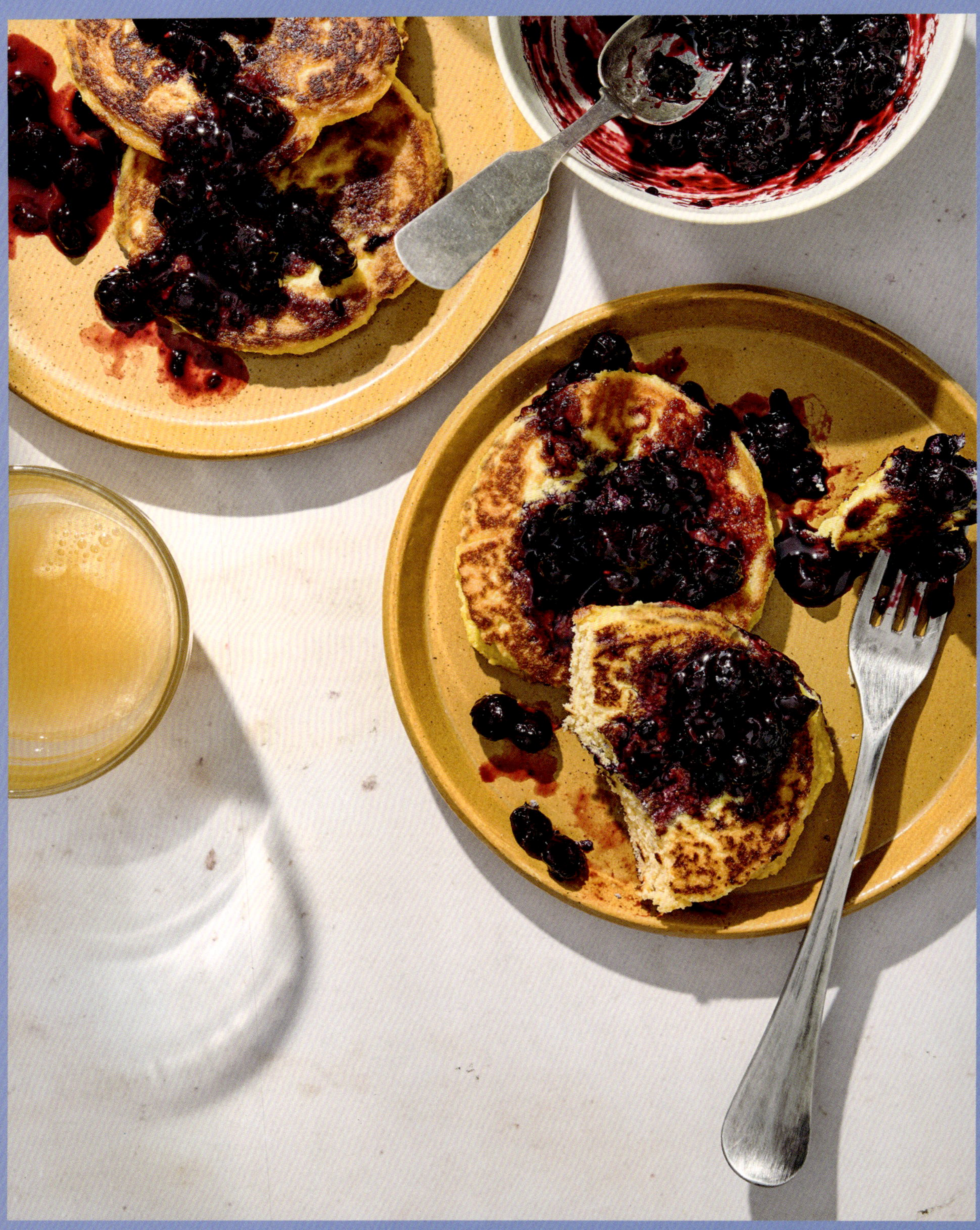

Breakfasts

Slow Mornings Sweet Potato and Kale Breakfast Hash

Serves 1
Prep Time: 10 minutes
Cook Time: 25 minutes

I first threw this together on a Sunday morning with a fridge full of leftovers, and it quickly became my go-to when I want something filling and delicious. The balance of crispy sweet potatoes and tender kale hits all the right textures. Sweet potatoes are a slow-digesting carb, which means they release energy gradually into the bloodstream. This helps stabilize blood sugar levels, reducing the fatigue and irritability that can peak during the luteal phase. The kale adds a boost of calcium and magnesium, which can ease muscle tension and support progesterone production. However, it's important to note that raw kale can be tough to digest and may cause bloating or discomfort during this time, so be sure to cook it. When I'm feeling adventurous, I swap the kale for Swiss chard or throw in some leftover roasted veggies, always finishing it off with a fun sauce like pesto (see recipe on page 109), salsa, or hot sauce!

1 tablespoon olive oil
1 medium sweet potato, diced
½ teaspoon smoked paprika, or more as desired
½ teaspoon salt
½ teaspoon freshly ground black pepper
1 cup stemmed and roughly chopped fresh kale
1 garlic clove, minced
2 large eggs
Hot sauce of choice (optional)

1 — Heat the olive oil in a medium skillet over medium heat. Add the sweet potato, ½ teaspoon smoked paprika, and the salt and pepper. Cook for 12 to 15 minutes, stirring occasionally, until the sweet potato is tender and slightly crisp on the edges.

2 — Add the kale and garlic to the skillet. Sauté for 3 to 4 minutes, stirring frequently, until the kale wilts and the garlic is fragrant.

3 — Make two small wells in the hash. Crack an egg into each well and reduce the heat to low. Cover the skillet and cook for 4 to 5 minutes, or until the eggs are set to your liking (soft yolks are highly recommended!).

4 — Serve warm, garnished with an extra pinch of smoked paprika or a drizzle of hot sauce, if desired.

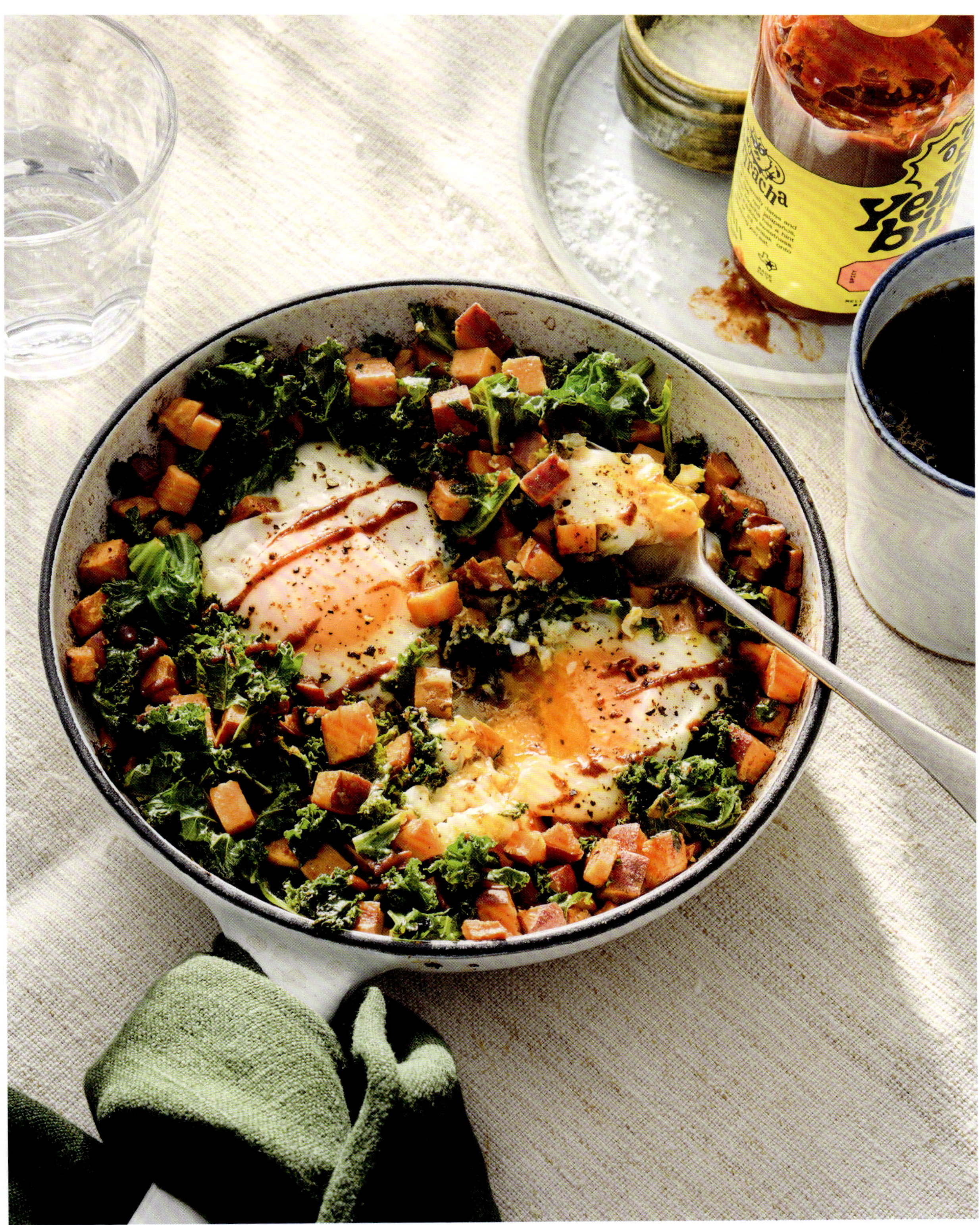

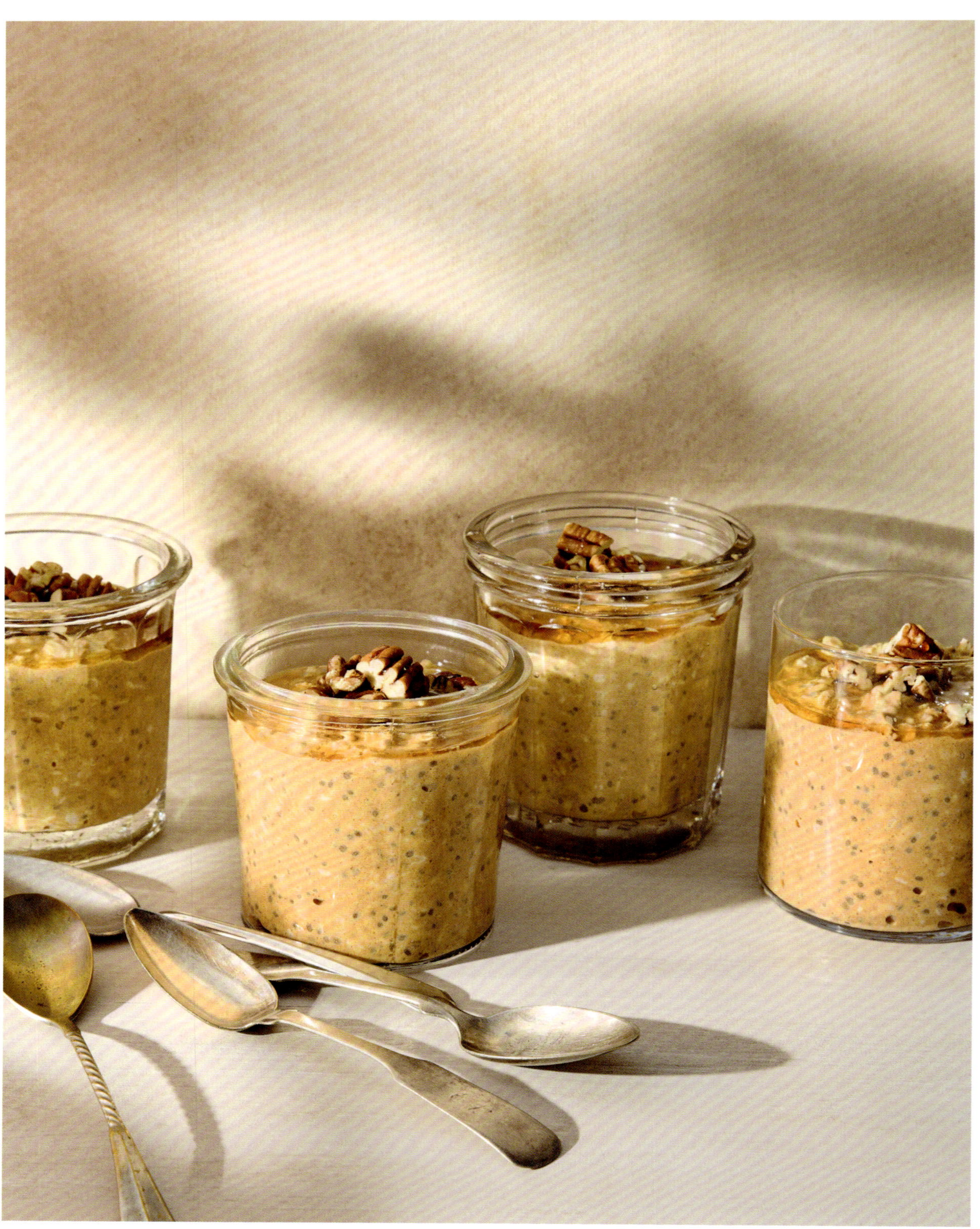

Pumpkin Spice Overnight Oats

Serves 4

Prep Time: 5 minutes, plus overnight chilling

Your luteal phase is like your inner autumn—a time to slow down, get cozy, and lean into foods that ground and nourish you. As with your favorite fall recipes, this one is packed with warming spices like cinnamon and pumpkin pie spice, enhancing circulation and supporting digestion, which can slow down due to rising progesterone. Pumpkin is rich in beta-carotene, encouraging progesterone production and overall hormone balance. Overnight oats are also a great option for meal prep, requiring virtually no effort in the morning, and so allowing you to sleep in a bit longer while still providing deep nourishment! This recipe will give you 4 servings. Continue to store them in the fridge until ready to eat, up to a week.

2 cups old-fashioned rolled oats
2 cups unsweetened almond milk
1 cup pumpkin puree
1 cup plain Greek yogurt (or dairy-free alternative)
2 teaspoons pumpkin pie spice
2 teaspoons ground cinnamon
4 tablespoons chia seeds
4 teaspoons pure maple syrup
¼ cup chopped pecans (optional)

1 — In a large bowl or container, combine the oats, almond milk, pumpkin puree, yogurt, pumpkin pie spice, cinnamon, chia seeds, and maple syrup. Stir well to ensure all the ingredients are evenly mixed.

2 — Divide the mixture evenly into 4 jars or containers. Cover and refrigerate overnight (or at least 6 hours).

3 — In the morning, grab a jar, give the oats a stir. Top with chopped pecans, if desired. Serve and enjoy!

Apple Cinnamon Quinoa Porridge

Serves 1
Prep Time: 5 minutes
Cook Time: 7 minutes

Mornings can be hectic, but I love having little rituals that make them feel special—especially during the luteal phase, when slowing down and nourishing my body are both key. This quinoa porridge is my way of diversifying beyond oats—and now it's a weekly staple! Cooking apples releases their pectin, a type of soluble fiber that not only supports digestion but also helps calm any bloating that can occur during this phase. The warmth of this dish is perfect for soothing PMS symptoms, improving circulation, and easing tension. There's just something about a comforting cinnamon-spiced bowl that makes everything feel a little easier. I love finishing it off with almond butter or toasted coconut for that extra cozy touch!

½ cup cooked quinoa
½ cup unsweetened almond milk
½ apple, cored and diced
½ teaspoon ground cinnamon
1 teaspoon honey
1 tablespoon chopped walnuts (optional)

1 — Add the quinoa, almond milk, apple, and cinnamon to a small saucepan and place over medium heat. Cook for 5 to 7 minutes, stirring occasionally, until warmed through and slightly thickened. Transfer to a medium bowl.

2 — Stir in the honey and top with the walnuts, if desired.

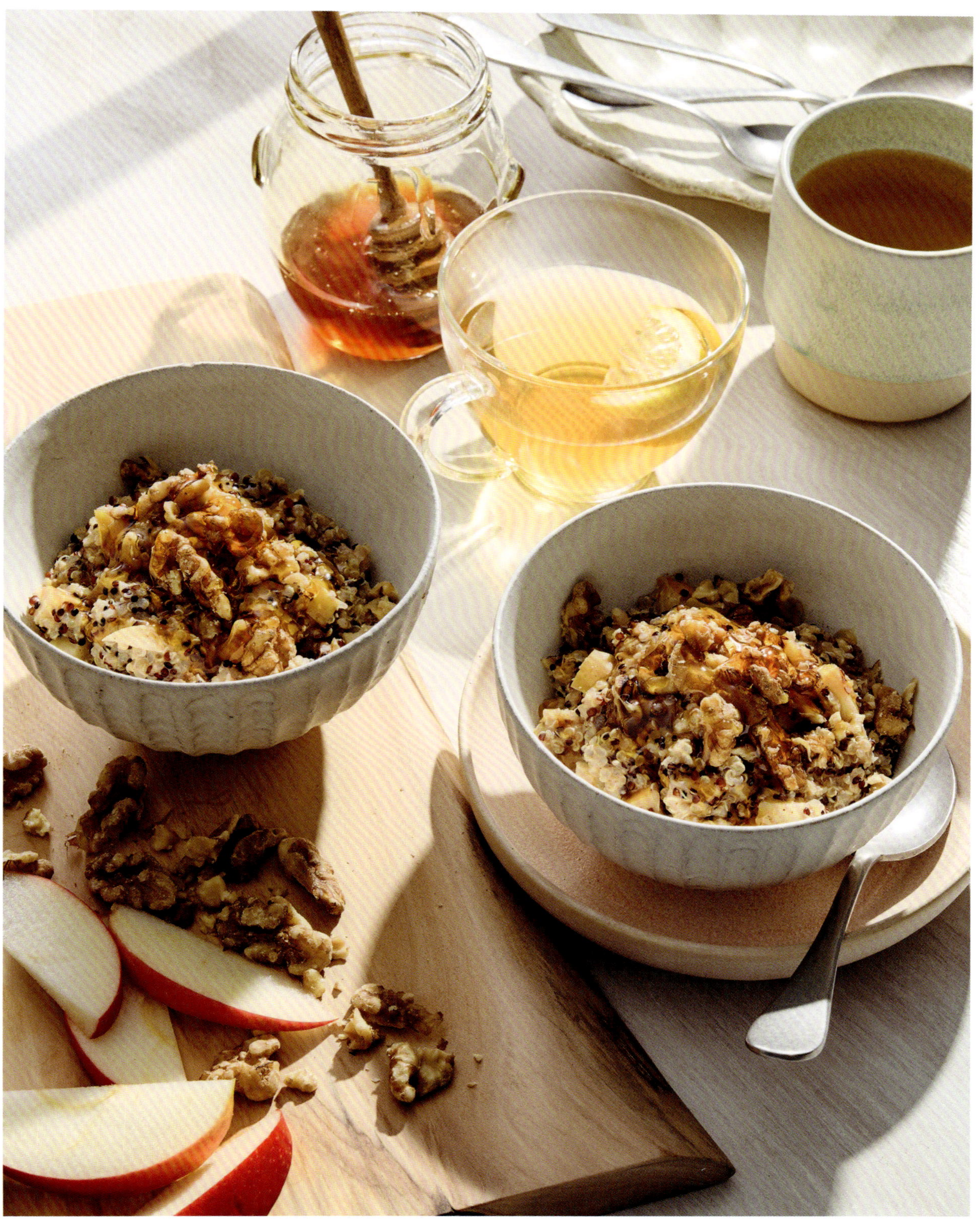

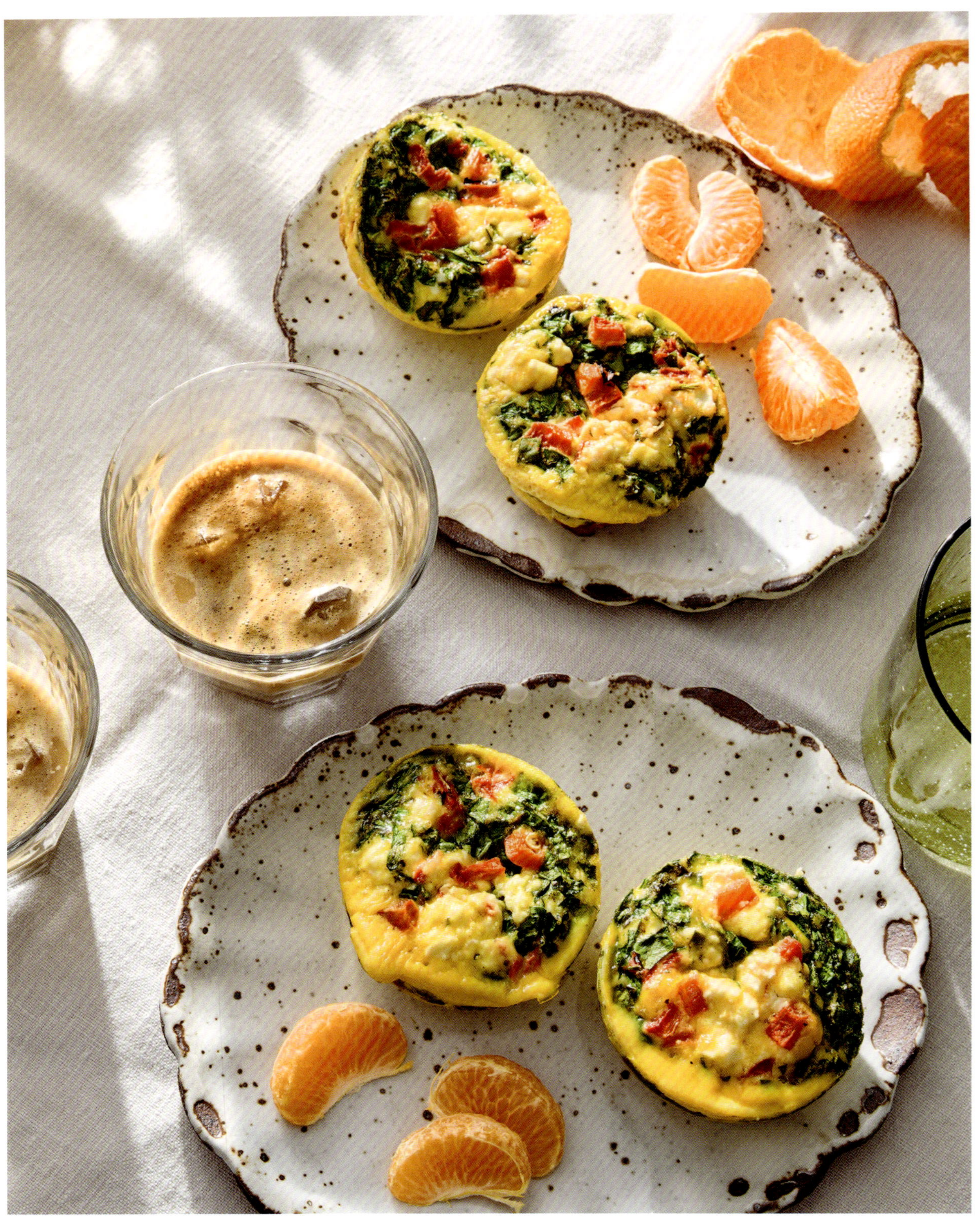

Rooted and Ready Egg Muffins

Makes 12 muffins
Prep Time: 10 minutes
Cook Time: 20 minutes

During the latter half of the luteal phase, when energy and motivation to cook in the morning are at a low, these egg muffins become such a lifesaver! The combo of eggs and spinach is perfect for those days when progesterone is on the rise, and your body craves protein and magnesium. Magnesium, found in spinach, helps ease muscle tension and supports hormone metabolism—both so important during this phase. The tangy feta adds a savory balance to the richness of the eggs. They take no effort: Just toss everything in a bowl, mix, and bake. I love making a batch on Sundays, so I have a protein-packed, grab-and-go breakfast ready for the busy week ahead! Note: A serving is 2 muffins.

12 large eggs
1½ cups chopped fresh spinach
½ cup crumbled feta cheese
½ cup finely chopped roasted red pepper
½ teaspoon garlic powder
1 teaspoon fresh thyme leaves (or ½ teaspoon dried thyme)
1½ teaspoons salt
1½ teaspoons freshly ground black pepper

1 — Preheat the oven to 375°F. Lightly grease a 12-cup muffin tin.

2 — In a large bowl, whisk together the eggs, spinach, feta, red pepper, garlic powder, thyme, salt, and pepper.

3 — Divide the mixture evenly among the 12 muffin cups and bake for 18 to 20 minutes, or until the eggs are set.

4 — Once cooled, remove from the tin and store in an airtight glass container in the refrigerator until ready to consume. Feel free to eat cold or reheat in the microwave or toaster oven.

Coconut Flour Collagen Pancakes with Mixed Berry Compote

Serves 2
Prep Time: 5 minutes
Cook Time: 25 minutes

My luteal phase makes me crave slow and cozy mornings, extra time in bed, a warm mug in hand, and pancakes. These pancakes, made with collagen and coconut flour, are light yet satisfying—nourishing without feeling heavy. Collagen is rich in amino acids like glycine and proline, which support gut health, lower inflammation, and help your body produce the hormones it needs during this second half of your cycle. Coconut flour is high in fiber and naturally low in carbs, making it great for stabilizing blood sugar! They pair beautifully with a spiced chai or warm cinnamon tea!

---

1 cup mixed fresh berries
2 teaspoons honey
½ cup coconut flour
1 teaspoon baking powder
4 large eggs
½ cup unsweetened almond milk
2 scoops collagen powder
1 tablespoon butter or coconut oil

1 — Add the berries and honey to a small saucepan and place over low heat. Allow the berries to cook for 8 to 10 minutes, gently mashing with a spoon and stirring as they cook. The berries will break down and begin to thicken, releasing their juices. You'll know it's ready when the mixture has thickened to a syrup-like consistency, but still has a little texture from the fruit (not too watery, but not totally smooth, either). If it's too runny, cook it a little longer until it thickens. Once done, remove from the heat and set aside.

2 — In a large bowl, combine the coconut flour, baking powder, eggs, almond milk, and collagen powder. Mix until smooth. The batter will be thicker than regular pancake batter, so don't be concerned if it feels dense—it's just the nature of coconut flour!

3 — Heat a large nonstick skillet over medium heat and lightly grease with the butter or coconut oil. Pour a few tablespoons of batter into the pan at a time, forming small pancakes. Cook for 2 to 3 minutes until golden brown. Flip carefully (since the pancakes can be a bit delicate) and cook the other side, another 2 to 3 minutes. Repeat with the remaining batter.

4 — Stack the pancakes on a plate and top with the warm berry compote. Enjoy!

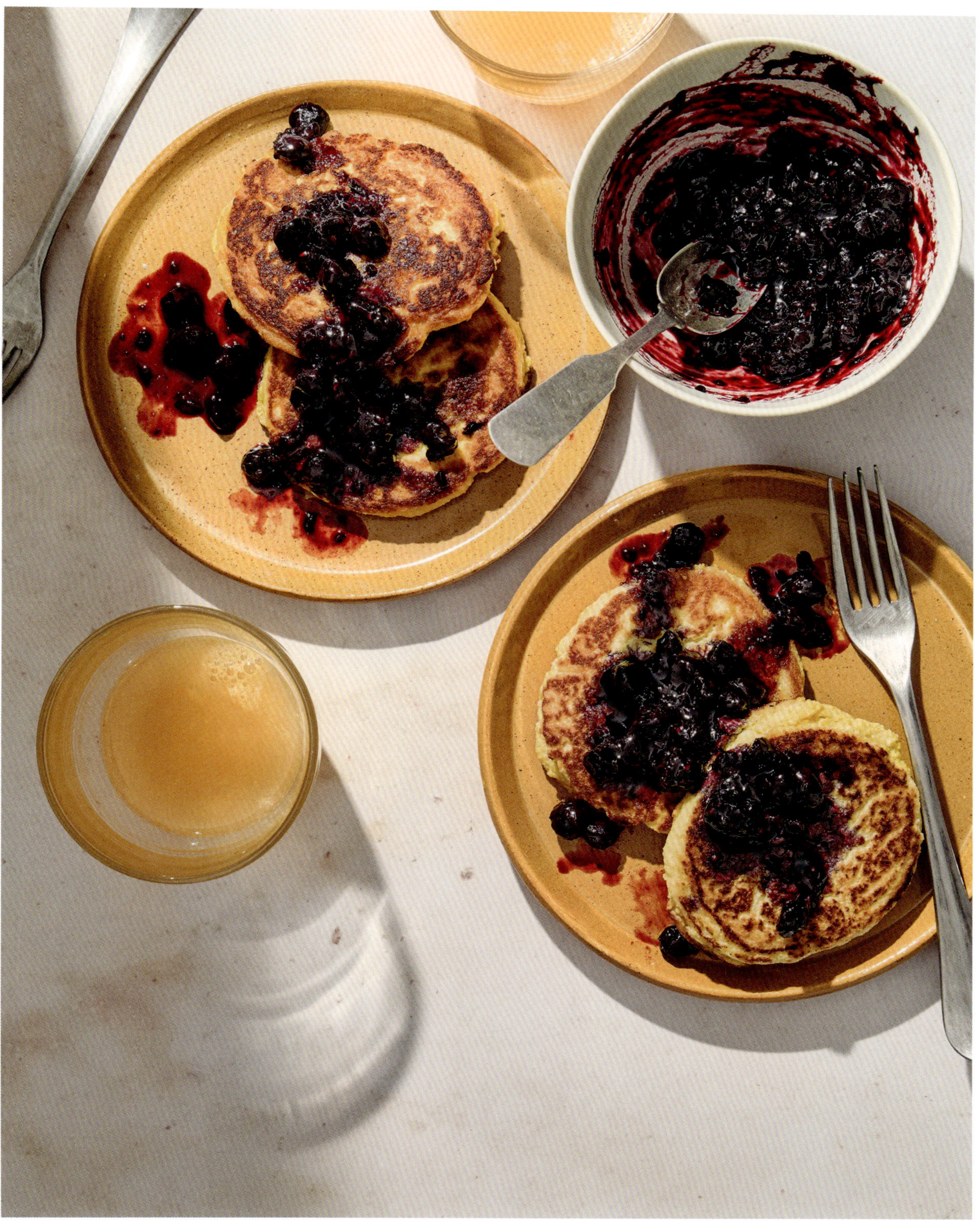

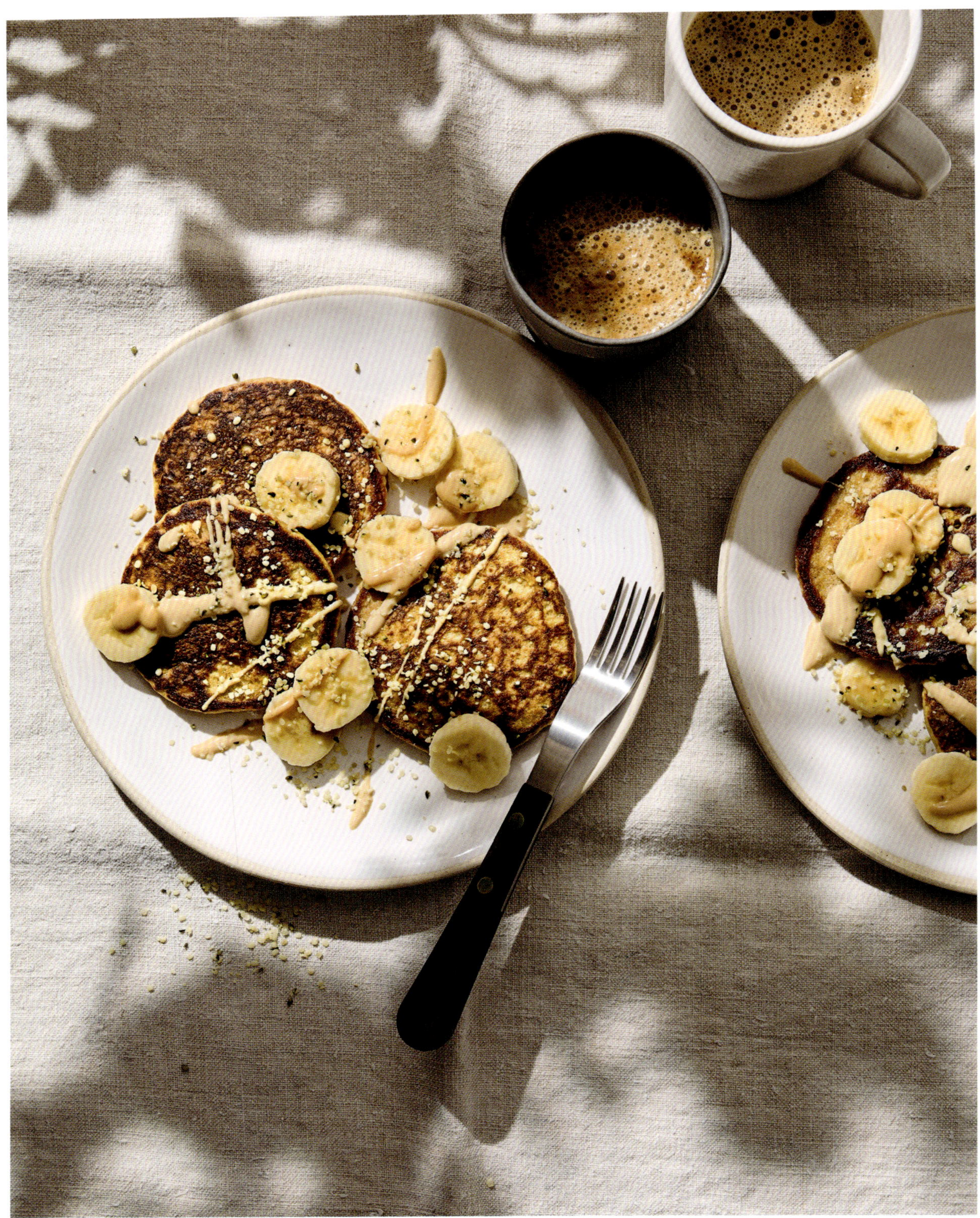

Banana-Oat Pancakes with Nut Butter Drizzle

Serves 2
Prep Time: 5 minutes
Cook Time: 10 minutes

In my opinion, you can never have enough pancakes for those slow, warming luteal phase mornings—that's why I'm including two recipes in this chapter! These are the best because you just throw everything in a blender—it's easy cleanup, minimal effort, and perfect when you just want a single-serve stack. Bananas are high in potassium, which helps counter bloating and water retention (luteal phase win); the complex carbs from the oats keep blood sugar stable, helping to prevent energy crashes; and the cinnamon adds that warmth element I like to talk about in this phase! These hit the spot every time!

1 ripe banana, mashed
2 large eggs
½ cup old-fashioned rolled oats
½ teaspoon ground cinnamon
½ teaspoon baking powder
½ teaspoon vanilla extract
Pinch of sea salt
1 tablespoon avocado oil or coconut oil
2 tablespoons almond butter or peanut butter
1 teaspoon pure maple syrup
1 tablespoon cacao nibs
1 tablespoon hemp seeds

1 — In a blender, place the banana, eggs, oats, cinnamon, baking powder, vanilla, and salt. Blend until smooth.

2 — Heat a large nonstick skillet over medium heat and add the avocado or coconut oil.

3 — Pour small rounds of batter into the skillet and cook for 2 to 3 minutes, until bubbles form on the surface. Flip and cook for another 1 to 2 minutes. Repeat with the remaining batter.

4 — Mix the nut butter with the maple syrup and microwave for about 10 seconds, until it reaches a sauce-like consistency.

5 — Drizzle the sauce over the pancakes and sprinkle with the cacao nibs and hemp seeds.

Flaxseed "Oatmeal" Bowl

Serves 1
Prep Time: 5 minutes
Cook Time: 5 minutes

Flaxseed "oatmeal" is one of my favorite ways to switch up my usual oatmeal bowl! It's grain-free, loaded with fiber to support digestion and hormone detox, and packed with omega-3s from flax seeds to help fight inflammation and support progesterone levels. I love topping mine with raspberries, blueberries, a drizzle of honey, and a big scoop of nut butter (coconut butter is my favorite for a rich and slightly sweet addition)!

---

2 tablespoons ground flaxseed

1 tablespoon chia seeds

½ cup unsweetened almond milk or full-fat coconut milk

½ teaspoon ground cinnamon

½ teaspoon vanilla extract

1 teaspoon pure maple syrup or raw honey (optional)

1 tablespoon almond butter, peanut butter, or coconut butter, or more as desired

¼ cup fresh berries

1 teaspoon hemp seeds, for topping (optional)

1 — In a small saucepan over low heat, combine the flaxseed, chia seeds, and milk. Stir well.

2 — Add the cinnamon, vanilla, and maple syrup (if using). Stir continuously for 2 to 3 minutes, until the mixture thickens.

3 — Remove the pan from the heat and stir in the almond butter for extra creaminess.

4 — Transfer to a bowl and top with the berries and hemp seeds, if desired. Enjoy warm with a spoonful of extra nut butter, if desired!

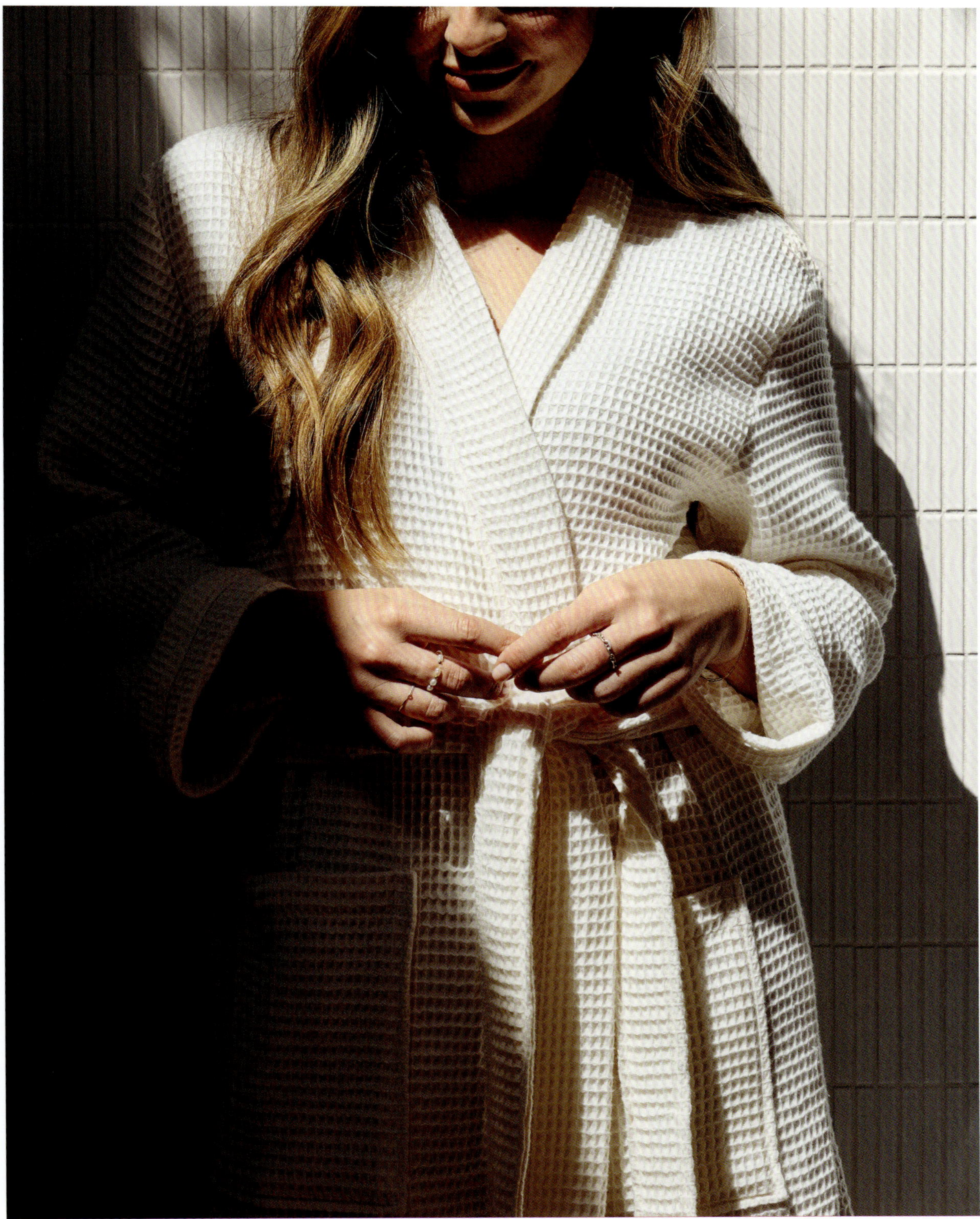

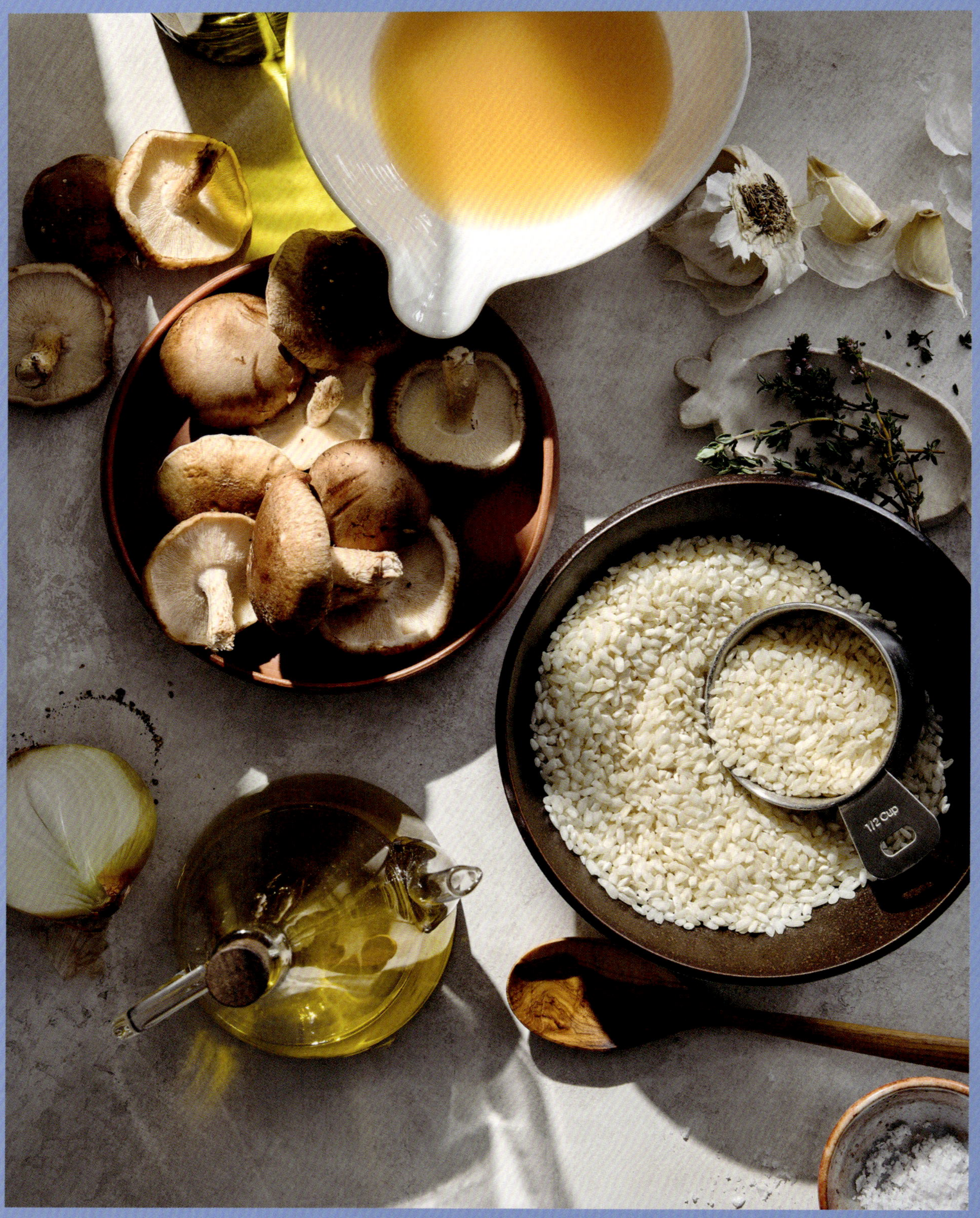
1/2 Cup

Lunches & Dinners

Warming Wild Mushroom Bowl

Serves 4

Prep Time: 10 minutes

Cook Time: 40 minutes

As my body shifts into its inner fall, I begin craving warming, comforting dinners. Risotto has always been one of my favorites, but the traditional version often leaves me feeling sluggish, so I created this nourishing, dairy-free take that's just as creamy and satisfying. Slow-cooked rice and mineral-rich bone broth make it easy on digestion while supporting gut health, and mushrooms provide selenium, a key mineral for progesterone production. The mix of earthy mushrooms, fresh thyme, and velvety texture makes this dish feel indulgent in the best way—comforting but never too heavy.

4 cups bone broth
1 tablespoon ghee (or olive oil)
1 small onion, finely chopped
2 garlic cloves, minced
1 cup arborio rice
½ cup dry white wine (optional)
Olive oil
2 cups sliced fresh mushrooms (such as cremini or shiitake)
1 teaspoon fresh or dried thyme leaves, or more as desired
Salt and freshly ground black pepper
2 tablespoons nutritional yeast (optional)

1 — In a medium saucepan, gently heat the bone broth over low heat while you prepare the rest of the dish. (Keeping the broth warm will help the rice absorb it more easily as you cook.)

2 — Heat the ghee in a large, deep saucepan over medium heat. Add the onion and cook for 4 to 5 minutes, until softened. Add the garlic and cook for an additional 1 to 2 minutes, until fragrant.

3 — Stir in the rice and cook, stirring constantly, for 1 to 2 minutes. This helps the rice release its starch and creates the creamy texture of risotto. If using wine, pour it in now and cook for 2 to 3 minutes, until absorbed.

4 — Begin adding the warm bone broth one ladleful at a time, stirring continuously. Allow each ladle of broth to be absorbed before adding more. Continue this process for 20 to 25 minutes, until the rice is tender and creamy, but still slightly firm to the bite. Stir occasionally to prevent sticking.

5 — While the rice is cooking, heat a large skillet over medium heat and add a splash of olive oil. Add the mushrooms and cook for 5 to 7 minutes, stirring occasionally, until golden and tender.

6 — When the rice is cooked, stir in the sautéed mushrooms, then the thyme and salt and pepper to taste. If you're using nutritional yeast, stir it in at this point for a savory, cheesy flavor.

7 — Spoon the risotto into bowls, garnish with extra thyme, if desired, and serve warm.

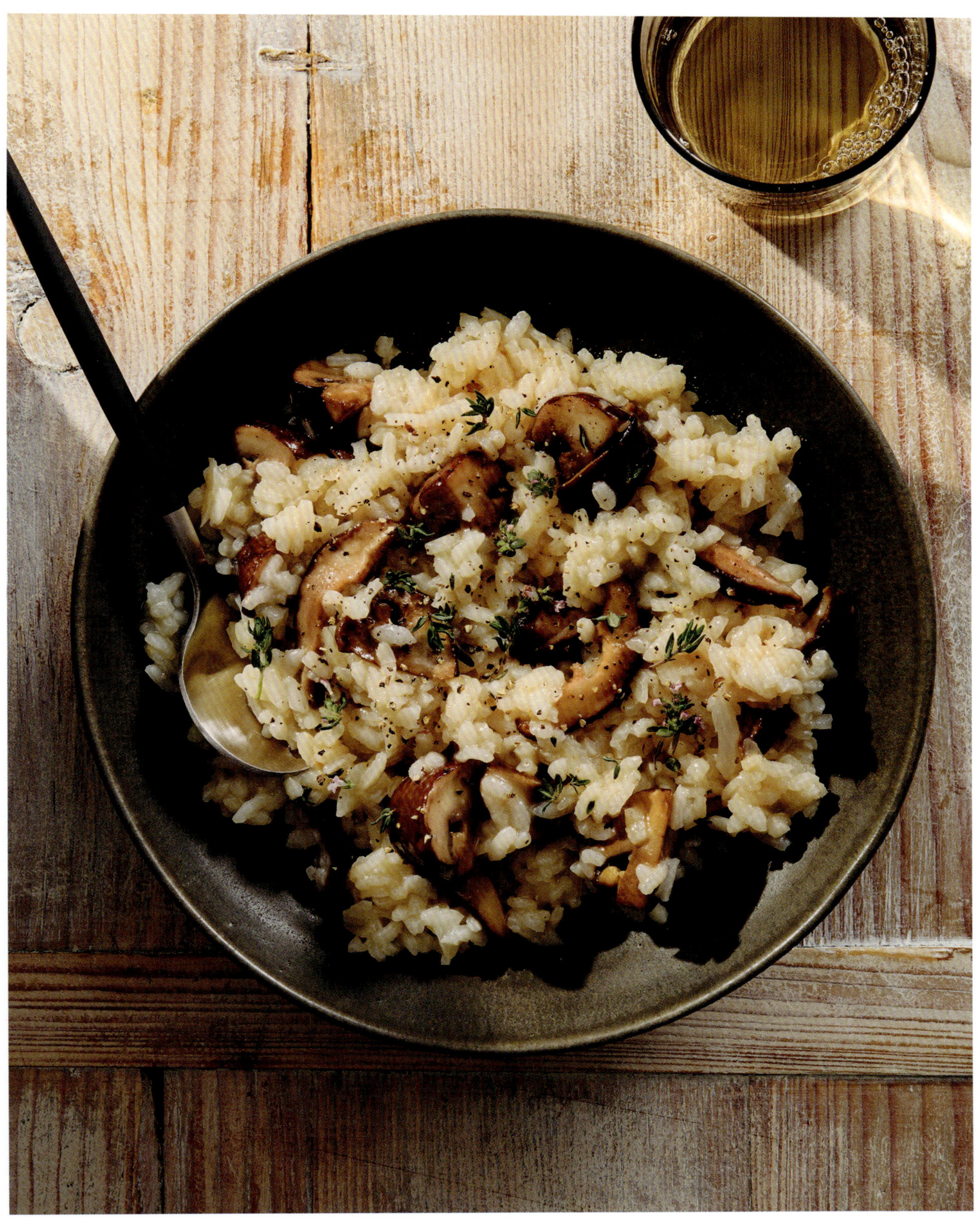

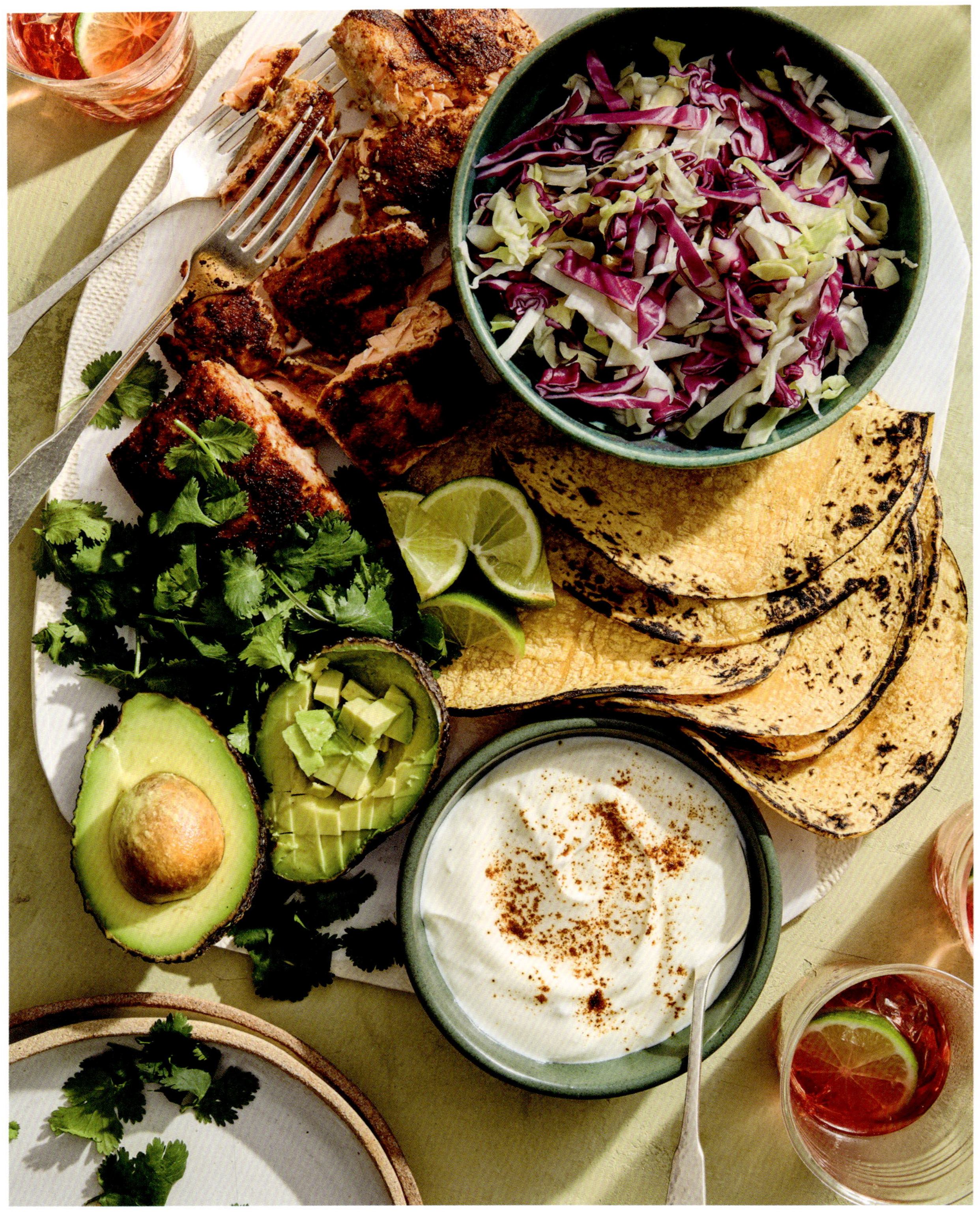

Soothe and Savor Salmon Tacos

This recipe was inspired by one of my favorite taco stands in San Diego, known for its incredible fish tacos. I love getting creative with how I use salmon, especially since I make a point of getting plenty of it during the luteal phase. Salmon is packed with omega-3s to help reduce inflammation and ease bloating, while the healthy fats and protein keep blood sugar steady—and that helps prevent the energy crashes and cravings that can hit during this time. The tangy lime juice boosts iron absorption, and the crisp cabbage brings fiber to support digestion and hormone detox. I love topping my tacos with avocado for extra creaminess and Greek yogurt for a gut-friendly sour cream swap. Pair these with a chilled hibiscus tea and pretend you're by the beach! Note: A serving is 2 tacos.

Serves 4
Prep Time: 10 minutes
Cook Time: 15 minutes

4 salmon fillets, about 4 ounces each
1 tablespoon olive oil
1 teaspoon chili powder
½ teaspoon smoked paprika
Juice of 1 lime
8 small (6-inch) corn tortillas
1 cup shredded red or green cabbage (red adds a pop of color and extra antioxidants!)
¼ cup cilantro leaves, chopped
Optional toppings: avocado slices, plain Greek yogurt

1 — Preheat the oven to 400°F. Line a baking sheet with parchment paper.

2 — Pat the salmon fillets dry and place them on the baking sheet. Brush with the olive oil, then sprinkle with the chili powder and smoked paprika. Add a squeeze of lime over the fillets.

3 — Bake for 12 to 15 minutes, until the salmon flakes easily with a fork. Let it rest for a few minutes, then use a fork to break it into bite-size pieces.

4 — Warm the tortillas by heating them in a dry skillet over medium heat for about 30 seconds per side, or by wrapping them in a damp paper towel and microwaving for 20 to 30 seconds.

5 — Fill each tortilla with some of the flaked salmon, then top each with some of the shredded cabbage and cilantro. Add the toppings, if desired. Serve immediately.

Moroccan Chickpea Tagine

Serves 4
Prep Time: 10 minutes
Cook Time: 30 minutes

At the beginning of this chapter, I talked about how warmth is the name of the game during the luteal phase, and one of the easiest ways to bring warmth to your meals is with spices. This cozy one-pot tagine is inspired by traditional Moroccan flavors, but has a few updates for weeknight cooking. And it's packed with cinnamon, cumin, and turmeric—all of which support circulation and digestion. Chickpeas and sweet potatoes provide fiber and slow-burning carbs to keep your energy stable, while the apricots add a natural sweetness and a boost of iron to support your body before your period. For the sweet potato, I recommend peeling it for a smoother texture, but you can leave the skin on, if you prefer more fiber and a slightly earthier taste. For serving suggestions, I love to top the tagine with a dollop of unsweetened yogurt for creaminess, fresh cilantro for brightness, or toasted almonds for extra crunch. Plus, it's an easy cleanup meal—because who has the extra brain space for dishes right now?

1 tablespoon olive oil
1 small onion, chopped
2 garlic cloves, minced
1 teaspoon ground cumin
1 teaspoon ground cinnamon
½ teaspoon ground turmeric
¼ teaspoon cayenne pepper (optional)
1 medium sweet potato, peeled and diced
1 (15-ounce) can chickpeas, drained and rinsed
1 (15-ounce) can diced tomatoes
¼ cup chopped dried apricots
½ cup bone broth
Salt and freshly ground black pepper
Optional toppings: plain Greek yogurt, chopped cilantro, sliced almonds

1 — Place a large pot over medium heat and add the olive oil. When the oil is hot, add the onion and garlic, cooking for 1 to 2 minutes, until softened.

2 — Stir in the cloves, cumin, cinnamon, turmeric, and cayenne (if using) and cook for 1 minute, until fragrant.

3 — Add the sweet potato, chickpeas, tomatoes, apricots, broth, and salt and pepper to taste. Stir and let simmer for 20 to 25 minutes, until the sweet potatoes are tender.

4 — Ladle into bowls and top with the optional yogurt, cilantro, or almonds, or enjoy as is!

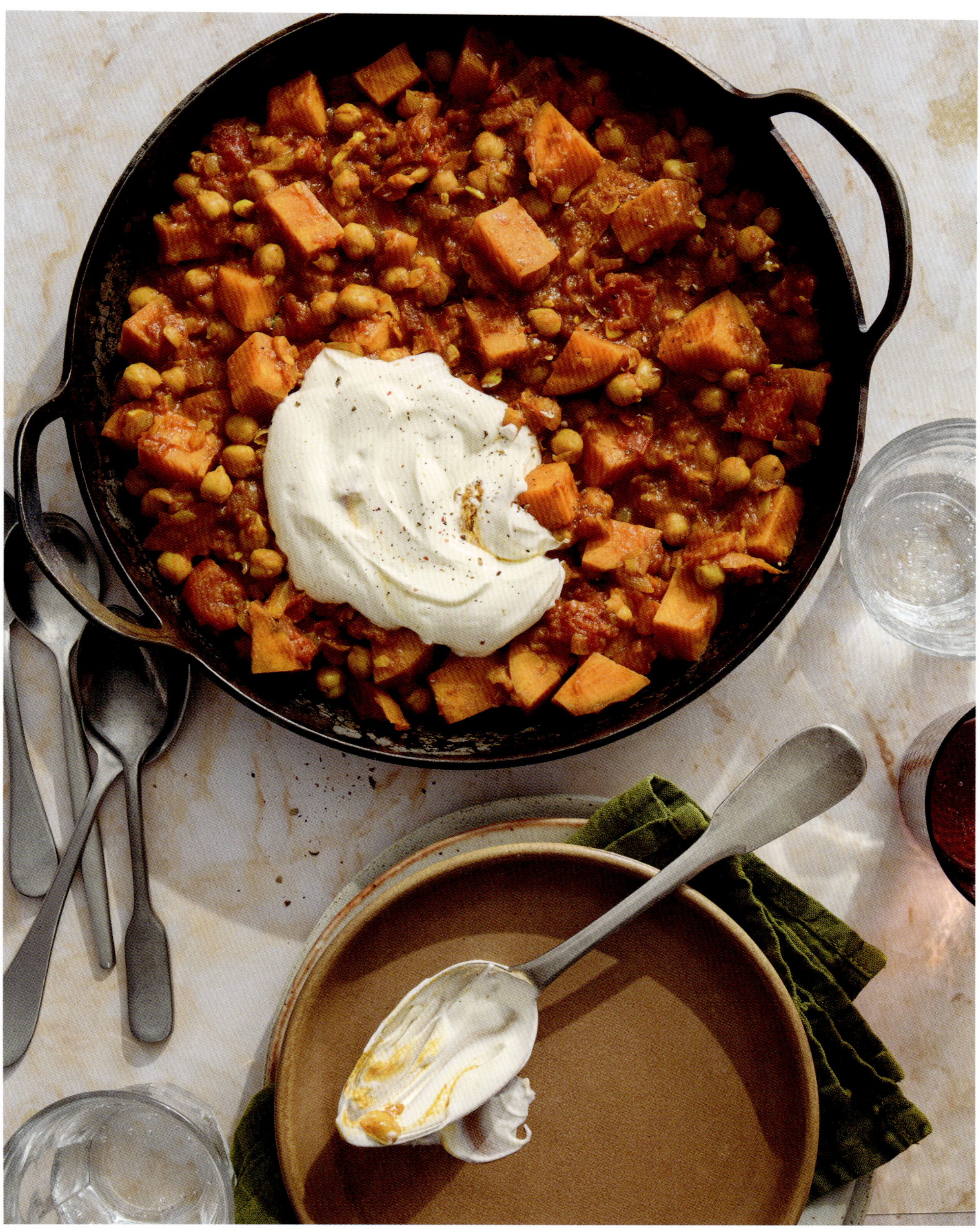

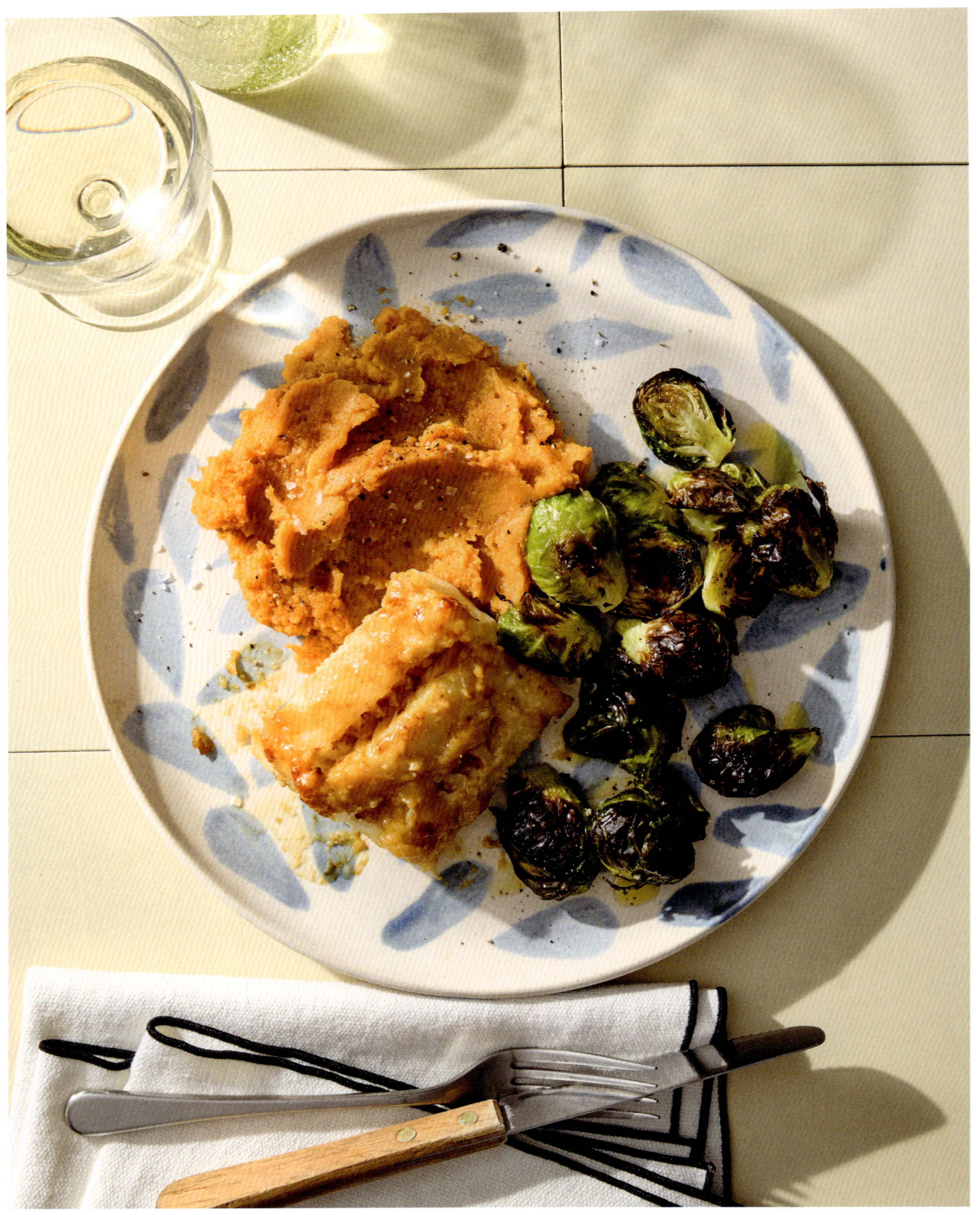

Baked Cod with Miso, Roasted Brussels Sprouts, and Sweet Potato Mash

Serves 4

Prep Time: 10 minutes

Cook Time: 55 minutes

This recipe came together one night when I realized how often I reach for sweet potatoes during my luteal phase—they're just so grounding and nourishing! Paired with fiber-packed Brussels sprouts and cod, which is rich in lean protein, this meal helps balance your blood sugar and keep your energy steady. The miso glaze brings out all the flavors and offers probiotics to support digestion, which is often sluggish in this phase. With a little sweetness from the maple syrup and a zing from the rice vinegar, this dish is comforting, easy to make, and supports everything your body needs during the luteal phase.

- 2 large sweet potatoes, peeled and cubed
- 2 tablespoons olive oil
- Salt and freshly ground black pepper
- 1 pound Brussels sprouts, trimmed and halved
- 2 tablespoons white miso paste
- 1 tablespoon pure maple syrup
- 1 tablespoon rice vinegar
- 4 cod fillets, about 4 ounces each

1 — Fill a large pot with water and bring to a boil. Add the sweet potatoes, reduce the heat to a simmer, and cook for 12 to 15 minutes, until fork-tender. Drain and transfer to a medium bowl, then mash with 1 tablespoon of the olive oil and salt and pepper to taste. Cover and keep warm.

2 — Preheat the oven to 400°F. Line a baking sheet with parchment paper for the sprouts. For the fish, have a greased baking dish handy.

3 — In a large bowl, toss the Brussels sprouts with the remaining tablespoon olive oil and some salt and pepper to taste, then spread the sprouts on the baking sheet. Place the baking sheet on the rack in the upper third of the oven. Roast for 25 minutes, turning halfway through.

4 — In a small bowl, mix the miso paste, maple syrup, and rice vinegar until smooth.

5 — Place the cod fillets in the baking dish and brush the miso glaze evenly over them. Place the baking dish on the rack in the lower third of the oven and bake for 12 to 15 minutes, until the fish flakes easily with a fork.

6 — Divide the sweet potato mash and Brussels sprouts among the serving plates, then top each with a cod fillet, and serve.

Chicken Meatball and Root Veggie Sheet-Pan Bake with Maple-Tahini Dressing

Serves 4
Prep Time: 15 minutes
Cook Time: 30 minutes

Clearly, easy cleanup is a big win during the luteal phase because, let's face it, our motivation can be low when we aren't feeling our best. That's why I rely on sheet-pan dinners! There's something nostalgic about roasted root veggies; they remind me of the cozy fall dinners I had when I was growing up, when the kitchen smelled like caramelized sweet potatoes and warm spices. Pairing the veggies with juicy, herby chicken meatballs makes this meal feel hearty without being heavy. And the maple-tahini dressing is the perfect mix of creamy, sweet, and nutty. This meal is another great one for meal prep; just store the extras in an airtight container and enjoy them throughout the week. This is comfort food with a hormone-supportive twist!

Meatballs

1 pound ground chicken
¼ cup almond flour
1 large egg
1 teaspoon garlic powder
1 teaspoon onion powder
½ teaspoon smoked paprika
Salt and freshly ground black pepper

Veggies

1 medium sweet potato, peeled and cubed
2 medium carrots, sliced
1 medium parsnip, peeled and cubed
1 tablespoon olive oil
Salt and freshly ground black pepper

Maple-Tahini Dressing

¼ cup tahini
1 tablespoon pure maple syrup
1 tablespoon freshly squeezed lemon juice
Pinch of salt
Chopped fresh parsley, for serving

1 — Preheat the oven to 400°F and line a sheet pan with parchment paper.

2 — Make the meatballs: In a large bowl, combine the chicken, almond flour, egg, garlic and onion powders, smoked paprika, and salt and pepper to taste. Mix with a wooden spoon or clean hands until well combined. Form into 1-inch meatballs and place the meatballs on one side of the sheet pan.

3 — Prepare the veggies: In a large bowl, toss the sweet potato, carrots, and parsnip with the olive oil and salt and pepper to taste. Spread the veggies on the other side of the sheet pan.

4 — Roast the meatballs and veggies for 25 to 30 minutes, flipping halfway through.

5 — Meanwhile, make the dressing: In a small bowl, whisk together the tahini, maple syrup, lemon juice, and a pinch of salt, then starting with about a teaspoon of water, thin to desired consistency.

6 — When the meatballs and veggies are finished, transfer them to serving plates and drizzle the dressing over them. Garnish with parsley, if desired, and serve.

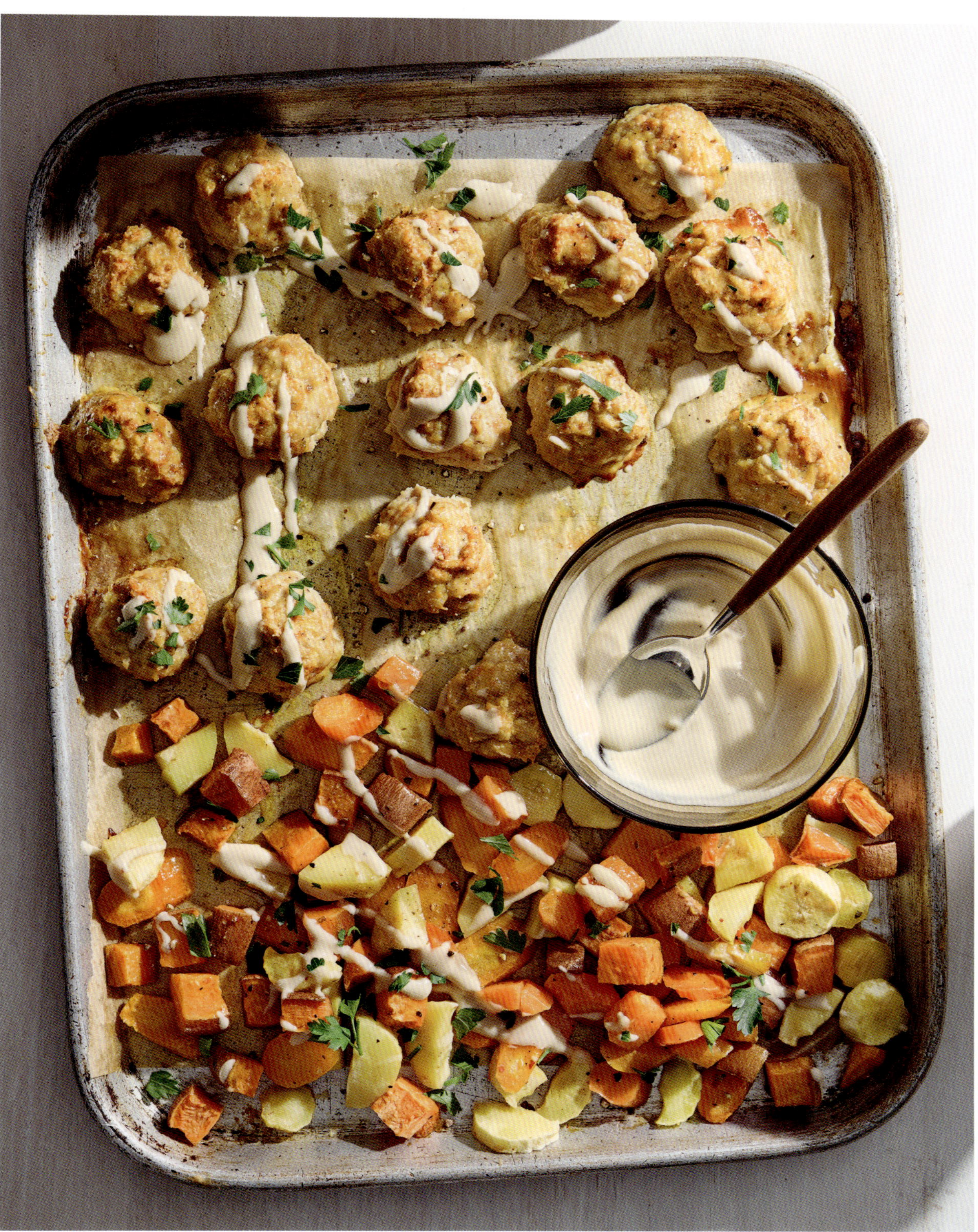

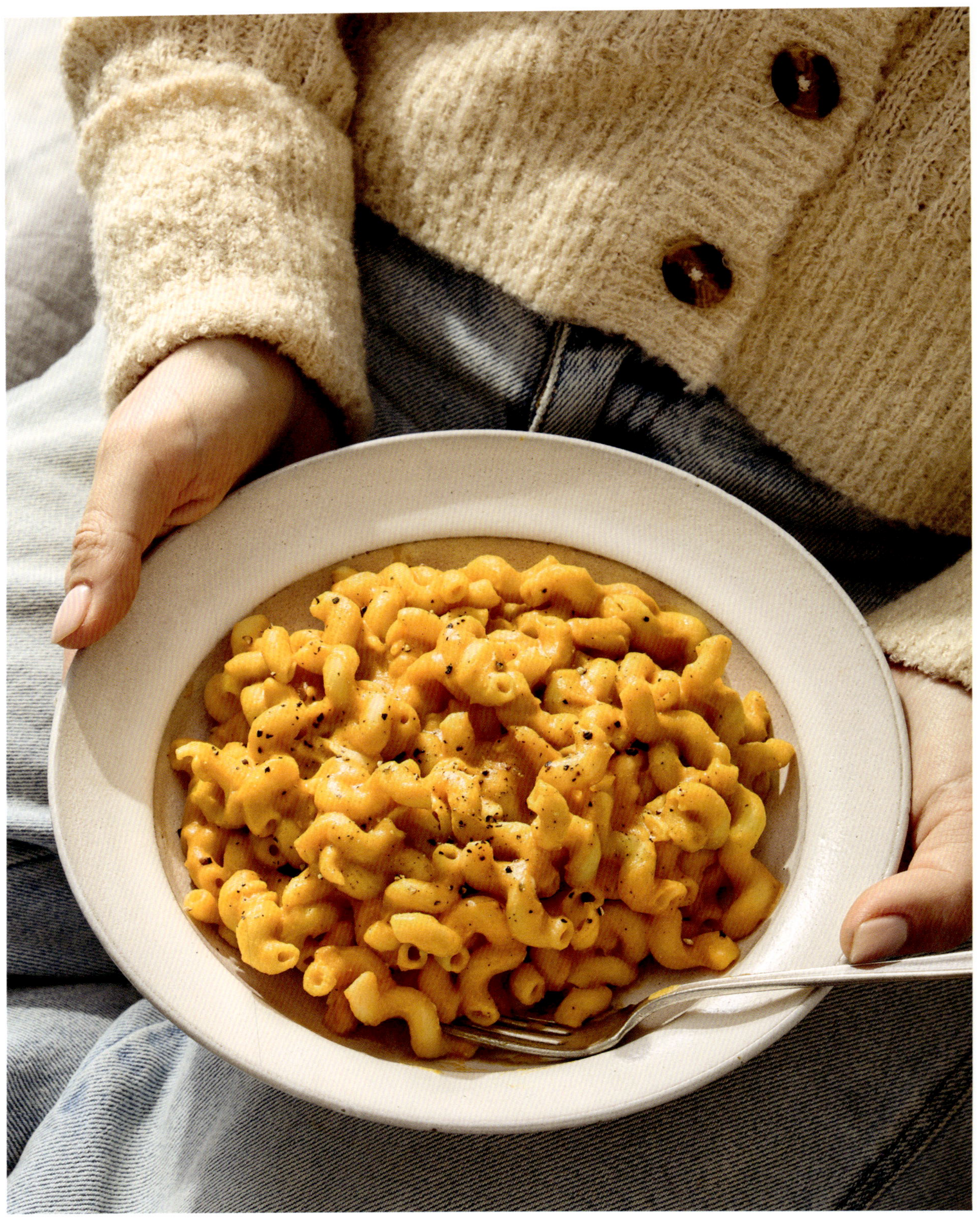

Creamy Butternut Squash Pasta

I used to think creamy pasta was a once-in-a-while indulgence, but this version with butternut squash changed the game. It's rich, velvety, and feels like comfort in a bowl—yet it's secretly packed with everything your body craves during the luteal phase. Fiber, protein, and warming spices work together to have you feeling full and grounded, while nutritional yeast adds a cheesy depth and a boost of B vitamins to support mood and energy. A hint of nutmeg brings that nostalgic, cozy fall flavor, making every bite feel like a hug. I love making this on a slower evening, lighting a candle, and fully embracing the wind-down energy of this phase.

Serves 4
Prep Time: 15 minutes
Cook Time: 20 minutes

1 (8-ounce) box chickpea pasta
1 tablespoon olive oil
1 small onion, chopped
2 garlic cloves, minced
2 cups cubed butternut squash
½ cup chicken bone broth
¼ cup nutritional yeast
¼ teaspoon grated nutmeg
Salt and freshly ground black pepper

1 — Cook the pasta according to package instructions. Drain and set aside.

2 — In a large, deep saucepan, heat the olive oil over medium heat. Add the onion and garlic and sauté for 1 to 2 minutes, until fragrant.

3 — Add the squash and broth to the pan, stirring. Reduce the heat and simmer for about 10 minutes, until the squash is tender.

4 — Blend the squash mixture until smooth:

Using an immersion blender: Blend directly in the pan until creamy.

Using a stand blender: Carefully transfer the mixture to a high-speed blender and blend until smooth. Be sure to vent the lid slightly to release steam. If using a NutriBullet, allow the mixture to cool slightly as hot ingredients can create pressure and seal it shut permanently!

5 — Stir in the nutritional yeast, nutmeg, and salt and pepper to taste.

6 — Add the cooked pasta to the pot. Toss to coat the pasta well. Serve warm.

Healthy Burrito Bowls with Cilantro-Lime Vinaigrette

Serves 4
Prep Time: 10 minutes
Cook Time: 20 minutes

There's something about a burrito bowl that always feels like a build-your-own feast. Maybe it's the endless topping possibilities or the way every bite is a little different, but I never get tired of them. During my luteal phase, I crave hearty meals that keep me full and steady, and this bowl delivers. The protein-packed turkey, fiber-rich beans, and warm, smoky spices make it so satisfying, while a squeeze of lime and fresh cilantro brighten everything up. I love to set out all the toppings and let everyone make their own bowl—because food should be fun, especially when your body needs a little extra care!

Burrito Bowls

1 pound ground turkey or chicken
1 teaspoon chili powder
1 teaspoon ground cumin
½ teaspoon smoked paprika
¼ teaspoon garlic powder
½ teaspoon salt
½ teaspoon freshly ground black pepper
2 cups cooked brown rice or quinoa
1 (15-ounce) can black beans, drained and rinsed
1 cup canned corn kernels
1 cup diced ripe tomatoes
2 cups chopped lettuce (or other leafy greens)

Vinaigrette

¼ cup olive oil
2 tablespoons freshly squeezed lime juice (from 1 lime)
1 tablespoon cider vinegar
1 teaspoon honey or pure maple syrup
½ teaspoon garlic powder
¼ teaspoon salt
¼ teaspoon freshly ground black pepper
¼ cup finely chopped cilantro

For Serving

¼ cup chopped cilantro
1 lime, cut into wedges

1 — Make the bowls: In a large skillet over medium heat, place the ground meat, chili powder, cumin, smoked paprika, garlic powder, salt, and pepper and cook for 15 to 20 minutes, stirring occasionally, until browned.

2 — Layer the brown rice or quinoa in the serving bowls as the base. Top each with some of the ground meat mixture, the black beans, corn, tomatoes, and chopped lettuce.

3 — Make the vinaigrette: In a small bowl, whisk together the olive oil, lime juice, vinegar, honey, garlic powder, salt, pepper, and cilantro until well combined.

4 — Serve the bowls: Drizzle the vinaigrette over the bowls. Top with the cilantro and add a squeeze of lime juice. Enjoy!

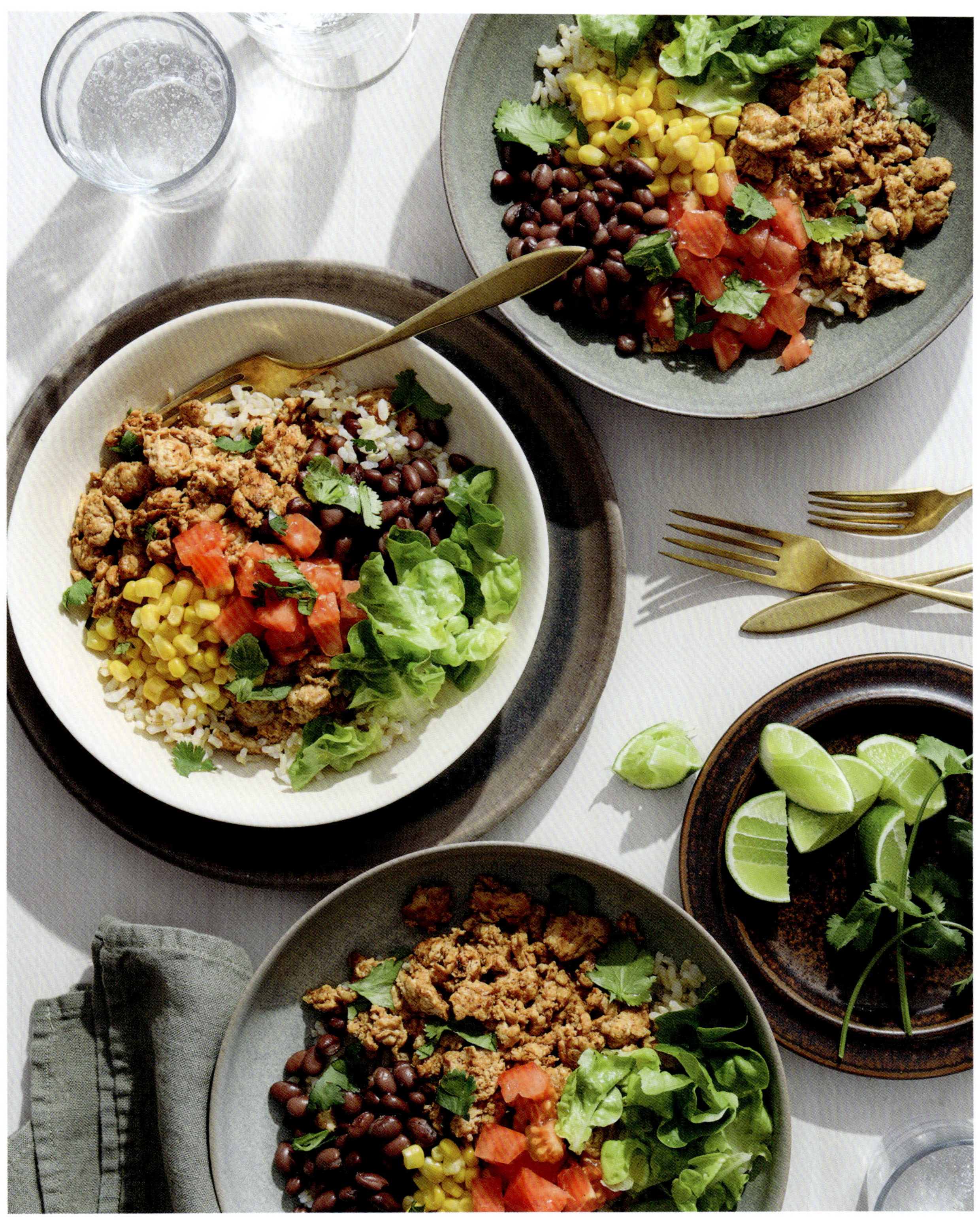

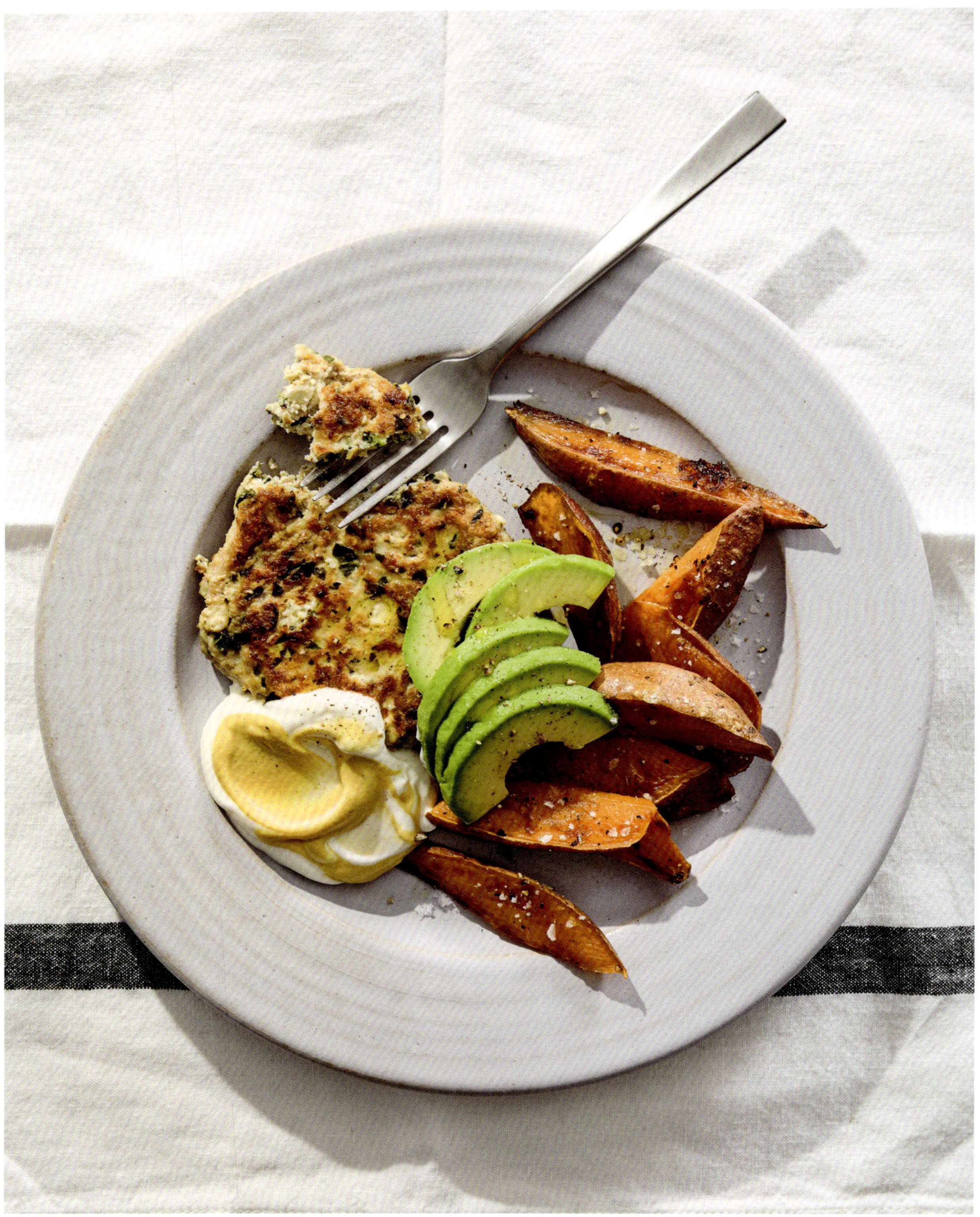

Bunless Spinach and Feta Turkey Burgers with Sweet Potato Fries

Serves 4
Prep Time: 10 minutes
Cook Time: 30 minutes

Burgers and fries—but make it hormone friendly! This bunless turkey burger is packed with spinach for a boost of magnesium to help relax muscles and calm the nervous system. Instead of a blood sugar–spiking bun, I'm all about pairing it with crispy sweet potato fries for slow-burning energy and fiber to support digestion and mood balance. The feta adds the perfect tangy bite, giving this a Mediterranean twist that keeps it from ever feeling boring. I love using ground turkey for variety, but beef or chicken works just as well!

Sweet Potato Fries

2 large sweet potatoes
1 tablespoon olive oil
½ teaspoon paprika
Salt

Burgers

1 pound ground turkey
½ cup chopped spinach
¼ cup crumbled feta cheese
1 teaspoon garlic powder
Salt and freshly ground black pepper
Olive oil or avocado oil, for frying

Optional accompaniments: avocado slices, mustard, dollops of plain Greek yogurt

1 — Preheat the oven to 425°F. Line a baking sheet with parchment paper.

2 — Prepare the fries: Cut the sweet potatoes into evenly sized wedges for even cooking. Toss with the olive oil, paprika, and salt, then spread in a single layer on the baking sheet. Roast for 25 to 30 minutes, flipping halfway through, until crispy and golden brown.

3 — Meanwhile, make the burgers: In a large bowl, combine the turkey, spinach, feta, garlic powder, and salt and pepper to taste. Mix gently with your hands until just combined—overmixing can make the burgers tough. Divide the mixture into 4 equal portions and shape into patties about ½ inch thick.

4 — Heat a large skillet over medium (or preheat a grill to medium-high). Lightly grease the skillet with olive oil or avocado oil. Add the patties and cook for 4 to 5 minutes per side, until fully cooked (internal temperature of 165°F).

5 — Plate the turkey burgers with the sweet potato fries alongside, and serve with your favorite condiments, like avocado, mustard, or a dollop of Greek yogurt for extra creaminess.

Soup Section

Soup is the ultimate comfort food, especially during the luteal phase, when your body craves warmth and nourishment. It's gentle on the digestive system, as the slow cooking process breaks down the ingredients, making them easier to absorb. The warmth of soup can also help relax the digestive tract, aiding in the reduction of bloating and discomfort. Plus, soups are a perfect way to sneak in nutrient-dense veggies without overwhelming your system, which is especially helpful during this phase, when cravings and sensitivities may be higher.

I love blending my soups with bone broth for an extra boost of protein and amino acids that support muscle repair and hormone balance, but feel free to use veggie broth if you're looking for a lighter, plant-based option. To make sure you're getting enough protein alongside your soup, try topping it with crunchy roasted chickpeas for a little texture (toss drained and rinsed chickpeas with some paprika, cumin, salt, and pepper and roast at 425°F for 20 minutes), stirring in some shredded rotisserie chicken, or adding crispy bacon bits. If you want something on the side, pair the soup with a turkey and cheese wrap, a hard-boiled egg with sea salt, or a slice of sourdough with hummus and hemp seeds for extra plant-based protein. Here, you'll find three of my go-to, simple soup recipes, each of them customizable with different veggies and spices to keep things fresh and exciting!

For Each
Serves 2 to 4
Prep Time: 10 minutes
Cook Time: 20 to 25 minutes

Butternut Squash Soup

1 tablespoon olive oil
1 medium onion, chopped
2 garlic cloves, minced
4 cups cubed butternut squash
3 cups bone broth, or more as needed
Salt and freshly ground black pepper
½ cup full-fat coconut milk

1 — Heat a large pot over medium heat. Add the olive oil, then stir in the onion and garlic. Sauté for 3 to 4 minutes, stirring occasionally, until the onion is translucent and fragrant.

2 — Add the squash to the pot and stir to coat it in the oil and aromatics. Pour in the 3 cups bone broth and add a generous pinch of salt. Bring the mixture to a gentle boil, then reduce the heat to low and let simmer for 15 to 20 minutes, or until the squash is very soft and easily pierced with a fork.

3 — Turn off the heat and blend until smooth using one of the following methods:

IMMERSION BLENDER Blend directly in the pot until completely smooth.

STAND BLENDER Carefully transfer the soup in batches to a high-speed blender, removing the center cap from the lid and covering

continued

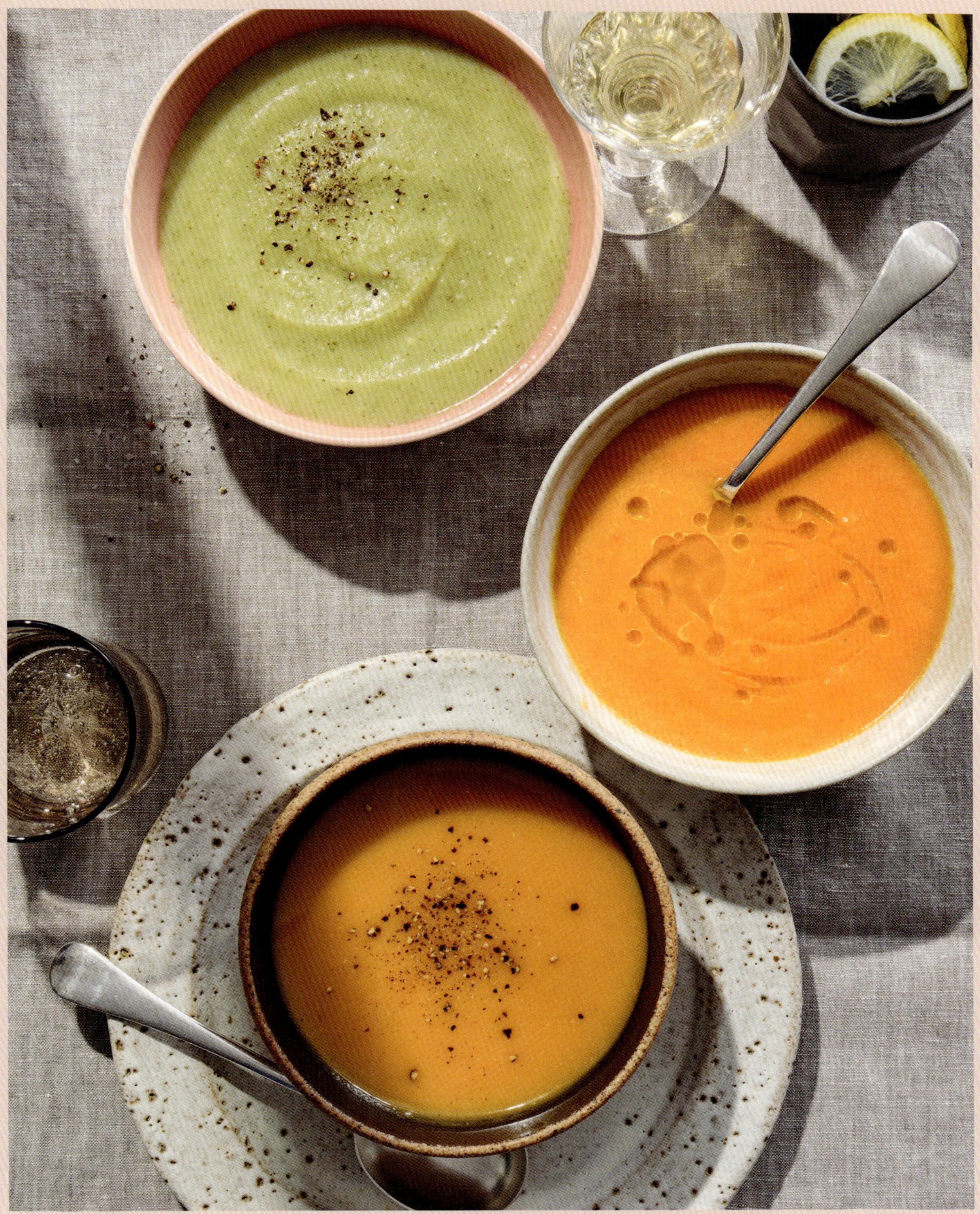

Butternut Squash Soup, *continued*

the opening with a kitchen towel to allow steam to escape. Blend until smooth, then return to the pot. If using a NutriBullet, allow the mixture to cool slightly, as hot ingredients can create pressure and seal it shut permanently!

4 — Stir in the coconut milk, then season the soup to taste with salt and pepper. Simmer on low for an additional 2 to 3 minutes to let the flavors meld. If the soup is too thick, add a splash of additional broth or water to reach your desired consistency.

5 — Serve warm and enjoy.

Carrot-Ginger Soup

1 tablespoon olive oil
1 medium onion, chopped
4 large carrots, sliced
1 tablespoon grated fresh ginger
4 cups bone broth
Juice of 1 orange
Salt and freshly ground black pepper

1 — Heat a large pot over medium heat and add the olive oil. When the oil is hot, add the onion and sauté for 3 to 4 minutes, until soft and translucent.

2 — Stir in the carrots and ginger, cooking for another 2 minutes to release their flavors.

3 — Pour in the bone broth, bring to a boil, then reduce the heat to a simmer. Let it cook for about 20 minutes, or until the carrots are tender and easily pierced with a fork.

4 — Blend until smooth using one of the following methods:

IMMERSION BLENDER Blend directly in the pot until the soup is silky smooth.

STAND BLENDER Let the soup cool slightly before transferring in batches to a blender. Remove the center cap from the lid and cover the opening with a towel to allow steam to escape safely. Blend until smooth, then return to the pot to reheat if needed. If using a NutriBullet, allow the mixture to cool slightly as hot ingredients can create pressure and seal it shut permanently!

5 — Stir in the orange juice, season to taste with salt and pepper, and serve warm.

Broccoli-Potato Soup

1 tablespoon olive oil
1 medium onion, chopped
3 medium potatoes, peeled and diced
3 cups broccoli florets
4 cups bone broth
½ cup unsweetened almond milk
Salt and freshly ground black pepper

1 — Heat a large pot over medium heat and add the olive oil. When the oil is hot, add the onion and sauté for 3 to 4 minutes, until soft and translucent.

2 — Add the potatoes and broccoli, stirring to coat them in the oil. Cook for another 2 minutes to enhance the flavors.

3 — Pour in the bone broth, bring to a boil, then reduce the heat to a simmer. Let it cook for about 20 minutes, until the potatoes and broccoli are tender and easily mashed with a fork.

4 — Blend until smooth using one of the following methods:

IMMERSION BLENDER Blend directly in the pot until the soup is creamy and smooth.

STAND BLENDER Allow the soup to cool slightly before transferring in batches to a blender. Remove the center cap from the lid and cover the opening with a towel to allow steam to escape. Blend until smooth, then return to the pot to reheat if needed. If using a NutriBullet, allow the mixture to cool slightly as hot ingredients can create pressure and seal it shut permanently!

5 — Stir in the almond milk, season to taste with salt and pepper, and serve warm.

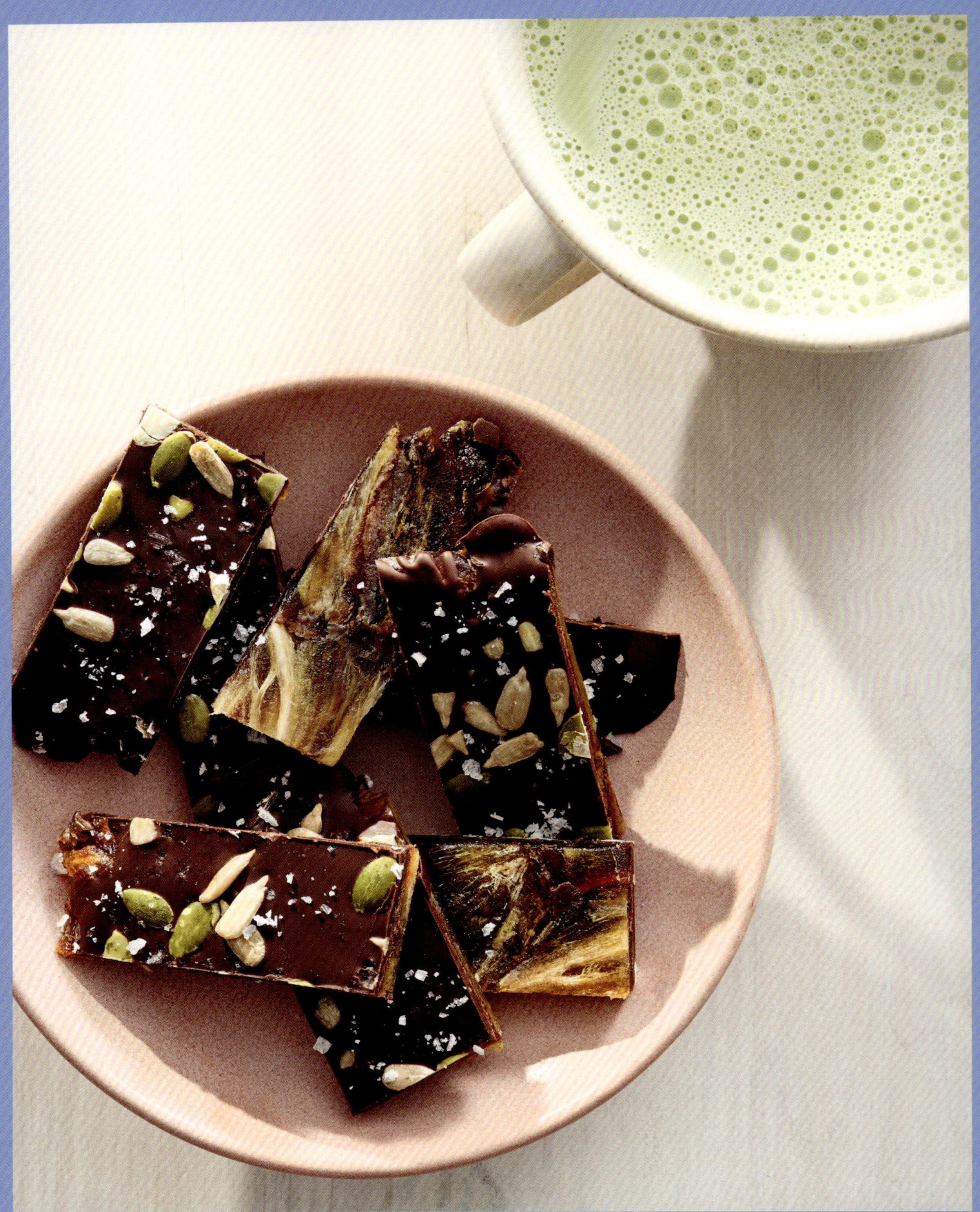

Snacks & Desserts

Homemade Hummus

Makes 1½ cups
Prep Time: 5 minutes

Homemade hummus is my favorite way to incorporate seed cycling into my luteal phase. Sesame seeds, found in tahini, are rich in zinc and calcium—two key minerals that support progesterone production and can help ease PMS symptoms like mood swings, bloating, and fatigue. Hummus is perfect for dipping fresh veggies, spreading on toast, or enjoying by the spoonful. I love adding dill for extra freshness, turmeric for an anti-inflammatory boost, or even cacao powder and honey for a dessert-style hummus. (When I do this, I omit the garlic, cumin, and lemon, of course!) I like to add a scoop of hummus on toast, in Buddha bowls, on roasted sweet potatoes, in sandwiches, and on avocado toast. Get creative and make it your own!

1 (15-ounce) can chickpeas, drained and rinsed
3 tablespoons tahini
2 tablespoons olive oil
Juice of 1 lemon
1 garlic clove, chopped
½ teaspoon ground cumin
Salt

1 — In a food processor, combine the chickpeas, tahini, olive oil, lemon juice, garlic, cumin, and salt to taste. Blend until smooth.

2 — Add 2 to 3 tablespoons of water, 1 tablespoon at a time, until you reach your desired consistency.

3 — Store in an airtight glass container in the refrigerator and consume within 5 days.

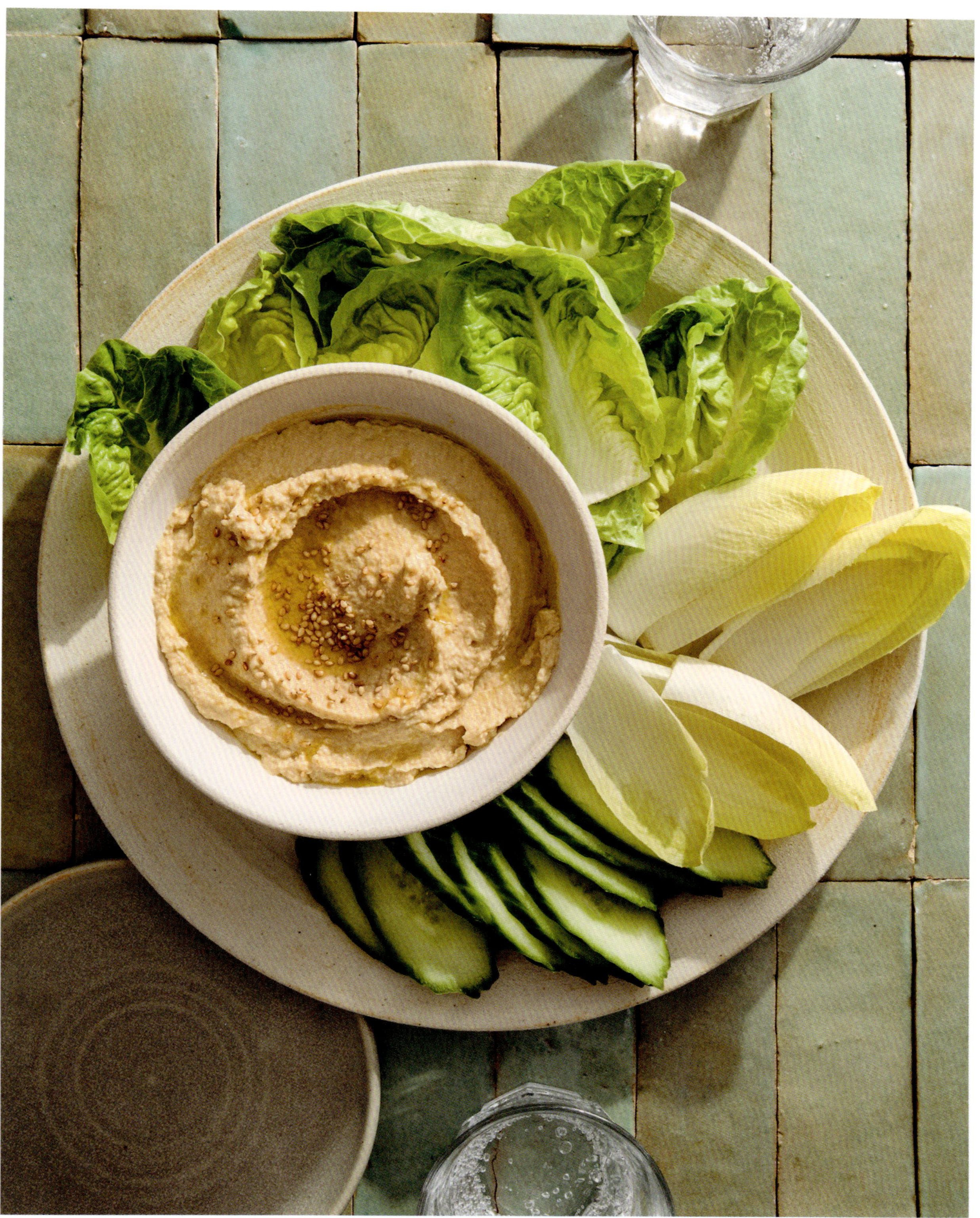

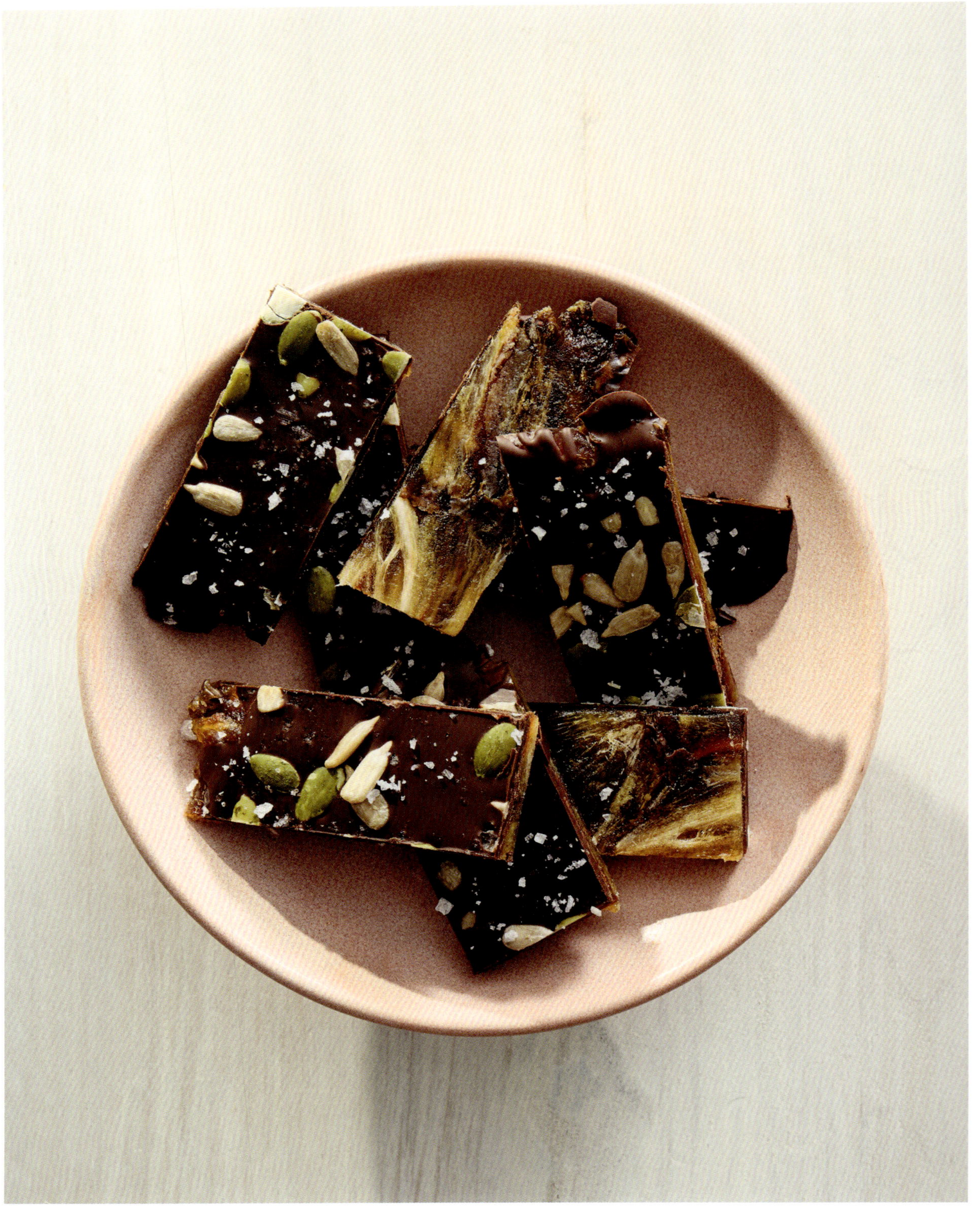

Pumpkin Seed Date Bark

Makes 8 to 10 pieces

Prep Time: 10 minutes, plus 1 hour chilling

This date bark is easily one of my top three favorite desserts in this book! It has the perfect mix of sweet, salty, crunchy, and chewy—everything I'm looking for when PMS cravings hit. Pumpkin seeds are packed with magnesium and zinc—two essential nutrients that support progesterone production and help ease bloating, mood swings, and fatigue during the luteal phase. Sunflower seeds provide a boost of vitamin E, which plays a key role in hormone balance and reducing inflammation. Plus, dates have a lower glycemic index, helping to keep blood sugar stable while still satisfying that natural sweet tooth. I love texture, so I often add extra toppings like shredded coconut, hemp seeds, or crushed nuts on top. I always keep a batch in my fridge or freezer for a post-meal treat or a late-night snack!

10 to 12 large medjool dates, pitted
½ cup 80% dark chocolate
1 tablespoon coconut oil
¼ cup pumpkin seeds
¼ cup sunflower seeds
Pinch of sea salt
¼ cup unsweetened coconut shreds (optional)

1 — Line a small baking dish with parchment paper.

2 — Press the dates down flat into an even layer, ensuring they are touching and form a solid base.

3 — In a small bowl, melt the chocolate and coconut oil in a microwave, heating in 30-second intervals, stirring until smooth.

4 — Pour the melted chocolate over the pressed dates, spreading it evenly with a spatula.

5 — Sprinkle the pumpkin seeds, sunflower seeds, sea salt, and, coconut, if using, over the top.

6 — Place in the refrigerator for about 1 hour, or until the chocolate is fully set. Once firm, cut into pieces and enjoy. (For storage, pack in an airtight container and store in the fridge for up to 1 week or in the freezer for 2 months.)

Balboa Bars–Style Banana Bites

Makes 15 to 20 bites

Prep Time: 10 minutes, plus 1 to 2 hours freezing

I grew up near a place called Balboa Island, in California, where we'd get Balboa Bars—chocolate-covered bananas coated and topped with all kinds of good things. I no longer live nearby, so I decided to re-create them at home, deconstructing them into bites and adding some luteal-phase love. Bananas are loaded with potassium, which helps reduce bloating and water retention, while dark chocolate is rich in magnesium, a key mineral for easing cramps, calming premenstrual tension, and stabilizing mood. One of my favorite tricks is adding a little sunflower seed butter (I get mine from Trader Joe's) on top of each banana slice before pouring over the chocolate. Plus, the healthy fats from the coconut oil and almonds provide slow-digesting energy to help keep blood sugar stable. These bites are ridiculously easy to make, store perfectly in the freezer, and bring a little taste of Balboa Island straight to your kitchen!

2 ripe bananas, sliced into coins

¼ cup sunflower seed butter (or peanut butter)

½ cup dark chocolate chips

1 teaspoon coconut oil

1 tablespoon sea salt

¼ cup crushed almonds or shredded coconut (optional)

1 — Line a baking sheet with parchment paper.

2 — Arrange the banana slices in a single layer on the baking sheet.

3 — Spread about ½ teaspoon of sunflower butter on each banana slice.

4 — Melt the chocolate and coconut oil in a microwave, heating in 30-second intervals, stirring until smooth.

5 — Drizzle the melted chocolate over the banana slices.

6 — Sprinkle the slices with some sea salt and add the almonds or coconut, if desired.

7 — Place in freezer for 1 to 2 hours, until firm. (Store pieces in an airtight container in the freezer for up to 6 months.)

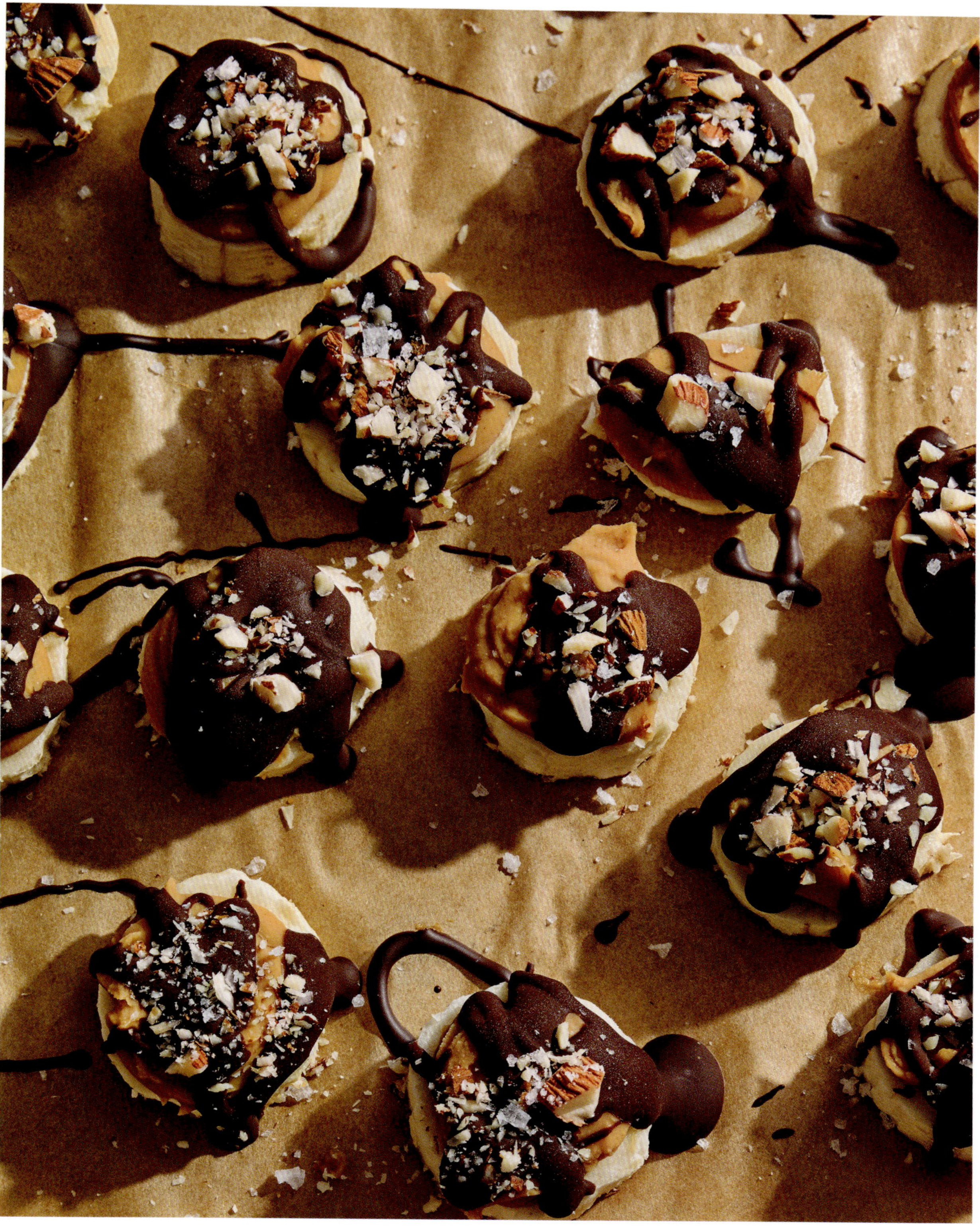

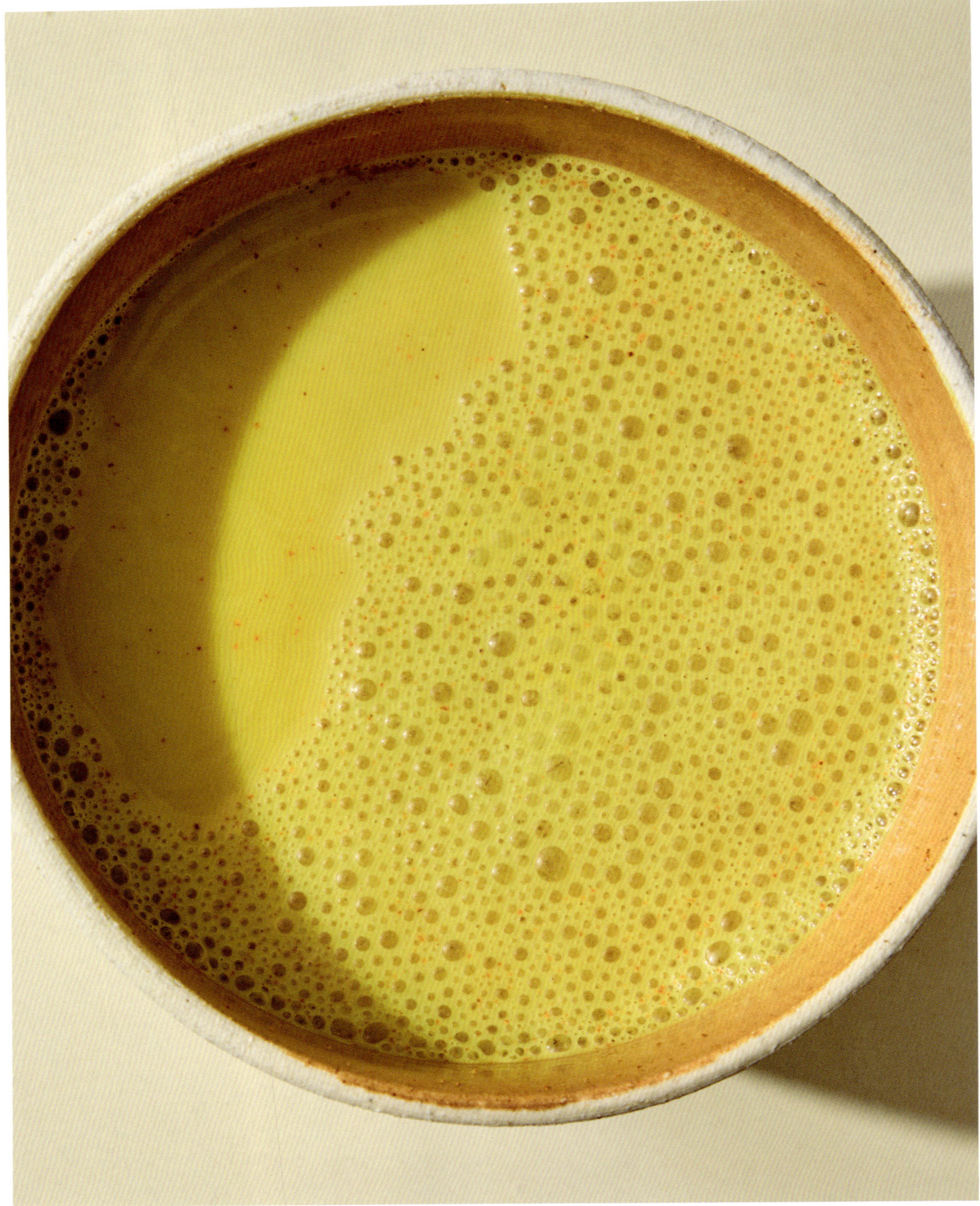

Turmeric Golden Milk

There's something about this golden milk that instantly makes me feel taken care of. Maybe it's the warmth, maybe it's the earthy spice blend, or maybe it's just knowing I'm giving my body exactly what it needs during the luteal phase. Turmeric is my go-to for soothing inflammation and fighting off those PMS aches. The ginger and cinnamon add a little heat, perfect for digestion and balancing blood sugar. And don't skip the black pepper; it helps your body absorb the turmeric, making this cozy drink as effective as it is comforting! I love sipping this at night as a way to slow down, reset, and remind myself to rest, because luteal phase me needs it.

Serves 1

Prep Time: 2 minutes

Cook Time: 5 minutes

---

1 cup unsweetened almond milk

½ teaspoon turmeric powder

¼ teaspoon ground ginger

½ teaspoon ground cinnamon

Pinch of freshly ground black pepper

1 teaspoon honey or pure maple syrup (optional)

1 — In a small saucepan, heat the almond milk over medium heat until warm, but not boiling.

2 — Whisk in the turmeric, ginger, cinnamon, and pepper until well combined.

3 — Stir in the honey or maple syrup, if desired, then pour into a mug and serve warm.

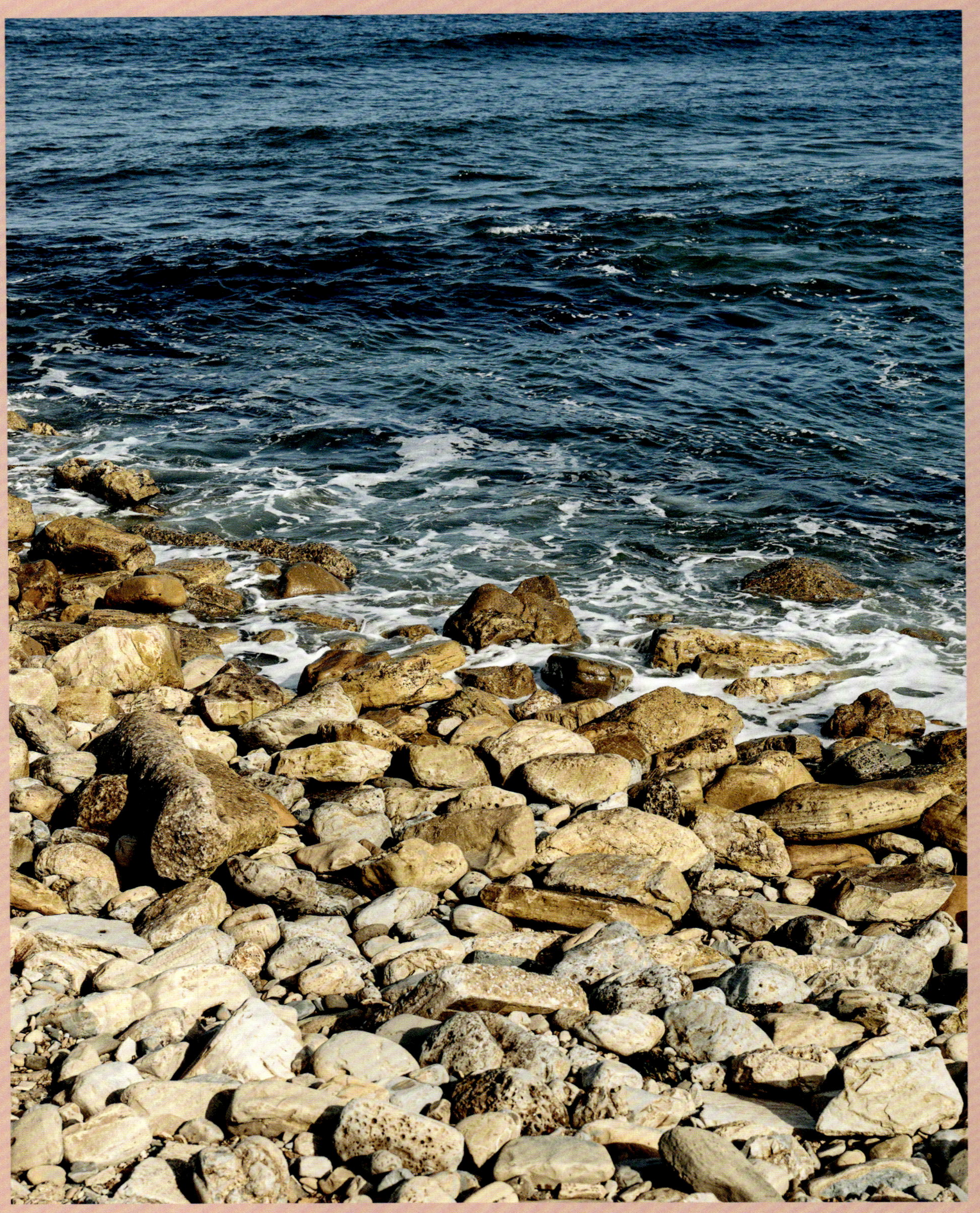

Acknowledgments

Writing this cookbook has been one of the most meaningful experiences of my life, and I'm so deeply grateful to every single person who helped make it a reality.

To Thea, my brilliant editor, thank you for believing in this vision from day one. Your insight, care, and encouragement shaped this book into something I'm incredibly proud of. To the entire team at Ten Speed Press, thank you for bringing this project to life with such heart and intention.

To Alix and Amy at DBA, thank you for being such steady supporters and advocates of my work. You've helped me build a brand and business that feels true to who I am, and I'm so lucky to have you in my corner. And to Lisa, my amazing agent at UTA, thank you for championing this idea and guiding me every step of the way.

To my parents and grandparents, your love, support, and encouragement mean more than I can ever put into words. Thank you for teaching me the value of nourishing others through food and for always cheering me on.

To my closest friends, you've been my sounding board, recipe testers, and biggest hype team. Thank you for the laughs, the honesty, and the endless support.

To my incredible followers, this book wouldn't exist without you. Thank you for trusting me with your health journeys, for being so engaged and curious, and for inspiring me to keep learning and sharing.

To my photography dream team, Kristin, Carrie, Joe, and Alicia, thank you for bringing these recipes to life so beautifully. Your creativity, talent, and eye for detail made this book truly shine.

And finally, to anyone navigating hormone imbalances or just trying to feel more at home in their body, this book is for you. I hope it nourishes you, supports you, and reminds you that food can be one of our most powerful forms of self-care.

With love and so much gratitude,

Paige

Index

Note: Page references in *italics* indicate photographs.

About the Author

PAIGE LINDGREN is a Los Angeles–based certified hormone specialist, holistic nutritionist, and social media creator with 550,000+ followers across Instagram, YouTube, TikTok, and Substack. She is on a mission to empower women with knowledge about their bodies, promote holistic well-being, and help them find balance in their lives. Lindgren has been featured on a number of podcasts, including *Pursuit of Wellness* and *Good Instincts,* to discuss women's health topics. Her expertise and contributions have been recognized and spotlighted in prestigious sources such as Well+Good, mindbodygreen, and *Yahoo News*.

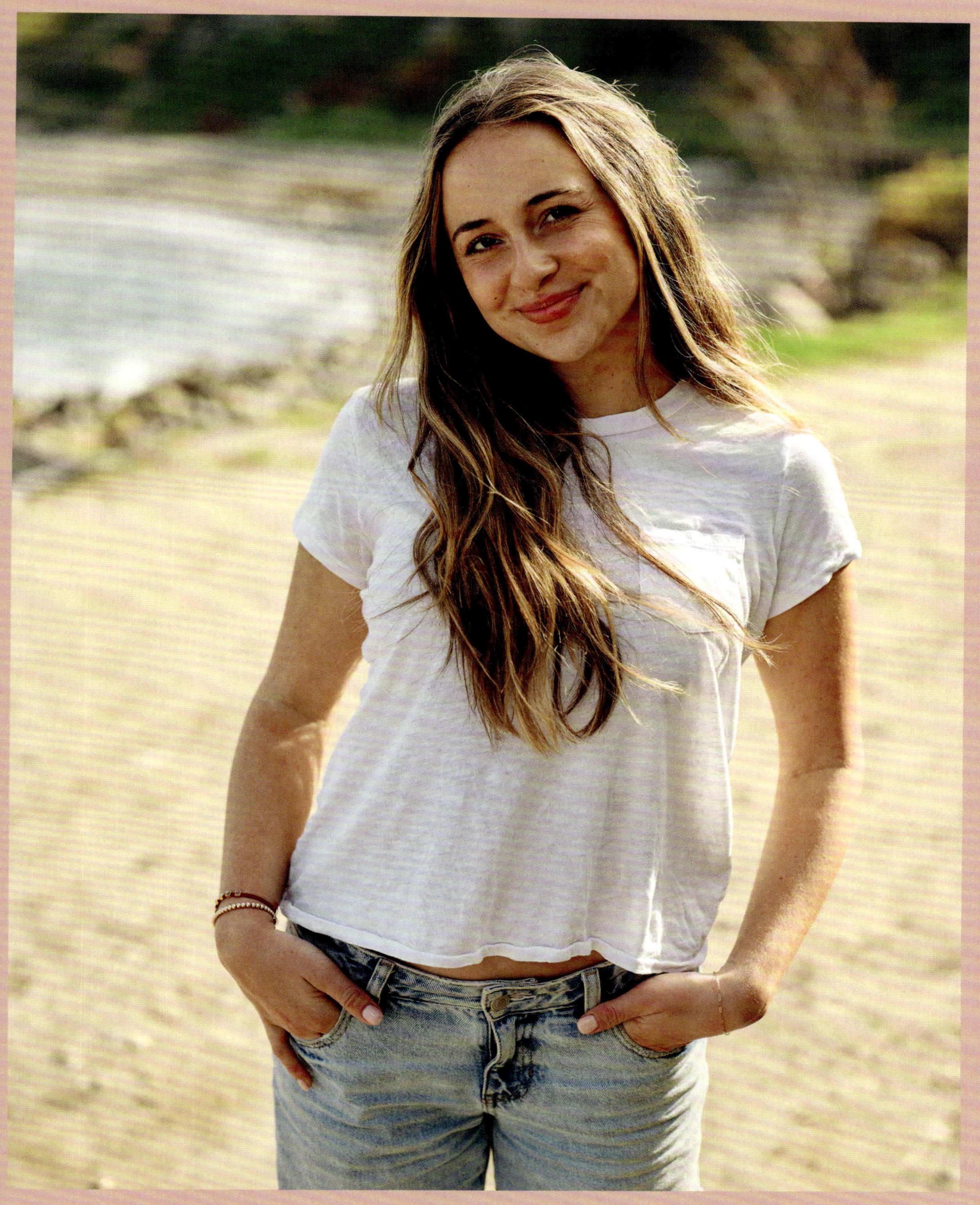

TEN SPEED PRESS
An imprint of the Crown Publishing Group
A division of Penguin Random House LLC
1745 Broadway
New York, NY 10019
tenspeed.com
penguinrandomhouse.com

Typefaces: Blaze Type's Inferi, and TypeType's TT Commons

Library of Congress Cataloging-in-Publication Data is on file with the publisher.

ISBN 978-0-593-83801-3
Ebook ISBN 978-0-593-83802-0

Editor: Thea Diklich-Newell | Production editor: Patricia Shaw
Designer: Annie Marino
Art director: Emma Boys Campion
Production designer: Mari Gill
Production: Serena Sigona | Prepress color manager: Jane Chinn
Food stylist: Carrie Purcell | Food stylist assistants: Ainhoa Hardy, Daniella Swamp
Prop stylist: Alicia Buszczak | Prop stylist assistant: Aubrey Devin
Photo assistant: Joe Elgar
Copy editor: Carole Berglie | Proofreaders: Diana Drew, Hope Clarke, Sigi Nacson
Indexer: Elizabeth T. Parson
Publicist: Natalie Yera-Campbell | Marketer: Natalie Portanova

Manufactured in China

10 9 8 7 6 5 4 3 2 1